Nuclear Medicine

A CORE REVIEW

Second Edition

Nuclear Medicine

A CORE REVIEW

Second Edition

Editors

Chirayu Shah, MD

Associate Professor
Department of Radiology
Nashville VA Medical Center
Vanderbilt University Medical Center
Nashville, Tennessee

Marques Bradshaw, MD, MSCR

Associate Professor
Department of Radiology
Nashville VA Medical Center
Vanderbilt University Medical Center
Nashville, Tennessee

Ishani Dalal, MD

Senior Staff
Department of Radiology
Henry Ford Hospital
Detroit, Michigan

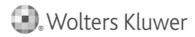 Wolters Kluwer

Philadelphia • Baltimore • New York • London
Buenos Aires • Hong Kong • Sydney • Tokyo

Acquisitions Editor: Nicole Dernoski
Development Editor: Eric McDermott
Editorial Coordinator: Vinoth Ezhumalai
Marketing Manager: Kirsten Watrud
Production Project Manager: Catherine Ott
Design Coordinator: Stephen Druding
Manufacturing Coordinator: Beth Welsh
Prepress Vendor: SPi Global

Second Edition

Cataloging-in-Publication Data available on request from the Publisher

ISBN: 978-1-9751-4792-1

To my parents, Yatin and Anjana Shah, whose unconditional love and support allowed me to follow my dreams. They worked hard so that we did not have to and put our needs before theirs so that we could flourish.

To my wife, Payal Shah, for being there for me in my time of need, for her continued love and support, and for allowing what appeared to be an eternity out of our personal time so that one of my aspirations could come to fruition.

To our children, Kavya and Rihaan, for coming into our lives and putting things in perspective.

To my mentors, coworkers, and residents at the Vanderbilt University Medical Center and the Nashville VA Hospital for their continued support and guidance. I say thank you.

—Chirayu Shah

To my parents, Joyce and James Bradshaw, who sacrificed and worked long hours so that I could achieve my dreams. To my family who always supported me and encouraged me to continue striving to be the best that I could be.

To my wife, Francesca Bradshaw, who loves me just because, who is always my rock, who makes sure things are taken care of at home, while I strive to be the best clinician-educator that I can be. To my children, Mckinley, Sydney, and Ethan, who allow me to just be dad, part-time superhero, and full-time playmate. For never complaining when daddy has to go to work.

To all of those who helped me along the way, be it getting into medical school, getting into residency, teaching me how to do research, giving me career advice, keeping me grounded, or merely being a friend in a time of need. I say thank you.

—Marques Bradshaw

To my parents, Purnima and Mahendrakumar Shah; without their love, sacrifice, and support, I could not have achieved my dreams.

To my loving husband, Bhavin Dalal, who is my guru and role model and provides me continuous support and guidance.

To my kids, Astha and Devarshi, for their unconditional love and understanding. To my family including my sister, Shivani, and my in-laws, Pushpa and Devesh Dalal, who have helped me through all my difficult times.

Last but not least, to my teachers, mentors, and my colleagues, who have taught me how to be compassionate and sympathetic in both my professional and personal life.

—Ishani Dalal

Contributors to the Second Edition

Keisha C. McCall, PhD

Nuclear Medicine Physicist
Department of Radiology
Henry Ford Health System
Detroit, Michigan

Joseph Steiner, PhD

Nuclear Medicine Physicist
Department of Radiology
Maine Medical Center
Portland, Maine

Matt Vanderhoek, PhD

Imaging Physicist
Department of Radiology
Henry Ford Health System
Detroit, Michigan

Contributors to the First Edition

Twyla Bartel, DO, MBA, FACNM

Associate Professor
Diagnostic Radiology
UAMS
Little Rock, Arkansas

Adam J. Bobbey, MD

Pediatric Radiology Fellow
Department of Radiology
Monroe Carell Jr. Children's Hospital at Vanderbilt
Nashville, Tennessee

Jonathan David Perry, MD

Resident Physician
Department of Radiology
Medical University of South Carolina
Charleston, South Carolina

SERIES FOREWORD

The second edition of the *Nuclear Medicine: A Core Review* builds on the success of the first edition by covering the essential aspects of nuclear medicine in a manner that serves as a guide for residents to assess their knowledge and review the material in a format that is similar to the ABR core examination. The print copy of the *Nuclear Medicine: A Core Review, 2nd edition*, still contains 300 questions but 100 new questions have been added when compared to the first edition. The 100 questions from the print copy of the first edition are still available but have been moved to the eBook of *Nuclear Medicine: A Core Review, 2nd edition*.

The coeditors, Chirayu Shah, Marques Bradshaw, and Ishani Dalal, have done an excellent job in producing a book that exemplifies the philosophy and goals of the *Core Review Series*. They have done a meticulous job in covering key topics and providing quality images. The questions have been divided logically into chapters so as to make it easy for learners to work on particular topics as needed. The questions are multiple-choice with each question having a single best answer. There is a brief post-question rationale as to why the correct answer is correct and why the other plausible answer choices are incorrect. There are also references provided for each question to allow one to delve more deeply into a specific subject matter.

The intent of the *Core Review Series* is to provide the resident, fellow, or practicing physician a review of the important conceptual, factual, and practical aspects of a subject with multiple-choice questions written in a format similar to the ABR core examination. The *Core Review Series* is not intended to be exhaustive but to provide material likely to be tested on the ABR core examination and that would be required in clinical practice.

As Series Editor of the *Core Review Series*, it has been rewarding to not only be a coeditor of one of the books in this series but to work with so many talented individuals in the profession of radiology across the country. This series represents countless hours of work and involvement by many, and it would not have come together without their participation. It has been very gratifying to receive many positive comments from residents of the difference they feel the series has made in their board preparation.

I would like to thank all the coeditors for their dedication to the series and for doing an exceptional job on the second edition. I believe *Nuclear Medicine: A Core Review, 2nd edition*, will serve as a valuable resource for residents during their board preparation and a useful reference for fellows and practicing radiologists.

Biren A. Shah, MD, FACR
Professor of Radiology
Wayne State University School of Medicine
Associate Residency Program Director
Section Chief, Breast Imaging
Detroit Medical Center

In this second edition of the book, we have tried to improve on the first edition based on the feedback received from the readers. The radiopharmaceuticals chapter was expanded to include examples of the commonly used agents, the oncology chapter was expanded to include new imaging agents as well as others that are in the pipeline, and the physics chapter was completely revamped with 35 new questions. Matt Vanderhoek, Keisha McCall, and Joseph Steiner at Henry Ford created new questions and helped improve the discussion of the old questions. There are a total of 100 new questions scattered throughout the book. In order to remain with the total of 300 questions, we have removed 100 questions from the first edition, which will be available online. We highly recommend that when using this study material that you also review the questions and discussions that were removed and placed online. We are honored and humbled to have produced the first edition, which has proven to be a reliable study tool for residents preparing for the Core Examination. We hope that this book will serve as a useful tool for residents not only to prepare for the board examination but also to help them become clinically competent as they prepare to achieve their career goals.

Sometimes focus on an intermediate goal can make us lose sight of the ultimate goal. The ultimate goal of every radiology resident should be to become the best radiologist possible. Unfortunately, this aim is often clouded by pressure to pass the Boards. However, if there is an appropriate focus on the ultimate goal, achieving that intermediate goal becomes less of an obstacle. With this in mind, we have created a text containing 300 selective ABR Core Exam styled questions covering basic concepts in Nuclear Medicine with which a resident would be expected to be familiar. The questions are supplemented with detailed explanations of the findings and diagnosis as well as differential diagnosis. Updated references are provided for each question for those wishing to delve more deeply into a specific subject. This format is also practical for radiologists preparing for Maintenance of Certification. Within the confines of the three hundred questions limit, we have tried to ensure that the major topics are addressed. Our hope is that the pearls provided in the explanations/discussions will not only help residents with the Core Exam but will also prove helpful in day-to-day practice.

Multiple colleagues have contributed to this publication. The quality and timely completion of this book would not have been possible without the efforts of each of these intelligent, talented, and committed individuals who took time from their busy lives to research, write, and submit material in a timely manner. To all who helped, we offer our heartfelt thanks. Additionally, we would like to extend thanks to the staff at LWW for this opportunity and for their guidance along the way. Finally, we are truly grateful to our families who have encouraged us through this long process and supported us each step along the way.

Chirayu Shah, MD
Marques Bradshaw, MD, MSCR
Ishani Dalal, MD

ACKNOWLEDGMENTS

We would like to extend our heartfelt appreciation to Matt Vanderhoek, Keisha McCall, and Joseph Steiner for their valuable contribution to the physics chapter. Their insight and hard work are highly appreciated. We would like to thank Dr. Biren Shah for his guidance and support throughout the process. We would also like to thank Dr. William H. Martin for sharing his precious teaching files with us. This book would not have been as robust without his help. We would like to thank Eric McDermott and Vinoth Ezhumalai at Lippincott for their help and support in the timely completion and publication of this book. We would also like to thank other staff members at Wolters Kluwer and SPi Global who were integral in getting this book from the digital word document format to the final finished product.

CONTENTS

1 Which one of the following photon energies is associated with this radiopharmaceutical?

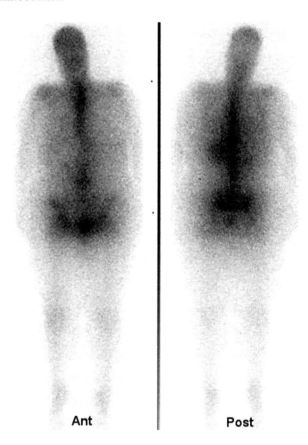

A. 69 to 83 keV (Hg x-rays)
B. 140 keV
C. 159 keV
D. 93, 185, 300, and 395 keV
E. 171 and 240 keV
F. 364 keV

2   What is the physical half-life of the following radiopharmaceutical?

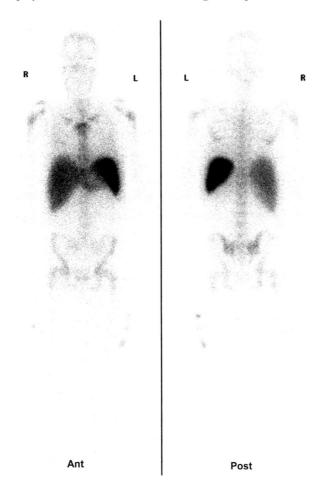

Ant   Post

   A. 6 hours
   B. 13 hours
   C. 2.8 days
   D. 3.0 days
   E. 3.2 days
   F. 8 days

3   Which of the following radiopharmaceuticals is least likely to localize within the myocardium as a part of normal physiologic uptake?

   A. Tc-99m tetrofosmin
   B. Tc-99m sestamibi
   C. Thallium-201
   D. I-123 MIBG
   E. F-18 florbetaben
   F. F-18 FDG

4   Which of the following radiopharmaceuticals is the best indicator of cellular proliferation?

   A. C-11 choline
   B. F-18 fluorothymidine (FLT)
   C. F-18 fluorodeoxyglucose (FDG)
   D. F-18 fluoromisonidazole (FMISO)

5 What is being measured when the activity in the Mo-99/Tc-99m generator eluate is measured in the dose calibrator before and after the placement of an eluate vial in a 6-mm-thick lead container?

A. Chemical impurity
B. Radiochemical impurity
C. Radionuclide impurity
D. Physical impurity

6 What is being measured when Mo-99/Tc-99m generator eluate is placed on a special test paper that changes color?

A. Chemical impurity
B. Radiochemical impurity
C. Radionuclide impurity
D. Physical impurity

7 What is being measured when the radiopharmacist performs thin-layer chromatography on Tc-99m MDP?

A. Chemical impurity
B. Radiochemical impurity
C. Radionuclide impurity
D. Physical impurity

8 If the biologic half-life of an isotope is 2 hours and the physical half-life is 6 hours, what is the effective half-life?

A. 1.5 hours
B. 2 hours
C. 4 hours
D. 6 hours

9 The following image is from a patient who underwent SPECT myocardial perfusion imaging. What is the critical organ for this radiopharmaceutical?

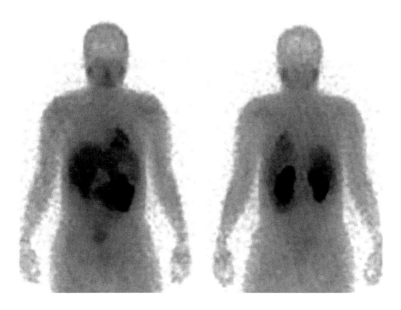

A. Myocardium
B. Bowel
C. Kidneys
D. Gallbladder
E. Urinary bladder

10 What type of collimator is used to image this radiopharmaceutical?

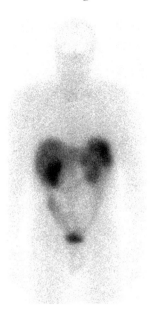

    A. Low energy high resolution (LEHR)
    B. Medium energy
    C. High energy
    D. Pinhole

11 A 2-year-old patient undergoes the following nuclear medicine examination for staging purposes. Assuming that the technical scanning parameters, scanning time, and injected radiopharmaceutical were appropriate, what is the principal photon energy associated with this radiopharmaceutical?

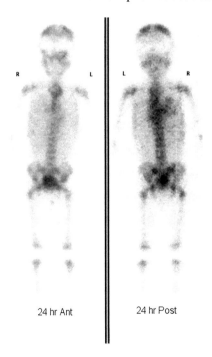

24 hr Ant   24 hr Post

    A. 140 keV
    B. 159 keV
    C. 185 keV
    D. 171 keV
    E. 245 keV

12 What is the most likely cause of abnormal biodistribution of I-123 MIBG in this patient?

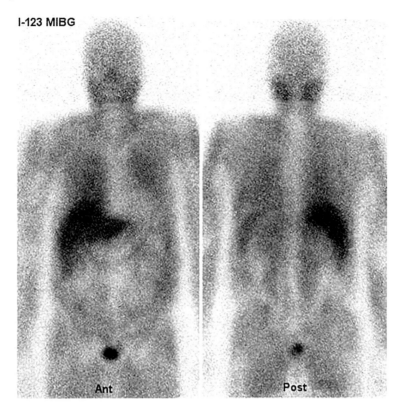

A. Renal failure
B. Contamination
C. Postprandial state
D. Competing medications
E. Images acquired too early

13 Cyclotron-produced SPECT radionuclides decay primarily by which one of the following mechanisms?

A. Alpha decay
B. Beta decay
C. Isomeric transition
D. Electron capture

14   What radiopharmaceutical was administered to the patient prior to acquiring the following images?

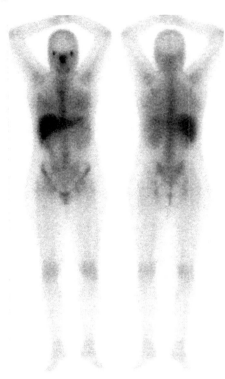

    A. I-131
    B. In-111 OctreoScan
    C. I-123 MIBG
    D. Gallium-67
    E. Tc-99m sestamibi

15   Identify the following positron emission tomography (PET) radiotracer based on its biodistribution.

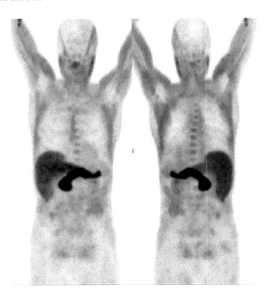

    A. Ga-68 DOTATATE
    B. F-18 FDG
    C. Ga-68 PSMA
    D. F-18 FACBC

ANSWERS AND EXPLANATIONS

1 **Answer B.** The image demonstrates distribution of a pharmaceutical to the skeleton and renal collecting system. The only radiopharmaceuticals that would demonstrate this pattern of distribution are bone scintigraphy agents Tc-99m MDP or Tc-99m HDP. The principal photon associated with Tc-99m is 140 keV. These images have poor resolution because they were acquired off-peak. The first image below is from the same patient acquired at 140 ± 20 keV window. The second image is also bone scintigraphy, but it was acquired earlier at 1.5 hours instead of 3, which explains the increased soft tissue and renal uptake.

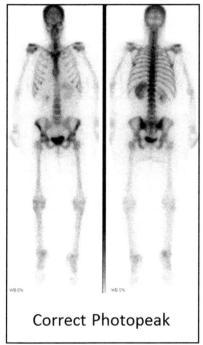

Correct Photopeak

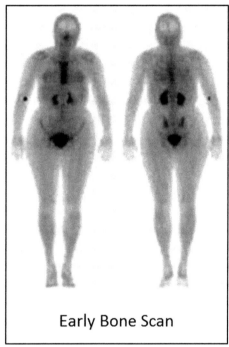

Early Bone Scan

Other radiopharmaceuticals that localize to the osseous skeleton include Ga-67, tagged leukocytes (In-111 or Tc-99m HMPAO), Tc-99m sulfur colloid, and F-18 FDG. The liver and spleen are part of the physiologic distribution of Ga-67, Tc-99m sulfur colloid, tagged leukocytes, and F-18 FDG. Since the liver and spleen are not visualized on this scan, they are excluded. I-123 and I-131 do not localize in the osseous skeleton as part of their normal physiologic distribution; their physiologic distribution is in the nasopharynx, salivary glands, thyroid, stomach, bladder, and bowel. The following table lists principle photon energies and physical half-lives of commonly used radiopharmaceuticals in nuclear medicine.

Radionuclide	Radiopharmaceutical	Scans	Energy (keV)	Physical Half-Life
Tl-201	Thallium chloride	Myocardial perfusion and viability scans	69–83 (Hg x-rays)	3.0 d
Xenon-133	Gas	Lung ventilation	81	5.2 d
Technetium-99m (Tc-99m)	Diphosphonate (MDP)	Bone	140	6 h
	DMSA	Renal cortical		
	DTPA	Renal (dynamic), brain		
	ECD	Brain death, Seizure		
	HMPAO	Brain death, seizure		
	HMPAO-labeled white cells	Tagged WBC (infection)		
	Labeled red cells	GI bleed, RVG		
	Macroaggregated albumin (MAA)	Lung perfusion		
	MAG3	Renal		
	Mebrofenin	HIDA		
	Pertechnetate	Thyroid, Meckel diverticulum		
	Sestamibi	Parathyroid, myocardial perfusion		
	Tetrofosmin	Myocardial perfusion		
Iodine-123	Sodium	Thyroid scintigraphy and uptake, whole-body radioiodine scans	159	13 h
	MIBG	Neuroblastoma and pheochromocytoma		
Indium-111	Oxine-labeled white cells	Tagged WBC	171, 245	2.8 d
	Pentetreotide	OctreoScan		
	DTPA	CSF flow studies		
	DTPA	CSF leak studies		
Gallium-67	Citrate	Gallium (infection)	93, 184, 296, 388	78 h
Iodine-131	Sodium	Thyroid uptake and whole-body radioiodine scans	364	8.1 d
	MIBG	Therapy for thyroid cancers		
		Imaging and treatment of neuroblastoma		

References: http://learnnuclearmedicine.com/introduction-to-radiopharmceuticals-studies/

Ziessman HA, O'Malley JP, Thrall JH. *Nuclear medicine: the requisites*, 4th ed. Philadelphia, PA: Saunders, 2014:3.

2 **Answer C.** Anterior and posterior whole-body images demonstrate the physiologic distribution of the radiopharmaceutical corresponding to the liver, spleen, and bone marrow. The spleen is the most intense organ. The degree of intensity from most intense to least is spleen > liver > bone marrow. The images appear coarse, suggesting that this is a polyenergetic medium-energy radiopharmaceutical. These images are from an In-111 oxine-labeled leukocyte scan. In-111 has a physical half-life of 2.8 days. Tc-99m HMPAO-labeled leukocytes scan would also have uptake in the liver and spleen; however, since the images are acquired earlier (4 hours vs. 24 hours) secondary to shorter half-life, more blood pool would be visualized. Also, the images would appear better than In-111 oxine-labeled leukocytes because of the better imaging characteristics of Tc-99m. One of the potential downsides of Tc-99m HMPAO labeled WBC imaging is that there is physiologic excretion into the GI tract and bladder. Other radiopharmaceuticals with distribution to the liver, spleen, and bone marrow include Tc-99m sulfur colloid and Ga-67 scans. On a traditional liver spleen scan performed with Tc-99m SC, the liver would be more intense than the spleen, and marrow would be hard to visualize unless there was a colloid shift. Physiologic distribution of Ga-67 includes the nasopharynx, lacrimal glands, salivary glands, liver, spleen, renal collecting system (first 12 to 24 hours), and bowel (after 24 hours). The liver is more intense on the Ga-67 scan than on leukocyte scans. Since gallium is a polyenergetic medium-energy radionuclide, the images produced are also coarse.

Reference: O'Malley JP, Ziessman HA, Thrall JH. *Nuclear medicine: the requisites*, 5th ed. Philadelphia, PA: Saunders, 2020:43–44.

3 **Answer E.** F-18 Florbetaben is used for the detection of beta amyloid plaques in the diagnosis of Alzheimer disease by PET imaging and does not demonstrate normal physiologic uptake in the heart. The utility of beta-amyloid agents in the evaluation of cardiac amyloidosis is being investigated. Tc-99m tetrofosmin and Tc-99m sestamibi are myocardial perfusion imaging agents that bind to the cytoplasmic mitochondria. These agents are excreted through the liver by the hepatobiliary system. As such, part of physiologic dissolution includes the hepatobiliary system and bowel. Thallium-201 is a K^+ analog that localizes within the cytoplasm of the myocardial cells by the sodium–potassium ATPase pump. Unlike Tc-99m-labeled myocardial perfusion agents, Tl-201 is excreted by the kidneys. The heart is also visualized on the I-123 MIBG scan as it is one of the sympathetically innervated organs. The heart can utilize glucose or fatty acids for metabolism and demonstrates variable F-18 FDG uptake.

Reference: O'Malley JP, Ziessman HA, Thrall JH. *Nuclear medicine: the requisites*, 5th ed. Philadelphia, PA: Saunders, 2020:364–365, 442–443.

4 **Answer B.** F-18 fluorothymidine (FLT) is a marker of cell proliferation. F-18 FDG is a marker of cellular glucose metabolism. F-18 fluoromisonidazole (FMISO) is used for the detection of hypoxia in tumors. C-11 choline is a radiolabeled analog of choline, a precursor molecule essential for the biosynthesis of cell membrane phospholipids; it has been approved by the FDA to evaluate prostate cancer.

Reference: O'Malley JP, Ziessman HA, Thrall JH. *Nuclear medicine: the requisites*, 5th ed. Philadelphia, PA: Saunders, 2020:66–69.

5 **Answer C.** Radionuclide impurity measures the fraction of total radioactivity that is present in the form of the undesired radionuclide. In the Tc-99m case, it is measured in the form of ratio of Mo-99 to Tc-99m. Mo-99 is the most important radionuclide contaminant in the Tc-99m based radiopharmaceutical. Its long half-life and beta emission result in a very high radiation dose. As such, a limit of 0.15 µCi of Mo-99 in 1 mCi of Tc-99m at the time of radiotracer administration has been set by the NRC. This test is performed by placing the vial of Tc-99m in a 6-mm-thick lead container, which is then measured in a dose calibrator. The vial of Tc-99m is measured again without the lead container. Relatively low-energy (140 keV) photons are reduced a million-fold by the lead container, compared to only a tenfold reduction in the higher-energy Mo-99 photons (366, 740, 778 keV). This allows for the determination of the ratio of Mo-99 to Tc-99m.

Reference: O'Malley JP, Ziessman HA, Thrall JH. *Nuclear medicine: the requisites*, 5th ed. Philadelphia, PA: Saunders, 2020:54.

6 **Answer A.** Chemical impurity measures the fraction of an unwanted chemical compared to a wanted chemical. In the Tc-99m case, the major chemical impurity is in the form of alumina breakthrough in the generator eluate. Excess aluminum can interfere with some labeling reactions resulting in radiochemical impurity. The maximum allowable limit for alumina breakthrough is 10 μg/mL of the eluate. This is measured by a qualitative colorimetric test where the generator eluate is placed on a special test paper chemically sensitive to the aluminum ion. Excessive amounts of aluminum capable of disturbing the radiochemical purity will turn the paper pink. The color is compared to a standard to estimate the aluminum amount. Excessive amounts of aluminum in the Tc-99m sulfur colloid kit results in diffuse lung uptake, while excessive amounts of aluminum in the standard Tc-99m MDP kit results in increased liver uptake.

Reference: O'Malley JP, Ziessman HA, Thrall JH. *Nuclear medicine: the requisites*, 5th ed. Philadelphia, PA: Saunders, 2020:54–55.

7 **Answer B.** Radiochemical impurity represents the fraction of radioactivity in a dose that is in the undesired chemical form. An example would be the fraction of the free Tc-99m pertechnetate and insoluble colloids in a Tc-99m MDP dose prepared for bone scintigraphy. Thin-layer chromatography is the most common method of testing radiochemical purity with Tc-99m-labeled compounds. The United States Pharmacopeia requires >95% of the compound to be in the desired chemical form (i.e., Tc-99m MDP).

Reference: O'Malley JP, Ziessman HA, Thrall JH. *Nuclear medicine: the requisites*, 5th ed. Philadelphia, PA: Saunders, 2020:55.

8 **Answer A.** Effective half-life = (physical half-life × biologic half-life)/(physical half-life + biologic half-life) = (12/8) = 1.5 hours.

Reference: Mettler FA, Guiberteau MJ. *Essentials of nuclear medicine imaging*, 7th ed. Philadelphia, PA: Saunders, 2019:5.

9 **Answer C.** Physiologic distribution is seen corresponding to the nasal mucosa, salivary glands, heart, kidneys, liver, and spleen. The only SPECT myocardial perfusion imaging agent that undergoes renal excretion is Tl-201. Also, the images are of poor quality secondary to higher attenuation of low-energy photon and lower dose due to 3-day half-life. The Tc-99m-labeled myocardial perfusion agents tetrofosmin and sestamibi are excreted through the hepatobiliary collecting system. As such, activity would be visualized within the liver and bowel (see below). Kidneys are the critical organ for Tl-201. The gallbladder is the critical organ for Tc-99m Sestamibi and wall of large intestine is the critical organ for Tc-99m Tetrofosmin.

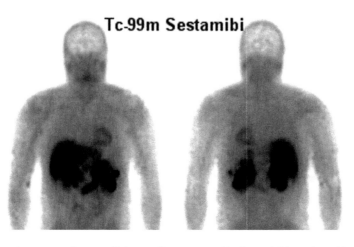

Tc-99m Sestamibi

Reference: SNMMI Nuclear Medicine Radiation Dose Tool. Available at http://www.snmmi.org/ClinicalPractice/doseTool.aspx?ItemNumber=11216&navItemNumber=11218

10 **Answer B.** This is an In-111-DTPA-pentetreotide (OctreoScan) that is used for the evaluation of neuroendocrine tumors such as carcinoid and gastrinoma with very high sensitivity. Planar images using a medium-energy collimator and symmetrical 20% energy window over 173 and 247 keV are acquired at 4 and 24 hours. SPECT-CT imaging of the appropriate regions may be acquired as indicated based upon the clinical history. Octreotide scans are readily identified by the intense activity within the bilateral kidneys and lack of myocardial uptake. With increased availability of PET somatostatin receptor imaging agents, OctreoScan is being replaced by PET agents such as Ga-68 DOTATATE.

Reference: Balon HR, Brown TL, Goldsmith SJ, et al. The SNM practice guideline for somatostatin receptor scintigraphy 2.0. *J Nucl Med Technol* 2011;39(4):317–324.

11 **Answer B.** This is an I-123 MIBG scan in a child with thoracic neuroblastoma and diffuse bone marrow involvement, which makes it look like a bone scan. The principal photon energy (PPE) of I-123 is 159 keV. While the normal physiologic distribution of I-123 MIBG would include organs innervated by the sympathetic nervous system such as salivary glands, myocardium, and liver (see answer 14), this normal physiologic distribution has been significantly altered due to high tumor burden. These images were acquired 24 hours after the intravenous administration of the radiopharmaceutical. Tc-99m MDP bone scintigraphy images would be acquired 3 to 4 hours after the IV administration and would also have images with better resolution due to the better imaging characteristics of Tc-99m (PPE 140 keV). While bone scintigraphy with an off-peak acquisition or wrong collimator may appear similarly, you are told that the technical scanning parameters were appropriate. Ga-67 (PPEs 83, 185, and 300 keV) and In-111 OctreoScan (PPEs 171 and 245 keV) would demonstrate physiologic activity within the liver and spleen, which is not seen in this patient.

Reference: O'Malley JP, Ziessman HA, Thrall JH. *Nuclear medicine: the requisites*, 5th ed. Philadelphia, PA: Saunders, 2020:43,346–351.

12 **Answer D.** Diffuse muscular uptake is identified on this I-123 metaiodobenzylguanidine (MIBG) scan. Normal physiologic distribution to organs rich in adrenergic innervation (i.e., salivary glands, heart, and liver) is altered (see the image in answer 14 for normal distribution of MIBG). MIBG scans are most commonly done to evaluate for neuroblastomas in children and pheochromocytomas/paragangliomas in adults. Medications are one of the most common causes of altered biodistribution of MIBG. As such, patients should be routinely screened for interfering medications prior to the injection of MIBG. This patient was taking one of the tricyclic antidepressants, which interfere with MIBG biodistribution. Known interfering medications with MIBG include the following:

> Antihypertensives: Labetalol and calcium channel blockers (i.e., diltiazem, nifedipine, verapamil)
> Tricyclic antidepressants: Amitriptyline, imipramine, doxepin, etc.
> Sympathomimetics (i.e., cold medications): Phenylephrine, pseudoephedrine, ephedrine, etc.
> Cocaine

References: O'Malley JP, Ziessman HA, Thrall JH. *Nuclear medicine: the requisites*, 5th ed. Philadelphia, PA: Saunders, 2020:346–348.

Saha GB. *Fundamentals of nuclear pharmacy*, 6th ed. New York, NY: Springer, 2010:370–371.

13 **Answer D.** Cyclotron-produced radionuclides are proton rich and decay by either positron emission or electron capture, which allows them to reduce their proton number and move closer to the line of stability. In positron (positively charged electron) emission, the nucleus emits a positron, which decreases the proton number relative to the neutron number. Isotopes such as F-18, N-13, and

Ga-68 decay by positron emission, a principle that is utilized in PET imaging. Similarly, in electron capture, the nucleus of the proton-rich radionuclide captures an inner-shell electron, which combines with a proton to form a neutron, resulting in one extra neutron and one fewer proton. Cyclotron-produced SPECT radiopharmaceuticals include I-123, Ga-67, Tl-201, and In-111. These decay by electron capture. The generator-produced radiopharmaceuticals, for example, Mo-99 or I-131, are neutron rich and decay by beta-decay. Alpha decay most often occurs in heavy radionuclides, for example, Ra-223 use in treating skeletal metastases of prostate cancer. Isomeric transition is a type of energy transformation where an excited nucleus of Tc-99m decays from one energy level to another, giving off a gamma ray in the process. A stable nucleus of Tc-99 is produced.

Reference: Mettler FA, Guiberteau MJ. *Essentials of nuclear medicine imaging*, 7th ed. Philadelphia, PA: Saunders, 2019:1–5.

14 **Answer D.** Anterior and posterior planar images demonstrate physiologic radiotracer uptake in the lacrimal glands, liver, spleen, bowel loops and mild diffuse activity in the bone marrow. Uptake in the liver is greater than that in the spleen. The images are photon deficient (noisy/coarse). The images are from a Ga-67 scan. The lacrimal gland uptake, when present, is a great clue in identifying gallium-67 scan, but it may not always be present.

Physiologic distribution of I-123 MIBG is in the nasal mucosa, salivary glands, heart, liver, spleen, adrenal glands, bowel, and bladder. The thyroid gland is typically not seen on the MIBG scan due to pretreatment with supersaturated potassium iodide (SSKI) solution. Myocardial uptake is a helpful clue in identifying I-123 MIBG scan. Radiotracers with myocardial uptake as part of physiologic distribution include Tc-99m tetrofosmin, Tc-99m sestamibi, Tl-201, F-18 FDG and I-123 MIBG. Physiologic distribution of In-111 OctreoScan (Question 10) includes the spleen greater than the liver, kidneys, bowel, and bladder. Bright kidneys on a whole-body scan is a clue that can be used to identify an In-111 OctreoScan. Occasionally physiologic gallbladder uptake can be seen on OctreoScan and should not be mistaken for malignancy. With I-123 or I-131, physiologic uptake is seen in salivary glands, thyroid gland, GI tract, and bladder. Liver uptake can be seen on more than 24 hours delayed imaging if there is functioning thyroid tissue as the thyroid hormone is metabolized in the liver. Please see below for labeled examples of I-131, In-111 OctreoScan, I-123 MIBG and Tc-99m sestamibi.

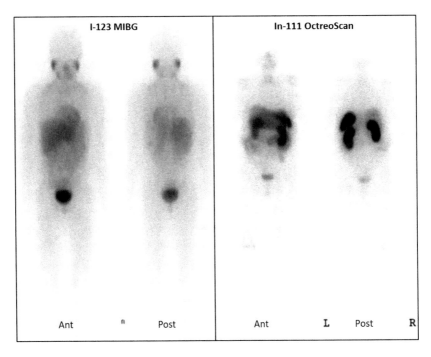

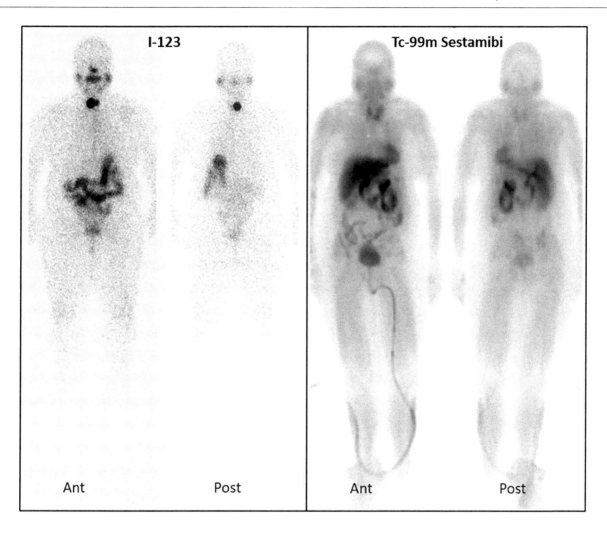

I-123	Tc-99m Sestamibi
Ant Post	Ant Post

Reference: O'Malley JP, Ziessman HA, Thrall JH. *Nuclear medicine: the requisites*, 5th ed. Philadelphia, PA: Saunders, 2020:168–171, 340–342, 346–351.

15 Answer D. Anterior and posterior MIP images demonstrate intense radiotracer uptake in the pancreas and moderate uptake in the liver. Mild to moderate uptake is seen in the marrow. Diffuse muscular activity is seen. Muscle activity is less in the lower body than in the upper body as the physiologic muscle uptake increases over time, and the scan is acquired bottom-up with the pelvis scanned first and the head scanned last. No brain activity is seen. This is an F-18 FACBC scan, also known as fluciclovine (Axumin®). Intense physiologic uptake in the pancreas is a helpful clue in identifying this radiotracer. Fluciclovine is an analog of L-leucine amino acid, which was approved by the FDA in 2016 for the diagnosis of suspected recurrent prostate cancer based on elevated blood PSA levels following prior treatment. The images are acquired approximately 4 minutes after the injection of 10 mCi of F-18 fluciclovine.

F-18 FDG has intense uptake in the brain and urinary tract, moderate uptake in the liver, and variable uptake in salivary glands, oropharynx, heart, and bowel.

Ga-68 DOTATATE has intense uptake in the pituitary, spleen, and kidneys. Moderate to intense uptake is seen in the adrenal glands and liver with variable mild uptake in the salivary glands, thyroid, and bowel. Pituitary uptake can be used as a clue to identify this tracer, and, unlike F-18 FDG, no uptake is seen in the brain. DOTATATE is used in the evaluation of neuroendocrine malignancies, which overexpress somatostatin receptors.

Ga-68 PSMA has high-intensity activity in the lacrimal glands, parotid glands, submandibular glands, and kidneys with no brain uptake; this combination is key to identify this novel radiotracer. Moderate uptake is seen in the liver and spleen. Ga-68 PSMA is excreted in saliva, which may result in oropharyngeal, laryngeal, or esophageal uptake as well. Intense uptake may also be seen in the small bowel, predominantly in the duodenum, where PSMA expression may facilitate absorption of dietary folates. PSMA targeting agents (PSMA-11, PSMA-617 and DCFPyL) have been extensively studied and successfully used in the diagnosis and treatment of prostate cancer in Europe and Australia. See labeled maximum intensity projection image examples below for biodistribution of F-18 FDG, GA-68 DOTATATE, and GA-68 PSMA.

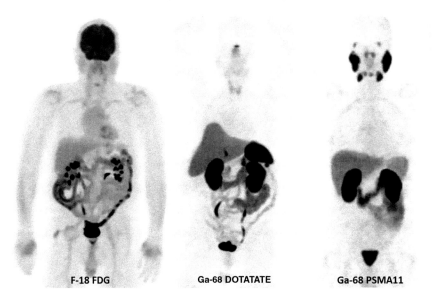

F-18 FDG   Ga-68 DOTATATE   Ga-68 PSMA11

Reference: O'Malley JP, Ziessman HA, Thrall JH. *Nuclear medicine: the requisites*, 5th ed. Philadelphia, PA: Saunders, 2020:67, 288–336, 352–353.

2 Endocrine System

1 What particulate emission during the radioactive decay of I-131 causes the destruction of the thyroid follicular cells?

A. Alpha
B. Beta
C. Gamma
D. Positron

2 What is the half-life of I-131?

A. 13 hours
B. 2.8 days
C. 3.2 days
D. 8.1 days
E. 13.2 days

3 You have 30 mCi of I-123 remaining in the radiopharmacy. A patient is scheduled to have I-123 scintigraphy approximately 2 days from now. How much I-123 would remain at the time of the scheduled examination?

A. 25.3 mCi
B. 18.9 mCi
C. 8.3 mCi
D. 2.3 mCi
E. 1.2 mCi
F. 0.646 mCi

4 Which of the following radiopharmaceuticals is trapped by the thyroid follicular cells but **NOT** organified?

A. Tc-99m pertechnetate
B. I-123 sodium iodide
C. I-131 MIBG
D. In-111 pentetreotide
E. Tc-99m sestamibi

5   A 67-year-old gentleman received 101 mCi of I-131 sodium iodide for the treatment of his differentiated thyroid carcinoma. Which of the following instruments would be typically used to measure the radioactivity emanating from the patient prior to his release?

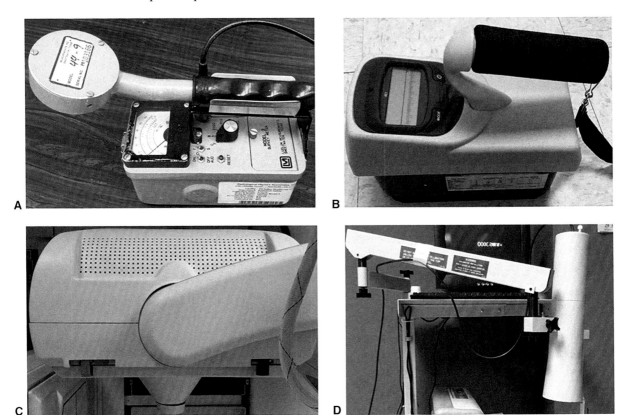

6   The following Tc-99m pertechnetate thyroid scintigraphy image is from a 25-year-old female with hyperthyroidism. What is the most likely 24-hour I-123 radioiodine uptake (RAIU) value for this patient?

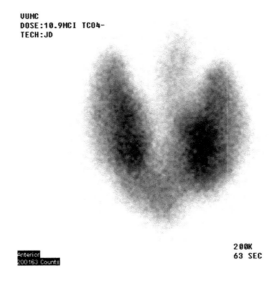

A. 5%
B. 15%
C. 30%
D. 60%

7a The following image is from a 21-year-old female with a recent history of viral upper respiratory infection who presents with complaints of palpitations and tremors. Which of the following is the most likely diagnosis?

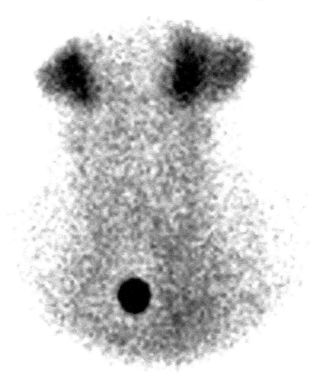

A. Plummer disease
B. Subacute thyroiditis
C. Graves disease
D. Acute suppurative thyroiditis
E. Primary hypothyroidism

7b What is the cause of hyperthyroidism in these patients?

A. Increased thyroid-stimulating immunoglobulins
B. Increased thyroid hormone production
C. Increased TSH secretion by the pituitary
D. Release of preformed thyroid hormone
E. Antithyroid peroxidase antibodies

8 What is the most appropriate I-131 dose to treat the patients with Graves disease?

A. 1 to 5 mCi
B. 10 to 20 mCi
C. 30 to 50 mCi
D. 100 to 200 mCi

9 Which of the following disease processes results in increased radioiodine uptake by the thyroid gland?

A. Viral thyroiditis
B. Iodine deficiency–induced hypothyroidism
C. Jod-Basedow phenomenon
D. Factitious hyperthyroidism

10 How long after the administration of I-131 radioiodine can the patient resume breast-feeding?

   A. 8 days
   B. 80 days
   C. 8 months
   D. Next pregnancy

11 What is the most accurate serum tumor marker to detect the recurrence of a well-differentiated papillary or follicular thyroid carcinoma?

   A. Triiodothyronine
   B. Thyroglobulin
   C. Thyrogen
   D. Thyroid peroxidase antibody
   E. Calcitonin
   F. Thyroid-stimulating immunoglobulin

12 Whole-body radioiodine scintigraphy is the most effective method for tumor detection and staging of which of the following malignancies?

   A. Medullary thyroid carcinoma
   B. Papillary thyroid carcinoma
   C. Hürthle cell thyroid carcinoma
   D. Anaplastic thyroid carcinoma

13 The following whole-body posttherapy I-131 scintigraphy was acquired in a patient with a history of high-risk, well-differentiated papillary thyroid carcinoma who was treated with 157 mCi of I-131 7 days ago. What is the significance of radiopharmaceutical uptake within the liver?

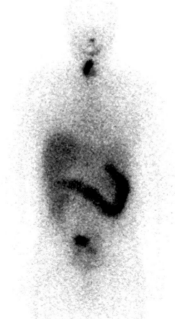

   A. Physiologic distribution
   B. Liver metastasis
   C. Fatty liver
   D. Hepatitis
   E. Cirrhosis

14 The following whole-body I-123 scintigraphy is of a patient who underwent thyroidectomy and radioiodine ablation for differentiated thyroid carcinoma 5 years ago. She now has progressively increasing serum thyroglobulin (Tg) levels, and her recent Thyrogen-stimulated Tg level was 23 ng/mL. What is the most appropriate next step?

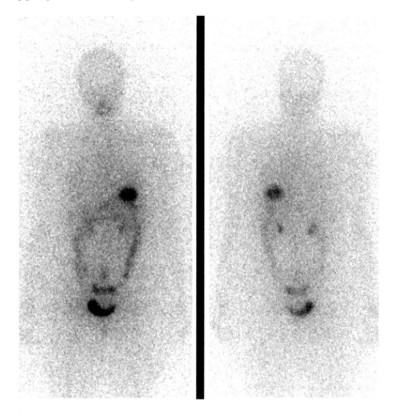

    A. Follow-up I-123 scan in 6 months
    B. Follow-up I-123 scan in 1 year
    C. CT of the abdomen
    D. I-131 therapy
    E. FDG PET/CT

15 A patient with high-risk differentiated thyroid carcinoma (DTC) is undergoing thyroid hormone withdrawal prior to radioiodine ablation therapy. Serum TSH value greater than what level is desirable to ensure the maximal effect of the ablation?
    A. 10 mIU/L
    B. 15 mIU/L
    C. 30 mIU/L
    D. 60 mIU/L

16 What is the MOST common cause of primary hyperparathyroidism?
    A. Multiple gland hyperplasia
    B. Parathyroid carcinoma
    C. Multiple adenomas
    D. Single adenoma

17 The patient is a 37-year-old lady with a clinical history of differentiated thyroid carcinoma status post thyroidectomy and radioiodine ablation approximately 4 years ago. Her Thyrogen-stimulated thyroglobulin level is 1.2 ng/mL. Based on the following 24-hour I-123 whole-body images, what is the most appropriate next step?

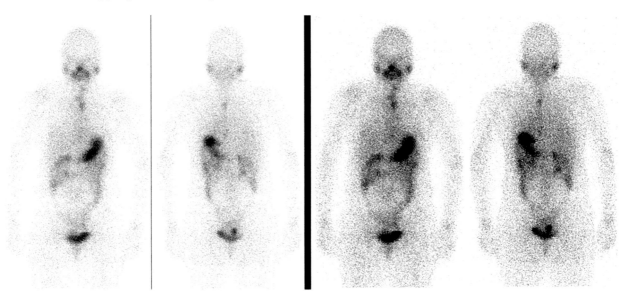

A. FDG PET/CT
B. Treatment with I-131 iodine
C. Contrast-enhanced CT of the chest
D. Reacquire images after water administration

18 A 68-year-old gentleman had the following incidental finding on his FDG PET/CT. What is the most likely chance of malignancy?

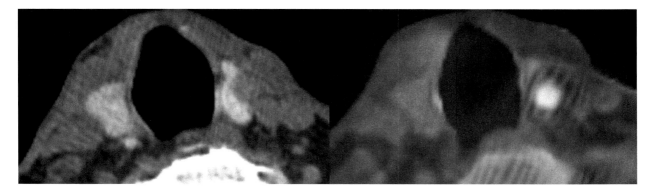

A. 1% to 10%
B. 10% to 20%
C. 30% to 40%
D. 60% to 80%

19 Dual-time imaging using which of the following radiopharmaceuticals is commonly used for the evaluation of primary hyperparathyroidism?

A. Tc-99m sestamibi
B. Tc-99m pertechnetate
C. Tl-201
D. Tc-99m tetrofosmin

20 Based on the following Tc-99m pertechnetate imaging, which of the following is the most likely diagnosis?

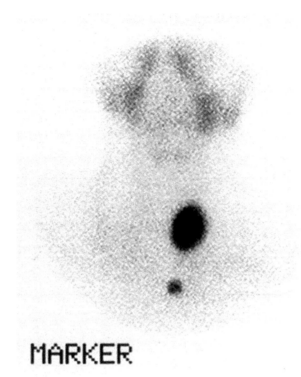

A. Thyroid carcinoma
B. Thyroid metastasis
C. Parathyroid adenoma
D. Parathyroid carcinoma
E. Hyperfunctioning thyroid adenoma

21 Which of the following is the most likely diagnosis?

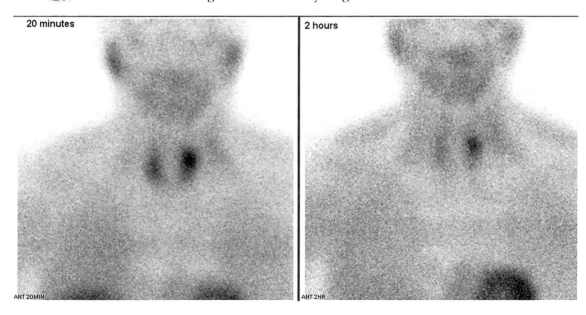

A. Thyroid metastasis
B. Thyroid carcinoma
C. Parathyroid adenoma
D. Parathyroid carcinoma
E. Hyperfunctioning thyroid adenoma

22 What is the most common cause of false-positive parathyroid scintigraphy?

A. Small size
B. Thyroid adenoma
C. Thyroid carcinoma
D. Thyroid metastases
E. Multigland hyperplasia

23 Metaiodobenzylguanidine (MIBG) is an analog of what naturally occurring substance in the body?

A. Norepinephrine
B. Somatostatin
C. Epinephrine
D. Serotonin
E. Guanine

24 What is the most common clinical presentation of patients with hyperparathyroidism?

A. Cramps
B. Bone pain
C. Renal stones
D. Asymptomatic
E. Generalized weakness

25 Which of the following is the most likely diagnosis?

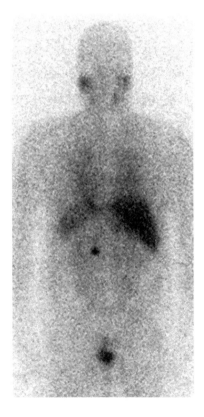
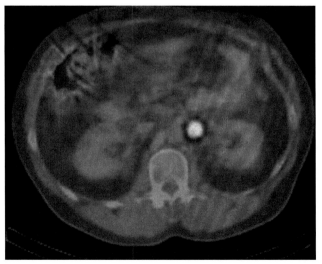

A. Lymphoma
B. Extra-adrenal paraganglioma
C. Metastatic testicular carcinoma
D. Benign adrenal pheochromocytoma

26 Which of the following classes of antihypertensive medications interfere with the uptake of metaiodobenzylguanidine (MIBG)?

A. Beta-blockers (except labetalol)
B. Calcium channel blockers
C. Alpha-blockers
D. ACE inhibitors
E. Diuretics

27 Which of the following receptors serves as the basis for In-111 pentetreotide (OctreoScan) uptake?

A. EGFR
B. Serotonin
C. Somatostatin
D. Growth hormone
E. Norepinephrine

28 The following CT scan and OctreoScan are from a 48-year-old gentleman suspected of having a pancreatic islet cell tumor. What is the most likely diagnosis?

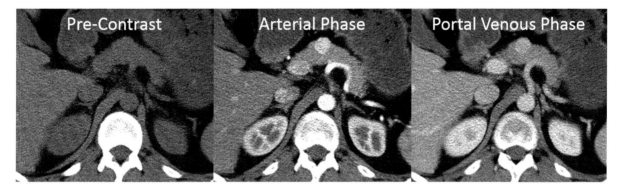

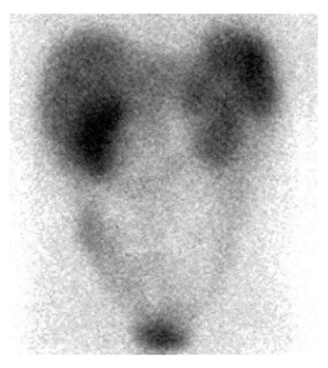

A. VIPoma
B. Insulinoma
C. Glucagonoma
D. Gastrinoma
E. Ectopic spleen

29 Based on the following anterior whole-body image, which of the following is the most likely diagnosis?

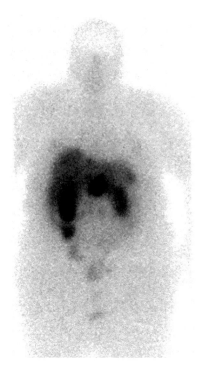

A. Hepatocellular carcinoma
B. Metastatic colon cancer
C. Metastatic gastrinoma
D. Metastatic carcinoid

30 What is the most likely diagnosis in this patient with a clinical history of MEN type I?

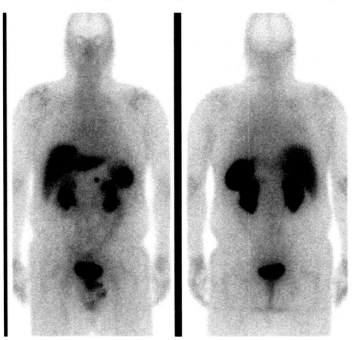

A. Carcinoid
B. Renal cell carcinoma
C. Pheochromocytoma
D. Pancreatic islet cell tumor

31 A 56-year-old lady with a recent diagnosis of papillary thyroid cancer has been referred for radioiodine ablation after undergoing complete thyroidectomy. The referring clinician noted that she had received intravenous iodinated contrast for a CT scan and asked what is the minimum wait time after the IV contrast administration to do the I-131 ablation.

   A. None
   B. 24 hours
   C. 2 weeks
   D. 4 weeks
   E. 4 months

32 A 33-year-old gentleman presents with a markedly elevated parathyroid hormone level of 807 pg/mL. Based on the following Tc-99m sestamibi scan below, what is the most likely diagnosis?

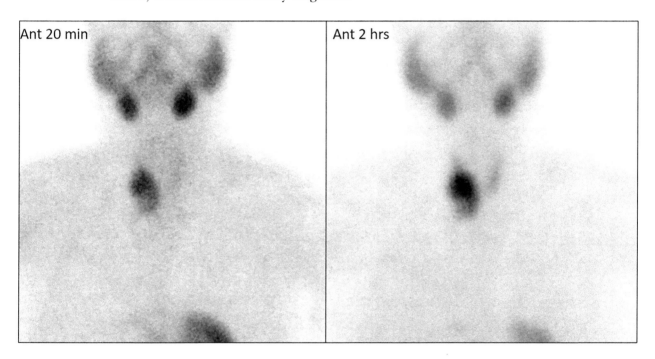

   A. Hyperfunctioning thyroid nodule
   B. Thyroid carcinoma
   C. Parathyroid adenoma
   D. Parathyroid carcinoma

33 A patient has persistent hyperthyroidism after undergoing radioactive iodine (RAI) ablation for Graves disease. How long should you wait prior to retreatment with I-131?

   A. 10 to 20 days
   B. 2 to 4 weeks
   C. 3 to 6 months
   D. 12 to 24 months
   E. Cannot retreat

34a A 58-year-old female with gradually progressive hyperparathyroidism undergoes a repeat parathyroid scintigraphy with Tc-99m sestamibi. What is the most appropriate next step?

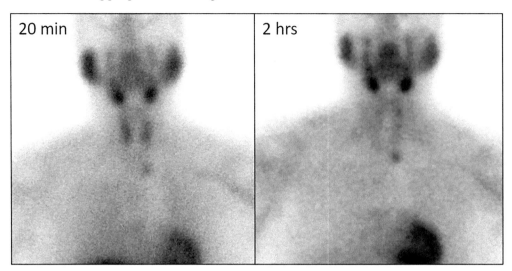

A. Neck ultrasound
B. SPECT/CT
C. PET CT
D. Chest CT
E. 4D contrast-enhanced neck CT

34b Based on the following SPECT/CT images, what is the most likely diagnosis?

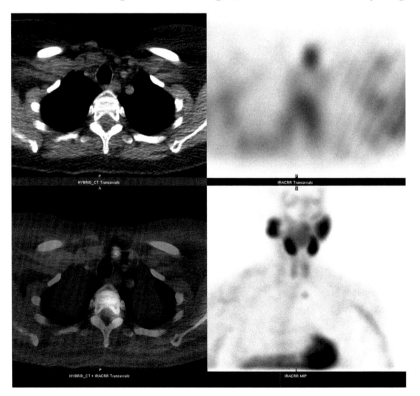

A. Parathyroid adenoma
B. Lymphoma
C. Brown fat
D. Atrial appendage
E. Thymic rebound

35 What is the most likely diagnosis in this 59-year-old lady with hyperparathyroidism?

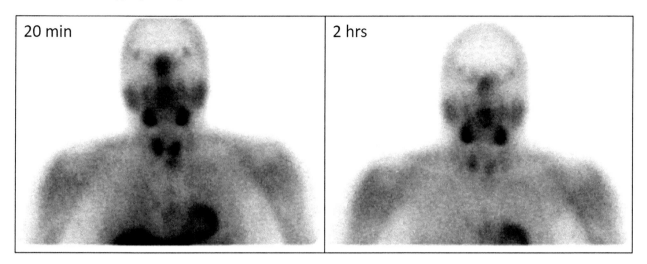

A. Thyroid carcinoma metastasis
B. Parathyroid adenoma
C. Parathyroid carcinoma
D. Esophageal duplication cyst
E. Lung cancer

36 A 35-year-old gentleman with chronic renal failure, hypothyroidism, hyperparathyroidism, and elevated calcium levels has the following imaging done. Based on the findings, what is the most likely diagnosis?

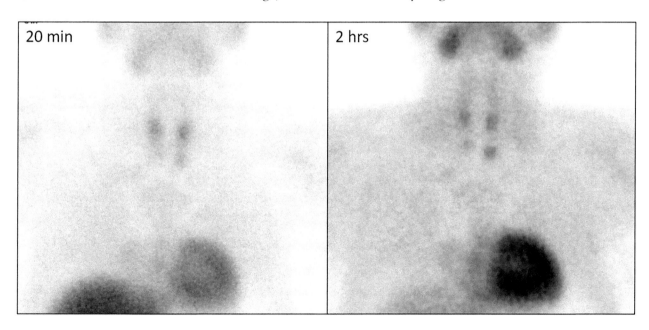

A. Multinodular goiter
B. Multigland hyperplasia
C. Parathyroid adenoma
D. Thyroiditis

ANSWERS AND EXPLANATIONS

1 **Answer B.** Iodine-131 (I-131) undergoes beta minus decay and emits a primary gamma photon of 364 keV as well as high-energy beta particles. Beta particles travel substantial distances in the air but only travel a few millimeters in tissue before getting absorbed. High radiation absorbed dose from beta particle emission combined with a long physical and biologic half-life of I-131 in the thyroid results in the gradual destruction of the thyroid follicular cells. Gamma and positrons are photons and not particles. Alpha particle is basically a helium nucleus consisting of two protons and two neutrons. Because of its heavy mass, it can only travel a few centimeters in air and is unable to penetrate a thin paper. Ra-223 (Xofigo) used in the treatment of metastatic prostate cancer emits alpha particles as it decays.

Reference: O'Malley JP, Ziessman HA, Thrall JH. *Nuclear medicine: the requisites*, 5th ed. Philadelphia, PA: Saunders, 2020:6–8, 152–154.

2 **Answer D.** I-131 has a half-life of 8.1 days. I-123 has a half-life of 13 hours. In-111 has a half-life of 67.2 hours (2.8 days), and Ga-67 has a half-life of 78 hours (3.2 days).

Reference: O'Malley JP, Ziessman HA, Thrall JH. *Nuclear medicine: the requisites*, 5th ed. Philadelphia, PA: Saunders, 2020:6–8, 152–154.

3 **Answer D.** Iodine-123 has a half-life of 13 hours. Two days (48 hours) is slightly less than four half-lives of 52 hours. So, the remaining activity would be slightly more than the residual activity of 1.8 mCi at 52 hours, making 2.3 mCi as the correct answer. Alternatively, this can be accurately calculated using the following formula:

$$A = A \times e^{(-0.693/\text{half-life}) \times (t)}$$

A = remaining activity; A_0 = activity at time 0; t = time of decay.

References: Mettler FA, Guiberteau MJ. *Essentials of nuclear medicine imaging*, 7th ed. Philadelphia, PA: Saunders, 2019:4–5.

O'Malley JP, Ziessman HA, Thrall JH. *Nuclear medicine: the requisites*, 5th ed. Philadelphia, PA: Saunders, 2020:8–9.

4 **Answer A.** "Trapping" refers to the intracellular concentration of a substance by the sodium–iodide symporter located on the cell membrane of the thyroid follicular cells. "Organification" refers to oxidation, iodination, and coupling of iodine to the tyrosine residues on thyroglobulin by the thyroid peroxidase enzymes. Tc-99m pertechnetate undergoes trapping without organification. As such, it can gradually wash out of the thyroid gland, requiring imaging at 20 minutes after IV administration. On the other hand, I-123 and I-131 are organified into T3 and T4 and stored in the colloid-filled follicular lumen. Antithyroid medication such as propylthiouracil and methimazole block this organification process. As such, they should be discontinued approximately 5-7 days prior to radioiodine uptake or therapy.

Reference: O'Malley JP, Ziessman HA, Thrall JH. *Nuclear medicine: the requisites*, 5th ed. Philadelphia, PA: Saunders, 2020:152–154.

5 **Answer B.** Ionization chambers (image B) are typically used to measure high exposure rates (range from 0.1 mR to 100 R), such as those from the patients receiving radioiodine therapy for cancer. If the patient receives more than 33 mCi of I-131 on an outpatient basis, then precautions are taken to ensure that no other person would receive more than 500 mrem (5 mSv) from exposure to the released patient. Activity is measured at 1 meter (m) and 3 m using an ionization chamber, and values are typically entered into a spreadsheet to generate a list of precautions to be discussed with the patient and the family members. Geiger-Müller counters (image A) are very sensitive and are used to detect a very small amount of radioactivity (i.e., contamination). Gamma camera (image C) and scintillation probe (image D) are used for scintigraphy and radioiodine uptake measurement, respectively.

The liquid scintillation counter (shown in the picture below) is utilized for detecting low-energy beta emitters such as hydrogen-3 (tritium), carbon-14, or sulfur-35. Due to low energy resulting in low penetration, B-particle emitters can be difficult to detect. With the liquid scintillation counter, a sample containing the isotope is placed in liquid organic scintillation material.

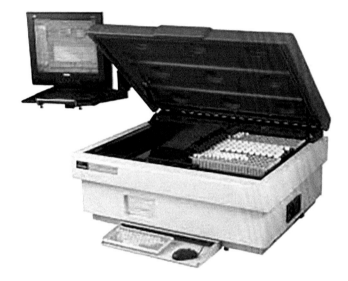

References: Mettler FA, Guiberteau MJ. *Essentials of nuclear medicine imaging*, 7th ed. Philadelphia, PA: Saunders, 2019:19–23.

O'Malley JP, Ziessman HA, Thrall JH. *Nuclear medicine: the requisites*, 5th ed. Philadelphia, PA: Saunders, 2020:14–17, 57–158.

6 **Answer D.** The 20-minute anterior image obtained after IV administration of 10.9 mCi of Tc-99m pertechnetate demonstrates an enlarged thyroid gland with convex borders. A linear focus of activity extending superiorly from the left isthmus is the pyramidal lobe. The absence of significant background activity and lack of visualization of the physiologic uptake in the salivary glands imply a marked increase in the radiopharmaceutical uptake. The findings are those of Graves disease.

Graves disease is caused by increased levels of thyroid-stimulating immunoglobulins (TSI), which cause marked overstimulation of the thyroid follicular cells. Typical 24-hour RAIU in these patients ranges from 50% to 80%. In comparison, the 24-hour RAIU in multinodular goiter and toxic autonomously functioning nodule ranges from 20% to 30% (upper limits of normal to mildly elevated). Normal % RAIU is 4% to 15% at 4 to 6 hours and 10% to 30% at 24 hours.

Reference: O'Malley JP, Ziessman HA, Thrall JH. *Nuclear medicine: the requisites*, 5th ed. Philadelphia, PA: Saunders, 2020:158–164.

7a **Answer B.** Absent or poor visualization of the thyroid gland and decreased RAIU are seen with primary or secondary hypothyroidism, thyroid gland destruction (acute phase of subacute thyroiditis, type II amiodarone toxicity), exposure to excess iodine (iodinated contrast, or type I amiodarone toxicity), or suppression of thyroid from excess exogenous thyroid hormone (struma ovarii or factitious hyperthyroidism). In this patient with a clinical history of recent URI and symptoms of hyperthyroidism, the diagnosis is subacute thyroiditis, specifically subacute granulomatous thyroiditis.

Acute suppurative thyroiditis is an extremely rare but potentially life-threatening bacterial infection; patients present with anterior neck swelling, pain, and fever. However, it typically does not result in significant hyperthyroidism. Plummer disease and Graves disease result in hyperthyroidism but demonstrate increased radioiodine uptake.

Reference: O'Malley JP, Ziessman HA, Thrall JH. *Nuclear medicine: the requisites*, 5th ed. Philadelphia, PA: Saunders, 2020:157–160.

7b **Answer D.** Subacute thyroiditis occurs secondary to the destruction of the thyroid follicular cells, which results in the spillage of preformed thyroid hormone into the bloodstream. Three forms of subacute thyroiditis are recognized: subacute granulomatous thyroiditis (aka painful or de Quervain thyroiditis), subacute lymphocytic thyroiditis (aka painless thyroiditis), and subacute postpartum thyroiditis. Increased thyroid-stimulating immunoglobulins (TSI) are seen with Graves disease. Antithyroid peroxidase antibodies are typically elevated with Hashimoto thyroiditis.

The specific diagnosis in patients with absent or markedly decreased radioiodine uptake and hyperthyroidism depends on their clinical presentation. Specific clinical inquiries regarding recent URI infection and neck pain, recent exposure to iodinated contrast, postpartum status, and amiodarone treatment would help establish a specific diagnosis of subacute granulomatous thyroiditis, Jod-Basedow syndrome, postpartum thyroiditis, and amiodarone toxicity, respectively.

References: Fatourechi V, Aniszewski JP, Fatourechi GZ, et al. Clinical features and outcome of subacute thyroiditis in an incidence cohort: Olmsted County, Minnesota, study. *J Clin Endocrinol Metab* 2003;88(5):2100–2105.

O'Malley JP, Ziessman HA, Thrall JH. *Nuclear medicine: the requisites*, 5th ed. Philadelphia, PA: Saunders, 2020:157–160.

8 **Answer B.** Most patients with Graves disease are effectively treated with I-131, with only 10% requiring retreatment. Symptomatic improvement is usually noted by 3 weeks with full therapeutic effect typically in 3 to 6 months. Some patients may experience an exacerbation of hyperthyroidism symptoms soon after the administration of I-131 due to spillage of preformed thyroid hormone. Elderly patients with cardiac history and pediatric patients may benefit from pretreatment with methimazole to "cool down" the thyroid gland and beta-blockade to prevent tachycardia.

One of the approaches to treating Graves disease is to use an empirical I-131 dose in the range of 8 to 15 mCi. Another approach takes into account the estimated size of the thyroid gland and 24-hour RAIU using the following formula: I-131 dose = (estimated thyroid gland size × 0.130 to 0.180 mCi/g of thyroid tissue)/24-hour RAIU.

Compared to Graves disease, hyperthyroidism from toxic multinodular goiter (MNG) and toxic autonomously functioning (AFN) thyroid nodule (shown in the image below) is generally more resistant to radioiodine therapy. This, combined with lower RAIU by the thyroid (typically 20% to 30%) in MNG, requires about twice the amount of I-131 compared to Graves disease. The typical empirical I-131 dose for these entities ranges from 20 to 30 mCi.

Doses of 30 to 50 mCi of I-131 are typically used in thyroid cancer patients with a low to moderate risk of recurrence to ablate the remnant thyroid tissue. Higher doses of 100 to 200 mCi of I-131 are utilized as adjuvant therapy after surgery in patients with moderate to high risk of recurrence or in patients with suspected recurrence.

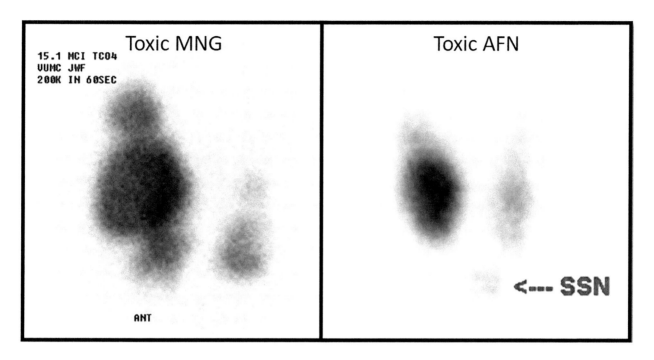

Reference: O'Malley JP, Ziessman HA, Thrall JH. *Nuclear medicine: the requisites*, 5th ed. Philadelphia, PA: Saunders, 2020:164–172.

9 **Answer B.** Iodine deficiency–induced hypothyroidism would result in elevated radioiodine uptake due to increased stimulation from elevated TSH levels. This is rarely seen in developed countries in the present day and age. The remaining choices demonstrate decreased or absent radioiodine uptake in the thyroid gland and would typically be associated with hyperthyroidism. In the Jod-Basedow phenomenon, thyrotoxic condition is caused by exposure to an increased amount of iodine, usually in patients with predisposing conditions such as subclinical multinodular goiter or Graves disease. In factitious hyperthyroidism, higher than normal thyroid hormone level is seen in blood from taking too much thyroid hormone medicine. This results in suppression of TSH and resultant decrease in the radioiodine uptake.

Reference: O'Malley JP, Ziessman HA, Thrall JH. *Nuclear medicine: the requisites*, 5th ed. Philadelphia, PA: Saunders, 2020:155.

10 **Answer D.** Iodine is concentrated in large amounts by the glandular tissue in the breast and is secreted in breast milk. As such, all lactating women undergoing I-131 therapy should be asked to stop breast-feeding to minimize the radiation dose to the sensitive breast tissue and to prevent the infant's exposure to I-131. Lactation and the ability of the breast tissue to concentrate a large amount of iodine stop 4 to 6 weeks after delivery or cessation of breast-feeding. As such, if possible, therapy should be delayed for approximately 6 weeks, and the patient should be initiated on dopamine agonist therapy to reduce the absorbed dose to the breast tissue. The patient should not resume breast-feeding for that child but may resume with the birth of another child.

Unlike I-131, Tc-99m pertechnetate and I-123 have short half-lives and do not emit beta radiation. As such, breast-feeding may be resumed 48 hours after administration of I-123 and 24 hours after administration of Tc-99m pertechnetate. The following I-123 whole body image from a postpartum lactating patient shows intense physiologic radiotracer activity in the glandular tissues of the breast.

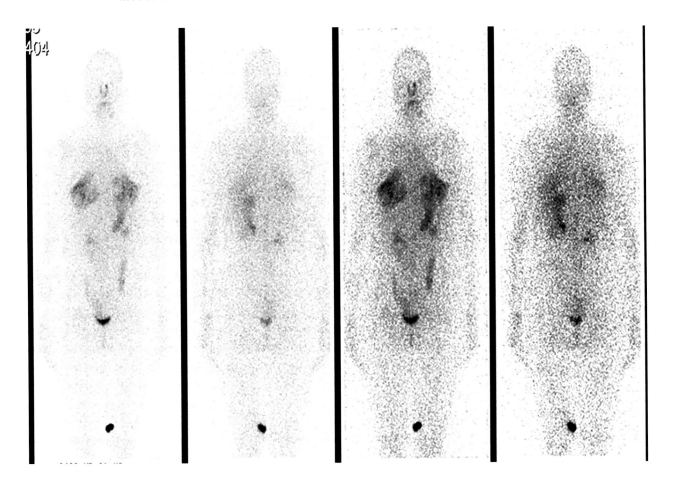

References: Baeumler GR, Joo KG. Radioactive iodine uptake by breasts. *J Nucl Med* 1986;27(1):149–151.

Oh JR, Ahn BC. False-positive uptake on radioiodine whole-body scintigraphy: physiologic and pathologic variants unrelated to thyroid cancer. *Am J Nucl Med Mol Imaging* 2012;2(3):362–385.

O'Malley JP, Ziessman HA, Thrall JH. *Nuclear medicine: the requisites*, 5th ed. Philadelphia, PA: Saunders, 2020:58.

11 **Answer B.** Serum thyroglobulin (Tg) is the most accurate tumor marker to detect the recurrence of well-differentiated thyroid carcinoma. It is not useful for poorly differentiated, anaplastic, or medullary forms of thyroid carcinoma. Please note that the presence of Tg antibody may compromise the accuracy of the Tg essay. Calcitonin levels are used to monitor medullary thyroid carcinoma as it is produced by the parafollicular cells (C cells) in the thyroid gland. Thyroid-stimulating immunoglobulins are elevated in Graves disease while thyroid peroxidase antibodies are elevated with any thyroid disease such as Hashimoto thyroiditis or Graves disease.

Reference: O'Malley JP, Ziessman HA, Thrall JH. *Nuclear medicine: the requisites*, 5th ed. Philadelphia, PA: Saunders, 2020:152.

12 **Answer B.** Papillary thyroid carcinoma is the most common thyroid malignancy and represents about 80% to 90% of well-differentiated thyroid cancers with follicular neoplasm accounting for the remaining percentage. Well-differentiated thyroid cancers are usually iodine avid but not FDG avid. Whole-body scan with radioiodine is the most effective method for tumor detection, staging, and treatment planning in patients with differentiated thyroid carcinoma (DTC).

F-18 FDG PET/CT has reduced sensitivity in the detection of DTC. As DTC cells dedifferentiate, their radioiodine uptake generally decreases, and their glucose metabolism/FDG uptake typically increases. FDG PET/CT is useful in the detection and localization of recurrent DTC only in patients with negative diagnostic radioiodine imaging despite elevated thyroglobulin levels. FDG PET/CT also has high sensitivity and specificity in the evaluation of recurrent Hürthle cell thyroid carcinoma (subtype of follicular carcinoma), undifferentiated/anaplastic thyroid carcinoma, and most cases of medullary thyroid carcinoma. These cancers are more aggressive and are associated with poorer prognosis than DTC. They are typically NOT iodine avid and are better evaluated with F-18 FDG PET/CT.

References: Marcus C, Whitworth PW, Surasi DS, et al. PET/CT in the management of thyroid cancers. *AJR Am J Roentgenol* 2014;202(6):1316–1329.

O'Malley JP, Ziessman HA, Thrall JH. *Nuclear medicine: the requisites*, 5th ed. Philadelphia, PA: Saunders, 2020:166–171, 172, 314.

13 **Answer A.** A large focus of intense activity within the right thyroid bed and a small focus of mild activity within the left thyroid bed likely represent remnant thyroid tissue in this patient with clean surgical margins on pathology. Physiologic radioiodine distribution is seen in the salivary glands, the oral cavity, liver, bowel, and bladder. Thyroid hormone undergoes conversion from T4 to T3 by type I iodothyronine deiodinase within the liver. Thus, the presence of liver uptake suggests evidence of functioning thyroid tissue elsewhere in the body. In this patient with remnant thyroid tissue in the neck, this finding is physiologic and requires no further workup.

References: Oh JR, Ahn BC. False-positive uptake on radioiodine whole-body scintigraphy: physiologic and pathologic variants unrelated to thyroid cancer. *Am J Nucl Med Mol Imaging* 2012;2(3):362–385.

Shapiro B, Rufini V, Jarwan A, et al. Artifacts, anatomical and physiological variants, and unrelated diseases that might cause false-positive whole-body 131-I scans in patients with thyroid cancer. *Semin Nucl Med* 2000;30(2):115–132.

14 **Answer E.** Delayed anterior and posterior whole-body images demonstrate physiologic radiotracer uptake within the nasal mucosa, oral cavity, stomach, bowel, renal collecting system, and bladder. There are no foci of abnormal activity identified. F-18 FDG uptake in differentiated thyroid carcinoma (DTC) is related to the loss of differentiation and transformation of the tumor into a higher grade. As such, FDG PET/CT is useful in the detection and localization of recurrent DTC in patients with negative diagnostic radioiodine imaging despite elevated thyroglobulin (Tg) levels; Centers for Medicare and Medicaid Services requires serum TG level of >10 ng/mL for approval of the procedure. The diagnostic accuracy of FDG PET/CT increases with increasing stimulated Tg levels and is most promising at levels >20 ng/mL.

References: Na SJ, Yoo IR, O JH, et al. Diagnostic accuracy of (18)F-fluorodeoxyglucose positron emission tomography/computed tomography in differentiated thyroid cancer patients with elevated thyroglobulin and negative (131)I whole body scan: evaluation by thyroglobulin level. *Ann Nucl Med* 2012;26(1):26–34.

O'Malley JP, Ziessman HA, Thrall JH. *Nuclear medicine: the requisites*, 5th ed. Philadelphia, PA: Saunders, 2020:172.

Schlüter B, Bohuslavizki KH, Beyer W, et al. Impact of FDG PET on patients with differentiated thyroid cancer who present with elevated thyroglobulin and negative 131I scan. *J Nucl Med* 2001;42:71–76.

15 **Answer C.** The patients undergoing radioiodine ablation therapy (RIAT) for DTC should undergo thyroid hormone withdrawal by stopping tetraiodothyronine (LT4, Synthroid) for 4 weeks or triiodothyronine (LT3, Cytomel) for 2 weeks before RIAT. The resultant elevation in the endogenous TSH levels ensures proper stimulation of the thyroid tissue to allow a poorly functioning or small amount of residual thyroid tissue to take up a maximal amount of radioiodine. Serum TSH value >30 mIU/L is desirable, and a level >50 mIU/L is optimal for this purpose. For patients who are unable to tolerate hypothyroidism or unable to generate an elevated TSH level, remnant ablation can be achieved with two doses of rh-TSH (Thyrogen) given intramuscularly 48 and 24 hours before RIAT.

References: Mettler FA, Guiberteau MJ. *Essentials of nuclear medicine imaging*, 7th ed. Philadelphia, PA: Saunders, 2019:107.

O'Malley JP, Ziessman HA, Thrall JH. *Nuclear medicine: the requisites*, 5th ed. Philadelphia, PA: Saunders, 2020:174.

16 **Answer D.** In a large meta-analysis, primary hyperparathyroidism was caused by a single adenoma in 89%, multiple gland hyperplasia in 6%, double adenomas in 4%, and carcinomas in <1% of the patients who underwent resection for primary hyperparathyroidism.

Tc-99m sestamibi scintigraphy with SPECT imaging has the highest positive predictive value of the available imaging techniques and is the preferred procedure to localize a parathyroid adenoma prior to surgery. It is usually supplemented with neck sonography and, in some cases, 4D CT of the neck/mediastinum with and without contrast.

References: Eslamy HK, Ziessman HA. Parathyroid scintigraphy in patients with primary hyperparathyroidism: 99mTc sestamibi SPECT and SPECT/CT. *Radiographics* 2008;28(5):1461–1476.

Lew JI, Solorzano CC. Surgical management of primary hyperparathyroidism: state of the art. *Surg Clin North Am* 2009;89(5):1205–1225.

O'Malley JP, Ziessman HA, Thrall JH. *Nuclear medicine: the requisites*, 5th ed. Philadelphia, PA: Saunders, 2020:173–174.

Ruda JM, Hollenbeak CS, Stack BC Jr. A systematic review of the diagnosis and treatment of primary hyperparathyroidism from 1995 to 2003. *Otolaryngology Head Neck Surg* 2005;132(3):359–372.

17 **Answer D.** Anterior and posterior whole-body images acquired at 24 hours after the oral administration of 5.3 mCi of I-123 demonstrate the presence of a linear focus of a mild to moderately increased activity within the midline of the upper thorax. This likely represents physiologic activity within the esophagus from the swallowed saliva or reflux. This can be confirmed by reacquiring images after the patient ingests some water to ensure that it clears (which was done for this patient; see image below). Alternatively, SPECT/CT images could be performed to confirm that the activity corresponds to the esophagus. FDG PET/CT is not indicated as the thyroglobulin (Tg) level is <10 ng/mL. The Thyrogen-stimulated Tg level of <2 is also reassuring for the absence of recurrence.

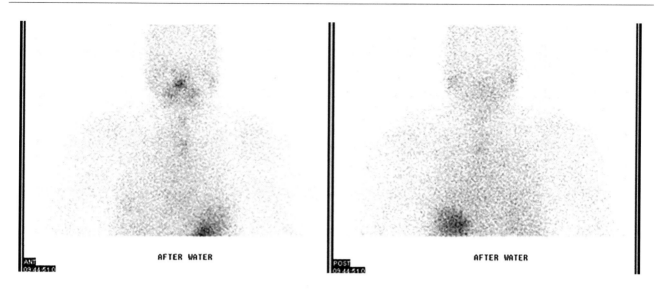

AFTER WATER   AFTER WATER

References: Knapska-Kucharska M, Makarewicz J. A case of iodine-131 retention in the esophagus mimicking a mediastinal metastasis in a patient with follicular thyroid carcinoma after gastric volume reduction operation. *Clin Nucl Med* 2011;36(9):817–818.

Oh JR, Ahn BC. False-positive uptake on radioiodine whole-body scintigraphy: physiologic and pathologic variants unrelated to thyroid cancer. *Am J Nucl Med Mol Imaging* 2012;2(3):362–385.

18 **Answer C.** CT and fused F-18 FDG PET/CT images demonstrate an intensely FDG-avid thyroid nodule in the anterior aspect of the left thyroid lobe. Thyroid incidentaloma (TI) is defined as an unsuspected, asymptomatic thyroid nodule detected on an imaging study or during an operation unrelated to the thyroid gland. The rate of detection of thyroid incidentaloma with FDG PET/CT is low at 1% to 3% (compared to 16% by CT and MRI and 9% by carotid duplex scan). However, FDG PET/CT–detected TI carries a higher risk of malignancy at about 33%, and the detected cancers are more aggressive. Because of this, when found, FDG-avid thyroid incidentaloma requires a prompt workup, preferably with an ultrasound-guided fine needle aspiration. On the other hand, diffuse increase in FDG uptake is benign, likely related to autoimmune thyroiditis, and does not require biopsy (see picture below).

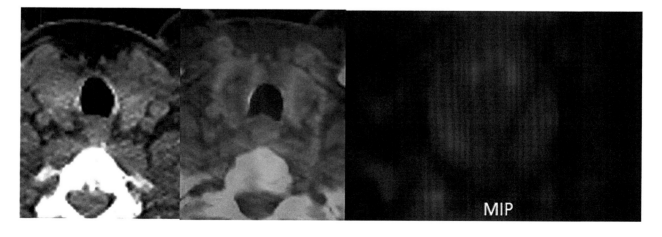

MIP

References: Are C, Hsu JF, Ghossein RA, et al. Histological aggressiveness of fluorodeoxyglucose positron-emission tomogram (FDG-PET)-detected incidental thyroid carcinomas. *Ann Surg Oncol* 2007;14(11):3210–3215.

Choi JY, Lee KS, Kim HJ, et al. Focal thyroid lesions incidentally identified by integrated 18F-FDG PET/CT: clinical significance and improved characterization. *J Nucl Med* 2006;47(4):609–615.

Jin J, Wilhelm SM, McHenry CR. Incidental thyroid nodule: patterns of diagnosis and rate of malignancy. *Am J Surg* 2009;197(3):320–324.

19 Answer A. Tc-99m sestamibi is a lipophilic cationic substance that crosses the cell membrane by passive diffusion and is concentrated within the mitochondria. Parathyroid adenomas are typically composed of chief cells (responsible for the synthesis and release of parathyroid hormone) and mitochondria-rich oxyphil cells, which accumulate the radiopharmaceutical in high concentrations. Immediate image acquired 20 minutes after the IV administration of Tc-99m sestamibi typically shows physiologic activity in the thyroid gland and in the parathyroid adenoma. On a 2-hour delayed image, activity from the thyroid is usually washed out with retention of activity in the parathyroid adenoma. Atypical parathyroid adenomas typically have a washout similar to that of the thyroid gland. Hence the need for dual-time imaging. While tetrofosmin localizes in both parathyroid and thyroid tissues, in contrast to sestamibi, there is no differential washout between the thyroid and parathyroid tissue. As such, dual-time imaging is not useful with tetrofosmin. Tc-99m pertechnetate is commonly utilized for thyroid scintigraphy and for the evaluation of Meckel diverticulum. Tl-201 is a potassium analog that is utilized in the evaluation of myocardial perfusion and viability.

References: Eslamy HK, Ziessman HA. Parathyroid scintigraphy in patients with primary hyperparathyroidism: 99mTc sestamibi SPECT and SPECT/CT. *Radiographics* 2008;28(5):1461–1476.

O'Malley JP, Ziessman HA, Thrall JH. *Nuclear medicine: the requisites*, 5th ed. Philadelphia, PA: Saunders, 2020:174–178.

20 Answer E. Single anterior pinhole collimation Tc-99m pertechnetate image demonstrates a large focus of intense activity within the left thyroid lobe. The remaining thyroid gland is not visualized. Findings are consistent with a toxic hyperfunctioning thyroid nodule or a toxic thyroid adenoma. This nodule represents less than a 1% chance of malignancy, and sonography and/or biopsy is not necessary for further workup. This is not a parathyroid adenoma or carcinoma as the supplied image is of Tc-99m pertechnetate and NOT Tc-99m sestamibi. Thyroid carcinoma usually presents as a cold nodule on Tc-99m pertechnetate or I-123 scintigraphy with preserved uptake in the normal surrounding thyroid gland.

Reference: O'Malley JP, Ziessman HA, Thrall JH. *Nuclear medicine: the requisites*, 5th ed. Philadelphia, PA: Saunders, 2020:174–178.

21 Answer C. Anterior early 20 minutes and 2.5-hour delayed images following the IV administration of Tc-99m sestamibi demonstrate a moderate-sized focus of persistent activity about the superior aspect of the left thyroid lobe. This is consistent with a parathyroid adenoma. A portion of the myocardium is usually included on these images for the purposes of quality control, as it should be visualized with Tc-99m sestamibi. Parathyroid carcinoma is rare and usually presents as a large sestamibi avid neck mass. Thyroid adenomas are a common cause of false-positive parathyroid scintigraphy, but most washout on delayed imaging. SPECT/CT imaging, as well as thyroid sonogram in this patient (shown below), confirmed a large parathyroid adenoma posterior to the upper pole of the left thyroid lobe.

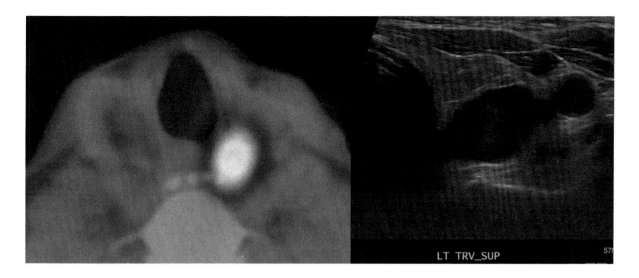

Reference: O'Malley JP, Ziessman HA, Thrall JH. *Nuclear medicine: the requisites*, 5th ed. Philadelphia, PA: Saunders, 2020:174–178.

22 **Answer B.** Thyroid follicular adenoma is the most common cause of false-positive parathyroid scintigraphy (see example below). When suspected, correlation with either SPECT/CT or thyroid sonogram should be considered for confirmation. While intrathyroidal parathyroid adenoma, thyroid carcinoma, and metastases may appear similarly, they are less common. Small size of the parathyroid adenoma and multigland hyperplasia are common causes of false-negative parathyroid scintigraphy.

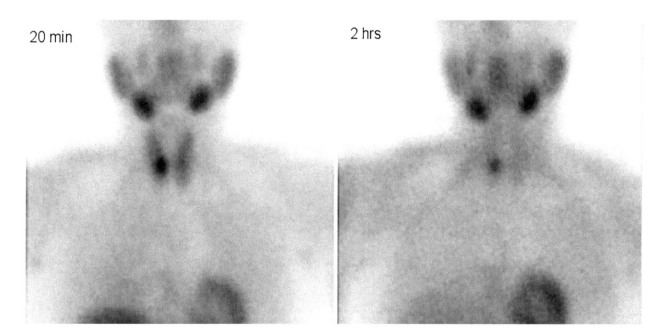

Reference: O'Malley JP, Ziessman HA, Thrall JH. *Nuclear medicine: the requisites*, 5th ed. Philadelphia, PA: Saunders, 2020:484.

23 **Answer A.** MIBG is an analog of norepinephrine. It localizes in the presynaptic neuron vesicles of the sympathetic nervous system (D in the image below) after getting transported intracellularly by an energy-dependent, active amine transport mechanism.

Free form of the I-123 or I-131 used to label MIBG will be taken up by the normally functioning thyroid gland, resulting in unnecessary radiation exposure. As such, the patients undergoing I-131 or I-123 MIBG are instructed to take a concentrated solution of potassium iodide (SSKI) or Lugol solution to block unwanted radioiodine accumulation in the normal thyroid gland. Similar precautions are taken with non-Hodgkin lymphoma patients undergoing radioimmunotherapy with I-131 tositumomab (Bexxar).

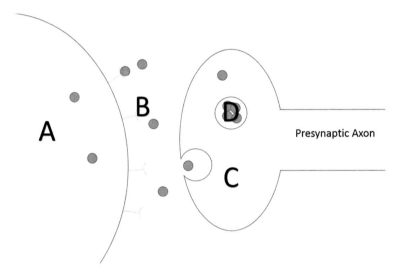

Reference: O'Malley JP, Ziessman HA, Thrall JH. *Nuclear medicine: the requisites*, 5th ed. Philadelphia, PA: Saunders, 2020:346–347.

24 **Answer D.** Today, the clinical diagnosis of primary hyperparathyroidism is predominantly based on serum laboratory test results, and the majority of these patients are asymptomatic. In the past, patients presented with secondary symptoms of hyperparathyroidism due to late diagnosis. These included brown tumors, nephrolithiasis, osteoporosis, pathologic fractures, as well as GI and neuropsychiatric symptoms.

Reference: O'Malley JP, Ziessman HA, Thrall JH. *Nuclear medicine: the requisites*, 5th ed. Philadelphia, PA: Saunders, 2020:173.

25 **Answer B.** A posterior I-123 MIBG image demonstrates a moderate-sized focus of intense activity within the left paraspinous region. The focus appears to be too low for the adrenal glands suggesting a paraganglioma. SPECT/CT confirmed that this was an extra-adrenal paraganglioma, which was responsible for the patient's symptoms. Testicular carcinoma and lymphoma do not demonstrate abnormal MIBG uptake and are not indications of performing an MIBG scan.

Anterior and posterior I-123 MIBG images in a different patient below show a small-sized focus of intense activity in the left adrenal bed, which corresponds to a left adrenal nodule on the SPECT/CT (white arrow), consistent with an adrenal pheochromocytoma.

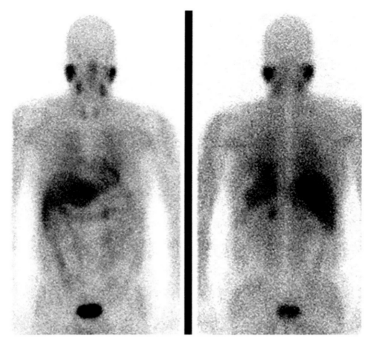

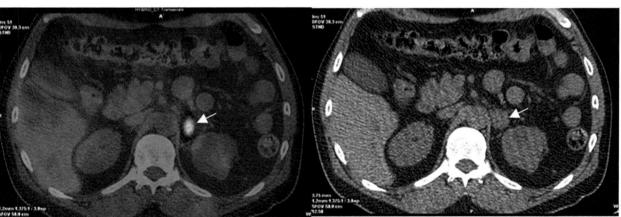

References: Mettler FA, Guiberteau MJ. *Essentials of nuclear medicine imaging*, 7th ed. Philadelphia, PA: Saunders, 2019:327.

O'Malley JP, Ziessman HA, Thrall JH. *Nuclear medicine: the requisites*, 5th ed. Philadelphia, PA: Saunders, 2020:346–348.

26 **Answer B.** Numerous medications interfere with the physiologic distribution of MIBG. As such, patients undergoing MIBG scan should be routinely screened for interfering medications prior to the initiation of the examination. Sympathomimetics such as phenylephrine, ephedrine, and pseudoephedrine are common ingredients in over-the-counter cold medications. These, along with tricyclic antidepressants, cocaine, insulin, some antipsychotics, and antihypertensives such as labetalol, calcium channel blockers, guanethidine, and reserpine, are expected to reduce MIBG uptake. Beta-blockers other than labetalol, alpha-blockers, ACE inhibitors, and diuretics are the class of antihypertensives that do not interfere with the MIBG uptake.

Reference: Mettler FA, Guiberteau MJ. *Essentials of nuclear medicine imaging*, 7th ed. Philadelphia, PA: Saunders, 2019:347.

27 **Answer C.** In-111 pentetreotide is an analog of octreotide, which binds with a high affinity to the somatostatin receptors type II and type V. It has a lesser affinity for type III receptors and does not bind to type I or IV receptors. Physiologic distribution of OctreoScan includes the liver, spleen, kidneys, and bowel on the 24-hour imaging. Although the main clearance of In-111-DTPA-pentetreotide (OctreoScan) is by the kidneys, about 2% of the radiopharmaceutical is cleared by the hepatobiliary system. Caution must be used to avoid misinterpreting physiologic gallbladder activity as hepatic metastases or primary gallbladder malignancy. Arrows in the below point to physiologic activity in the gallbladder, which should not be confused with liver metastasis. If indicated, this can be confirmed with SPECT/CT imaging. Meningioma is also a common cause of false-positive findings on OctreoScan. Other nonneuroendocrine tumors, which express somatostatin receptors and are positive on OctreoScan, include lymphoma, low-grade gliomas, renal cell carcinoma, and breast cancer. Remember that small cell carcinoma is a poorly differentiated neuroendocrine tumor and be positive on OctreoScan. Recently, OctreoScan has been largely replaced by somatostatin receptor binding positron emission tomography agents such as Ga-68 DOTATATE, DOTATOC, or DOTANOC.

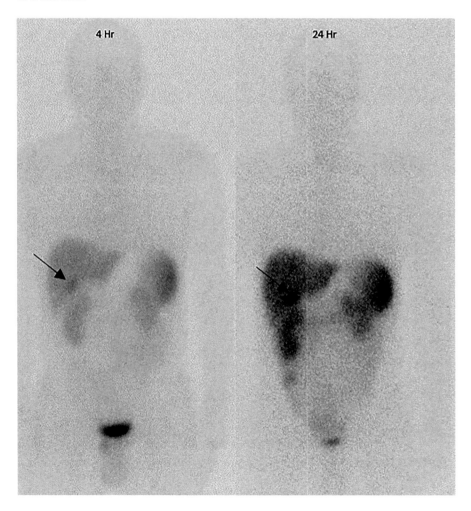

Reference: Mettler FA, Guiberteau MJ. *Essentials of nuclear medicine imaging*, 7th ed. Philadelphia, PA: Saunders, 2019:316–318.

28 **Answer B.** The CT scans show a hyperenhancing lesion in the pancreatic body. However, OctreoScan is normal. Of the neuroendocrine tumors, In-111 OctreoScan has the least sensitivity for insulinoma (25% to 70%) and medullary thyroid carcinoma (50% to 75%). Insulinoma is typically small in size at the time of diagnosis, secondary to an early symptomatic presentation. Small size, along with the lack of type II somatostatin receptors, are thought to be the reason why OctreoScan is less sensitive for its evaluation and may be falsely negative.

References: Mettler FA, Guiberteau MJ. *Essentials of nuclear medicine imaging*, 7th ed. Philadelphia, PA: Saunders, 2019:339–340.

O'Malley JP, Ziessman HA, Thrall JH. *Nuclear medicine: the requisites*, 5th ed. Philadelphia, PA: Saunders, 2020:339–344.

29 **Answer D.** The anterior In-111 OctreoScan images demonstrate a large focus of intense activity within the right lower quadrant (seen inferolateral to the right kidney) accompanied by a large focus of intense activity within the left hepatic lobe. The distribution pattern is typical for that of the metastatic carcinoid. Carcinoid is a slow-growing neuroendocrine tumor that typically originates in the GI tract or lungs. Since it overexpresses somatostatin receptors, OctreoScan and now Ga-68 DOTATATE or DOTATOC are very sensitive in its evaluation.

Reference: O'Malley JP, Ziessman HA, Thrall JH. *Nuclear medicine: the requisites*, 5th ed. Philadelphia, PA: Saunders, 2020:346–348.

30 **Answer D.** The anterior and posterior In-111 OctreoScan images demonstrate a small focus of intense activity superior and medial to the left kidney, which is seen on the anterior image and not on the posterior. In this patient with a history of MEN I, the findings are most compatible with a pancreatic neuroendocrine tumor. While a pheochromocytoma would be intensely avid on OctreoScan, it would appear more intense on the posterior image. Also, I-123 MIBG is typically utilized for the evaluation of pheochromocytoma and not OctreoScan. Contrast-enhanced CT demonstrated a hyperenhancing lesion in the pancreatic tail (arrow below). An area of photopenia along the lateral aspect of the left kidney corresponded to a renal cyst on the CT (not shown).

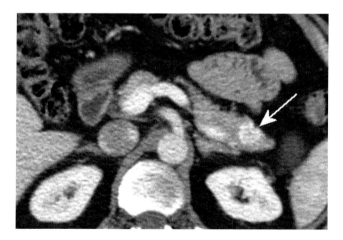

Reference: O'Malley JP, Ziessman HA, Thrall JH. *Nuclear medicine: the requisites*, 5th ed. Philadelphia, PA: Saunders, 2020:346–348.

31 Answer D. Intravenous iodinated contrast agents contain a lot of iodine, which will compete and interfere with subsequent whole-body scans or radioactive iodine treatment, potentially making thyroid ablation with I-131 ineffective. In patients with normal renal function, it takes approximately 1 month for the urinary iodine levels to return to baseline after the administration of intravenous iodinated contrast agents. As such, at least 4 weeks of wait is desired prior to the administration of radioiodine for thyroid ablation or whole-body thyroid scans.

Reference: O'Malley JP, Ziessman HA, Thrall JH. *Nuclear medicine: the requisites*, 5th ed. Philadelphia, PA: Saunders, 2020:155.

32 Answer D. Anterior 20 minutes and 2 hours delayed images show a large mass with intense sestamibi uptake in the right lower neck with a small area of photopenia along its inferolateral aspect. The large size of the lesion, intense uptake (greater than the submandibular gland activity on the delayed image), and markedly elevated parathyroid hormone (PTH) level favor this to be a parathyroid carcinoma over a parathyroid adenoma. Marked elevation in PTH level can also be seen with tertiary hyperparathyroidism in patients with chronic renal failure; however, a large mass would not be expected in that case. Also, parathyroid scintigraphy is not sensitive in the evaluation of multigland hyperplasia resulting from tertiary hyperparathyroidism. Thyroid carcinomas and hyperfunctioning thyroid nodules may present similarly but would not be associated with an increased parathyroid hormone level.

Parathyroid carcinomas are an uncommon cause of primary hyperparathyroidism, with an incidence of <1%. They should be suspected in patients with markedly high PTH levels (>500) with a large sestamibi-avid lesion. Correlating sonographic images of this lesion (below) show a 4.3 × 2.5 cm hypoechoic, hypervascular mass inferior to and invading the inferior pole of the right thyroid lobe.

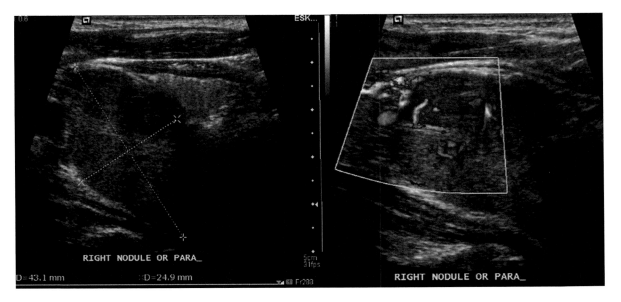

References: Cheon M, Choi JY, Chung JH, et al. Differential findings of Tc-99m sestamibi dual-phase parathyroid scintigraphy between benign and malignant parathyroid lesions in patients with primary hyperparathyroidism. *Nucl Med Mol Imaging* 2011;45(4):276–284.

Mettler FA, Guiberteau MJ. *Essentials of nuclear medicine imaging*, 7th ed. Philadelphia, PA: Saunders, 2019:111.

O'Malley JP, Ziessman HA, Thrall JH. *Nuclear medicine: the requisites*, 5th ed. Philadelphia, PA: Saunders, 2020:173.

33 **Answer C.** While the majority of the administered I-131 localizes in the thyroid gland within 24 hours, it destroys thyroid follicular cells gradually over several weeks. Symptomatic improvement is generally seen in about 3 weeks after the treatment; however, the full effect may take 3 to 6 months. Approximately 10% of patients may require retreatment. These patients should wait approximately 4 to 6 months after the initial treatment to evaluate its efficacy. For this reason, patients of childbearing age should be advised to avoid conception for at least 6 months after the initial treatment.

Radioiodine ablation (RAI) is the most widely used, effective treatment for Graves disease in the United States. Medical treatment with methimazole or propylthiouracil has variable control and is associated with poor compliance. Also, since these agents work by blocking the organification process, they do not offer a permanent solution. Surgical resection is uncommon and typically reserved in cases of uncontrolled thyrotoxicosis in pregnancy or large goiter resulting in significant airway narrowing/obstruction.

References: Mettler FA, Guiberteau MJ. *Essentials of nuclear medicine imaging,* 7th ed. Philadelphia, PA: Saunders, 2019:104–105.

Ziessman HA, O'Malley JP, Thrall JH. *Nuclear medicine: the requisites,* 4th ed. Philadelphia, PA: Saunders, 2014:267–268.

34a **Answer B.** Early and delayed anterior planar images show a small focus of moderate to severely increased activity in the anterior mediastinum to the left of the midline (arrow below). In this patient with persistent hyperparathyroidism and prior negative workup, findings are highly suspicious for an ectopic mediastinal parathyroid adenoma. Further evaluation with SPECT/CT would help confirm the diagnosis and better localize its location to facilitate preoperative planning.

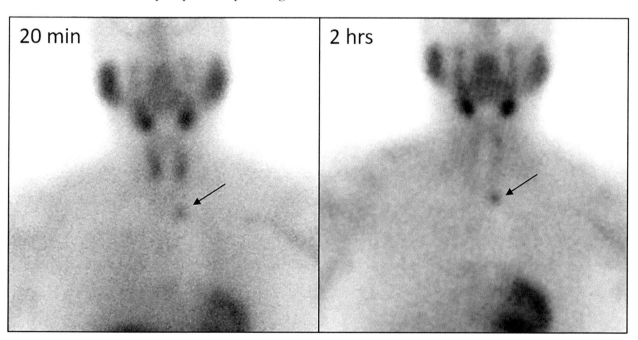

References: Mettler FA, Guiberteau MJ. *Essentials of nuclear medicine imaging,* 7th ed. Philadelphia, PA: Saunders, 2019:111–112.

O'Malley JP, Ziessman HA, Thrall JH. *Nuclear medicine: the requisites,* 5th ed. Philadelphia, PA: Saunders, 2020:174–179.

34b **Answer A.** SPECT images confirm a small focus of moderate to intense activity in the superior anterior mediastinum, which corresponds to a 4-mm soft tissue nodule on CT scan (arrow below). The findings are consistent with an ectopic inferior parathyroid adenoma.

The superior parathyroid glands originate from the fourth branchial pouch and descend with the thyroid glands, while the inferior glands originate from the third branchial pouch and descend with the thymus. Because the inferior glands descend a greater distance with the thymus, they have a more variable location and are typically present anywhere from the posterior aspect of the inferior thyroid lobe superiorly to the thymus in the anterior mediastinum inferiorly (as seen on image 2 from a different patient's SPECT/CT) as well as along the course of the thyrothymic ligament in between (our patient, image 1). While 90% of the superior parathyroid glands tend to be eutopic, only 61% of the inferior parathyroid glands are eutopic. The majority (~26%) of the ectopic inferior parathyroid glands are located in the thyrothymic ligament/cervical thymus, with about 4% to 5% located in the anterior mediastinum. The graphic below from an excellent RadioGraphics article best summarizes the ectopic locations of parathyroid glands.

An atrial appendage is a common cause of abnormal sestamibi uptake in the mediastinum. Along with its location and shape, SPECT/CT helps localize this physiologic uptake to the atrium. The classic thymic rebound has a triangular configuration in the anterior mediastinum, which has uptake seen mainly on FDG PET CT and not on the sestamibi scan. Brown fat uptake is generally seen in supraclavicular regions and in a paraspinal location, not in the anterior mediastinum, and should not have any soft tissue correlation on CT.

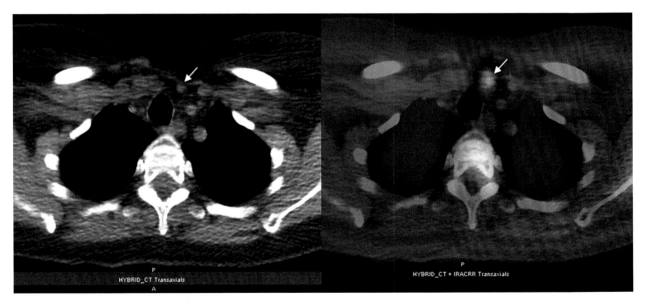

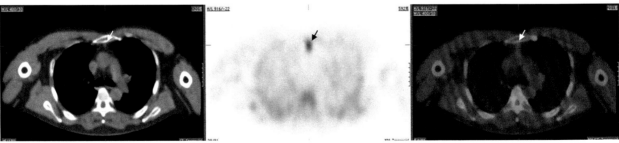

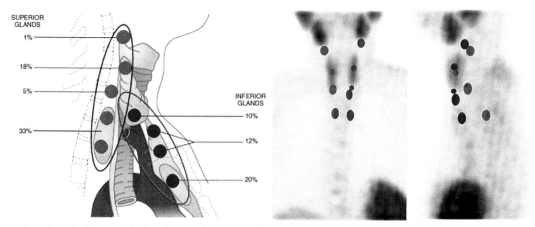

SUPERIOR GLANDS
1%
18%
5%
33%
INFERIOR GLANDS
10%
12%
20%

Reprinted with permission from Eslamy HK, Ziessman HA. Parathyroid scintigraphy in patients with primary hyperparathyroidism: 99mTc sestamibi SPECT and SPECT/CT. *Radiographics* 2008;28(5):1461–1476.

References: Eslamy HK, Ziessman HA. Parathyroid scintigraphy in patients with primary hyperparathyroidism: 99mTc sestamibi SPECT and SPECT/CT. *Radiographics* 2008;28(5):1461–1476.

Mettler FA, Guiberteau MJ. *Essentials of nuclear medicine imaging*, 7th ed. Philadelphia, PA: Saunders, 2019:111–112.

O'Malley JP, Ziessman HA, Thrall JH. *Nuclear medicine: the requisites*, 5th ed. Philadelphia, PA: Saunders, 2020:174–179.

35 **Answer B.** The 20-minute anterior planar image acquired after the IV administration of Tc-99m sestamibi demonstrates a moderate-sized focus of moderate to intense radiotracer uptake in the left lower neck inferior to the left thyroid lobe (arrow in the image below). This focus is not visualized on the 2-hour delayed images. In the setting of hyperparathyroidism, this abnormality is most consistent with an ectopic parathyroid adenoma with an early washout. While the majority of the parathyroid adenomas exhibit delayed washout pattern (retention of radiotracer on the 2 hours delayed imaging), early washout defined as minimal or no retention of radiotracer in the parathyroid gland on delayed imaging is also observed frequently (as in this case). As such, close evaluation of both early and delayed images is warranted. The delayed washout pattern provides additional diagnostic information when the activity in the adenoma is either contiguous or overlaps that in the thyroid gland; As such, the underlying adenoma is more conspicuous on delayed images upon normal washout from the overlying or adjacent thyroid gland. In order to avoid missing early washout parathyroid adenoma, some clinicians prefer SPECT/CT imaging soon after the 20-minute planar imaging is completed.

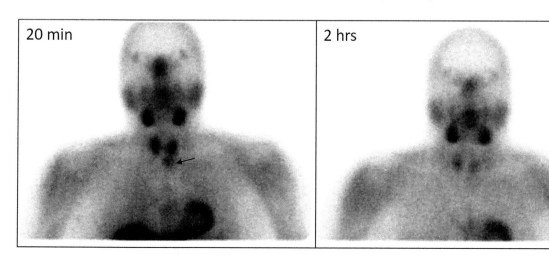

20 min

2 hrs

References: Eslamy HK, Ziessman HA. Parathyroid scintigraphy in patients with primary hyperparathyroidism: 99mTc sestamibi SPECT and SPECT/CT. *Radiographics* 2008;28(5):1461–1476.

Mettler FA, Guiberteau MJ. *Essentials of nuclear medicine imaging*, 7th ed. Philadelphia, PA: Saunders, 2019:111–112.

O'Malley JP, Ziessman HA, Thrall JH. *Nuclear medicine: the requisites*, 5th ed. Philadelphia, PA: Saunders, 2020:174–179.

36 Answer B. Four small foci of mild to moderate sestamibi uptake are present, two in the upper neck and two in the lower neck on the delayed images (arrows on the images below). These are in the expected location of parathyroid glands. The findings are most consistent with multigland hyperplasia in this patient with a history of chronic kidney disease and tertiary hyperparathyroidism. Multigland hyperplasia is typically difficult to detect with sestamibi scans secondary to the smaller size of the hyperplastic glands compared to a solitary enlarged parathyroid adenoma. Parathyroid adenoma would present with a solitary area of retained uptake on delayed images. Reduced physiologic radiotracer uptake in the thyroid gland in this patient with hypothyroidism is likely secondary to atrophy from chronic thyroiditis. Subtle but decreased physiologic uptake within thyroid on early images washes out on the delayed images; given the clinical history and these findings, multinodular goiter is less likely. In addition, multinodular goiter and thyroiditis would not explain the patient's hyperparathyroidism.

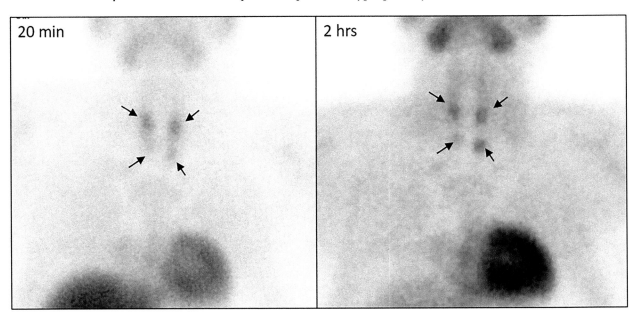

References: Eslamy HK, Ziessman HA. Parathyroid scintigraphy in patients with primary hyperparathyroidism: 99mTc sestamibi SPECT and SPECT/CT. *Radiographics* 2008;28(5):1461–1476.

Pitt SC, Sippel RS, Chen H. Secondary, and tertiary hyperparathyroidism, state of the art surgical management. *Surg Clin North Am* 2009;89(5):1227–1239.

3 Musculoskeletal System

QUESTIONS

1 Excessive aluminum in the technetium generator eluate during the preparation of Tc-99m MDP will result in localization of the radiopharmaceutical in which of the following organs?

A. Brain
B. Stomach
C. Lungs
D. Liver

2 Given the following 3-hour delayed Tc-99m MDP images, what is the most likely diagnosis?

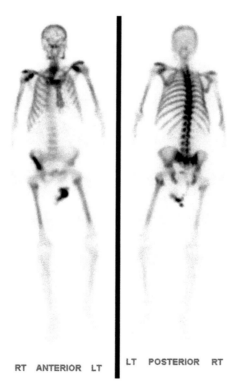

RT ANTERIOR LT   LT POSTERIOR RT

A. Renal failure
B. Normal study
C. Diffuse metastasis
D. Hypertrophic osteoarthropathy

3 A 13-year-old presents with right lower extremity pain. What is the most likely diagnosis?

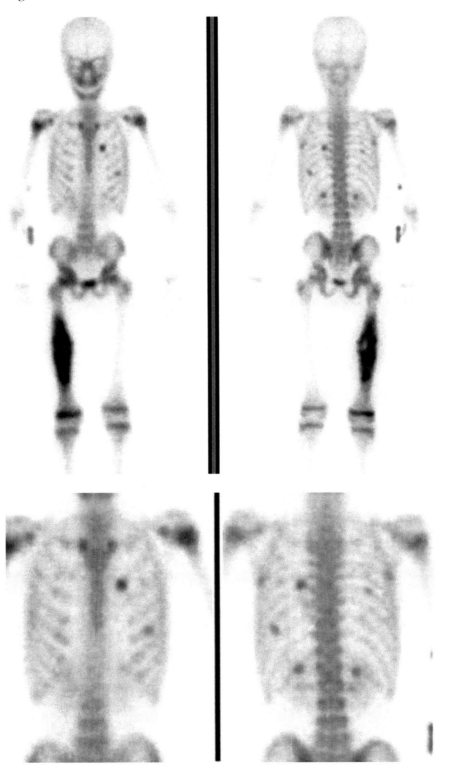

A. Paget disease
B. Osteosarcoma
C. Osteomyelitis
D. Fibrous dysplasia
E. Ewing sarcoma
F. Severely comminuted fracture

4 A 12-year-old boy presents with severe right knee pain that is worse at night. Based on the following scintigraphic and CT findings, what is the most likely diagnosis?

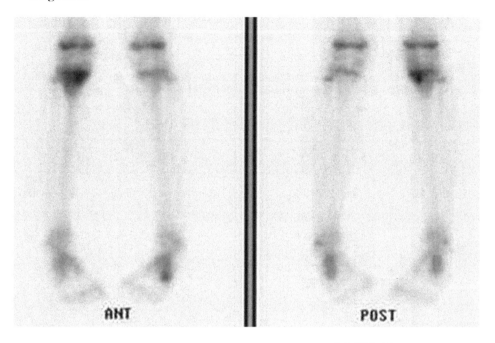

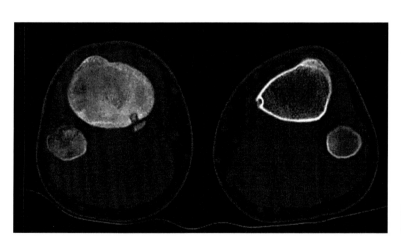

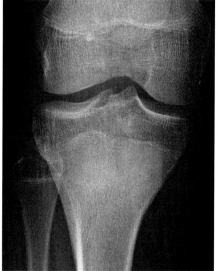

A. Stress fracture
B. Bone island
C. Osteosarcoma
D. Osteoid osteoma
E. Metastatic neuroblastoma

5 A 56-year-old male with a history of prostate cancer presents for further evaluation with bone scintigraphy in the setting of elevated alkaline phosphatase levels. Based on the bone scan and pelvic radiograph images, what is the most likely diagnosis?

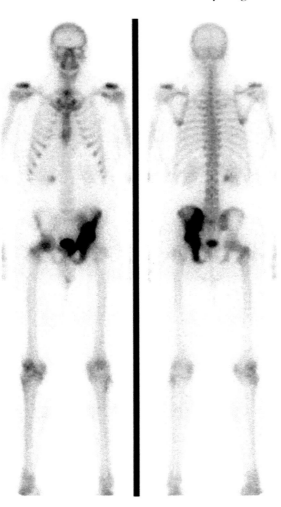
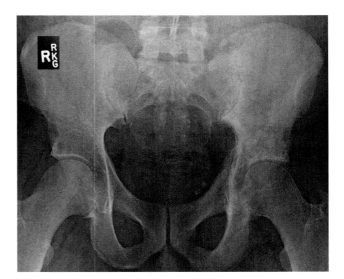

A. Metastasis
B. Fibrous dysplasia
C. Paget disease
D. Osteosarcoma

6 Which of the following statements is LEAST accurate regarding nuclear medicine imaging of complications related to hip replacement?

A. Activity surrounding a cemented prosthesis resolves within 1 year.
B. A diffuse increase in activity surrounding the stem suggests hardware infection.
C. A focal increase in activity at the tip and intertrochanteric regions suggests hardware loosening.
D. F-18 FDG-PET imaging is the method of choice for the evaluation of suspected prosthetic infection.

7 A 21-year-old patient with a history of hyperthyroidism presents with bone pain. Based on the supplied images below, what is the most likely diagnosis?

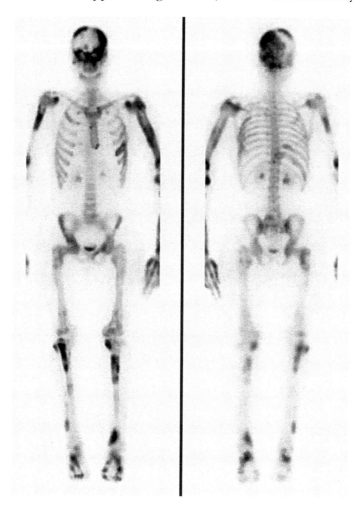

A. McCune-Albright syndrome
B. Fanconi syndrome
C. Polyostotic Paget disease
D. WAGR syndrome
E. Ollier disease

8 Which of the following statements is MOST accurate regarding the measurement of bone mineral density (BMD) using dual x-ray absorptiometry (DEXA) scan?

A. T-score represents the standard deviation by which the patient's BMD differs from the mean BMD of a healthy population of the same age, gender, and ethnicity.
B. Z-score represents the standard deviation by which the patient's BMD differs from the mean BMD of a young adult reference population of the same gender and ethnicity.
C. The hip (including total hip and proximal femur) is not a reliable site for measurement in children.
D. When the spine or hips cannot be evaluated, the distal one-third (33% radius) of the dominant forearm is the region of choice in the assessment of osteoporosis.
E. The femoral neck is the most reproducible measurement of the hip.

9   A 60-year-old male presents with diffuse bone pain and the following bone scintigraphy. What is the most appropriate next step?

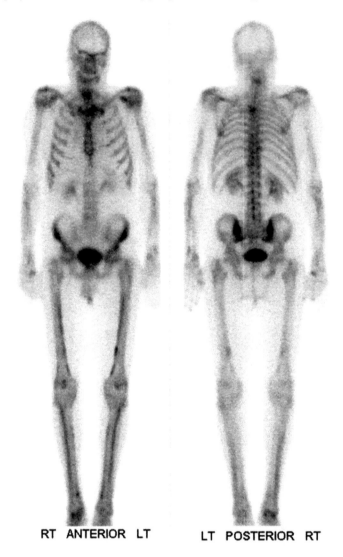

RT ANTERIOR LT   LT POSTERIOR RT

A. Venous duplex sonogram of bilateral lower extremities
B. Radiographs of bilateral lower extremities
C. Computed tomography of the chest
D. MRI of the thoracolumbar spine
E. MRI of bilateral lower extremities

10 What particle emission is responsible for the relief of painful osseous metastasis in a patient treated with radium-223 chloride?

A. Alpha
B. Beta
C. Gamma
D. Positron

11 A 67-year-old gentleman presents for the second dose of treatment with Xofigo (radium-223) for metastatic prostate cancer. Which of the following lab values is a contraindication for the second dose administration?

A. Hemoglobin 9 g/dL
B. Platelets 40×10^9
C. ANC 1.5×10^9
D. PSA 40 ng/mL

12 The following patient presents with fatigue, bone pain, hypoalbuminemia, and renal insufficiency. What is the most likely diagnosis?

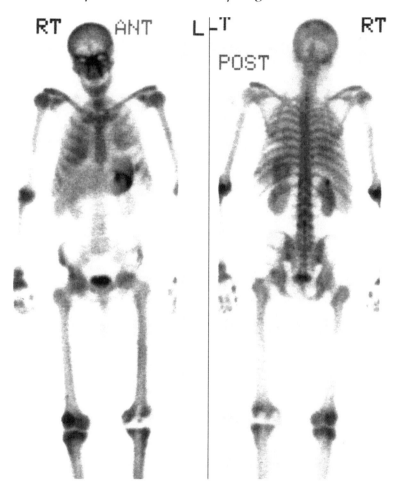

A. Free pertechnetate
B. Metastatic calcification
C. Hypertrophic osteoarthropathy
D. Metastatic lung cancer
E. Nephrogenic systemic fibrosis

13 A 52-year-old postmenopausal female undergoes a dual x-ray absorptiometry (DEXA) scan that reveals a T-score of −1. Based on this result, which is the most appropriate conclusion?

A. Normal
B. Osteopenia
C. Osteoporosis
D. Osteopetrosis

14 The following 3-hour delayed images were acquired after intravenous administration of Tc-99m MDP. Which of the following is most likely associated with this patient?

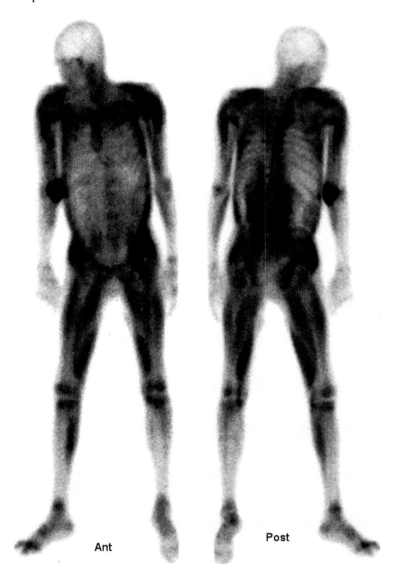

Ant   Post

A. End-stage renal disease with exposure to gadolinium-based contrast agents
B. Elevated creatine phosphokinase levels and renal failure
C. Wrong radiopharmaceutical administration
D. Markedly elevated serum calcium levels

15 What is the most likely diagnosis in this patient with the following bone scintigraphic and CT findings?

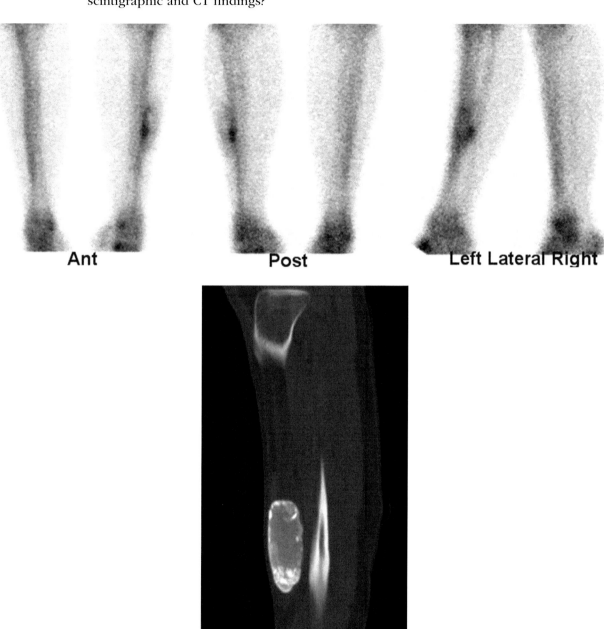

A. Rhabdomyolysis
B. Myositis ossificans
C. Tibial stress fracture
D. Parosteal osteosarcoma
E. Periosteal osteosarcoma

16 A 29-year athlete presents with bilateral lower extremity pain. Based on the following blood pool and delayed images, what is the most likely diagnosis?

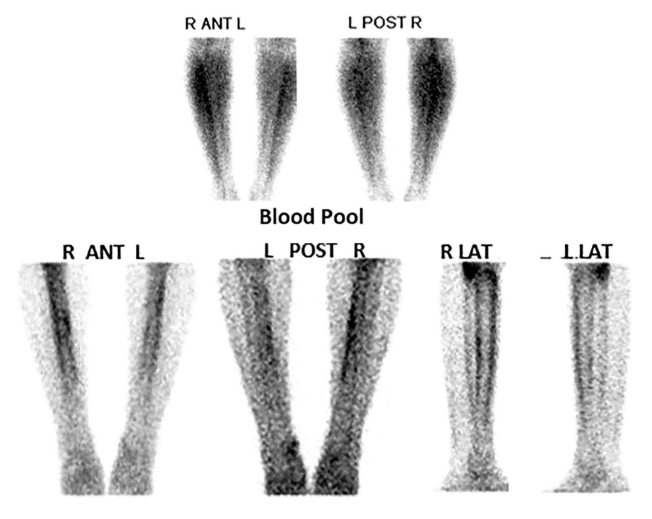

A. Hypertrophic pulmonary osteoarthropathy
B. Metastatic disease
C. Shin splints
D. Stress fractures

17 A 36-year-old lady undergoes whole-body bone scintigraphy secondary to diffuse bone pain. Based on the findings, what is the most appropriate next step?

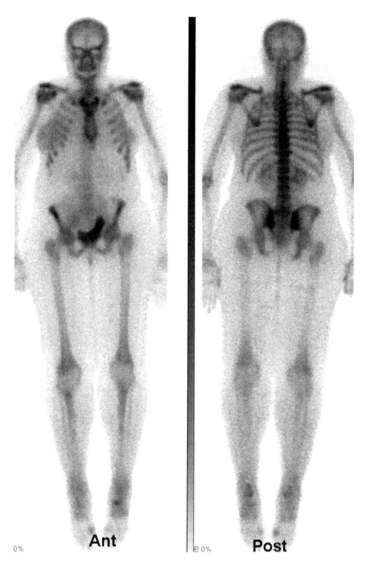

A. Chest radiograph
B. Mammogram
C. Lumbar spine radiographs
D. DEXA scan
E. Serum parathyroid hormone level

18 What is the most likely diagnosis in this 2-year-old with the following bone scintigraphy?

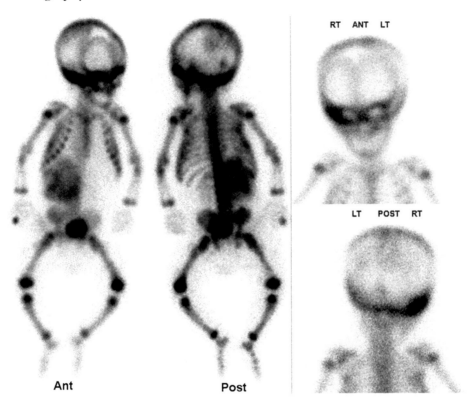

A. Nonaccidental trauma
B. Rhabdomyosarcoma
C. Fibrous dysplasia
D. Wilms tumor
E. Neuroblastoma
F. Paget disease

19 Based on the imaging findings shown below, what is the most likely etiology of this patient's lower back pain?

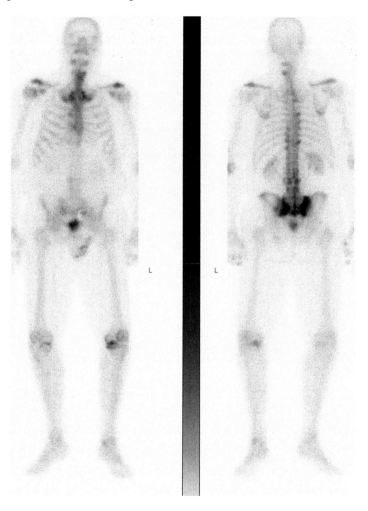

A. Primary bone malignancy
B. Osteoporosis
C. Metastatic disease
D. Benign metabolic bone disease

20 Which FDA-approved bone targeting radiopharmaceutical used in the treatment of refractory painful metastasis can also provide images similar to bone scintigraphy?

A. Radium-223 chloride
B. Strontium-89 chloride
C. Phosphorus-32 sodium orthophosphate
D. Samarium-153 EDTMP

21 A 58-year-old male underwent the following dual x-ray absorptiometry scan for the evaluation of bone mineral density. Which of the following statements is most accurate?

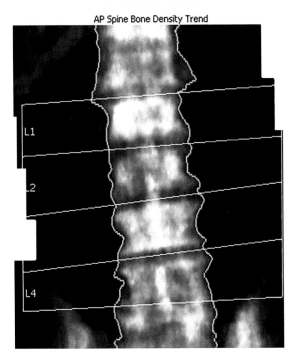

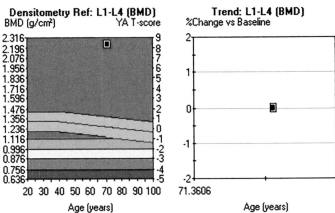

AP Spine Bone Density Trend

Region	BMD¹ (g/cm²)	Young-Adult² T-score	Age-Matched³ Z-score
L1	2.570	11.4	11.3
L2	1.892	5.3	5.2
L3	2.367	8.9	8.7
L4	2.112	6.6	6.5
L1-L4	2.232	8.0	7.9

Image not for diagnosis

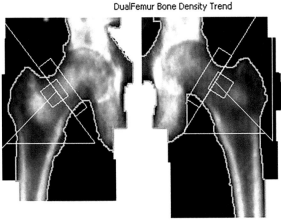

DualFemur Bone Density Trend

Region	BMD¹ (g/cm²)	Young-Adult²,⁷ T-score	Age-Matched³ Z-score
Neck			
Left	1.553	3.7	5.0
Right	1.863	6.1	7.4
Mean	1.708	4.9	6.2
Difference	0.310	2.4	2.4
Total			
Left	1.422	2.2	3.0
Right	1.713	4.2	5.0
Mean	1.567	3.2	4.0
Difference	0.291	2.0	2.0

Trend: Total Mean

Measured Date	Age (years)	BMD¹ (g/cm²)	Change vs Previous (g/cm²)	Previous (%)
5/29/2015	71.3	1.567	-	-

COMMENTS:

A. The patient should be initiated on bisphosphonate therapy.
B. No therapy is necessary; a follow-up is recommended in 1 year.
C. No therapy is necessary; a follow-up is recommended in 3 years.
D. No therapy is necessary; correlation with radiograph should be considered.
E. No therapy or follow-up is necessary.
F. The patient should be initiated on calcium and vitamin D.

22 A 22-year-old female with a clinical history of a prior car accident presents with continuing pain in the right lower extremity. Based on the following three-phase bone scintigraphy images, which of the following is the most likely diagnosis?

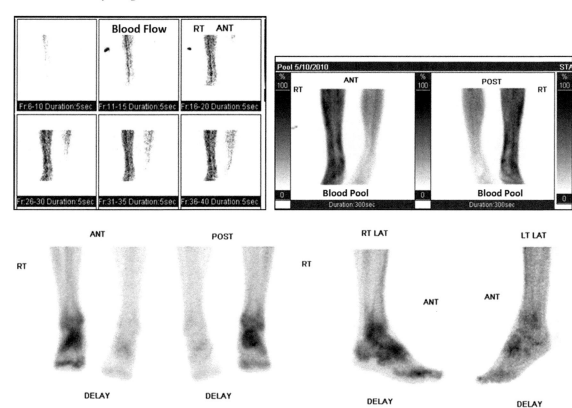

A. Right lower extremity deep venous thrombosis
B. Right lower extremity cellulitis
C. Right lower extremity complex regional pain syndrome
D. Right lower extremity Charcot arthropathy

23 Based on the findings on the following whole-body bone scan, what is the most likely diagnosis?

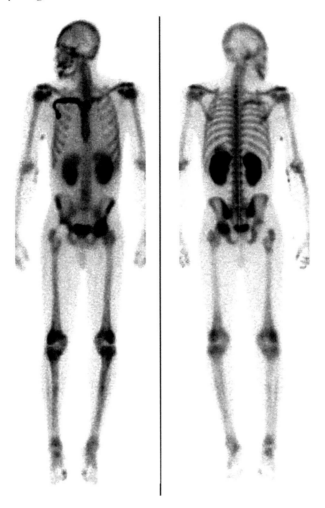

    A. Port infection
    B. Sickle cell anemia
    C. Renal obstruction
    D. Adrenal metastasis

24 Which of the following is an advantage of F-18 sodium fluoride PET/CT scan over the whole-body bone scan?

    A. Shorter uptake time
    B. Decreased radiation dose
    C. Increased sensitivity for lesions in the extremities
    D. Lack of uptake in degenerative changes

25 Which of the following is the most likely diagnosis in the following 58-year-old patient who presents for evaluation of metastatic prostate cancer with bone scintigraphy?

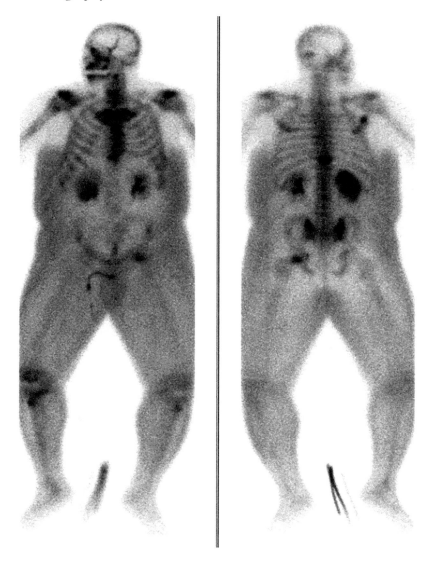

A. SVC obstruction
B. IVC obstruction
C. Cellulitis
D. Rhabdomyolysis

26 The following bone scintigraphy was done on a 75-year-old female with a history of breast cancer. What is the most likely diagnosis?

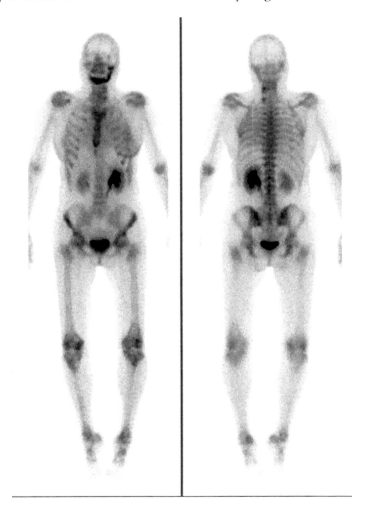

A. Osseous metastasis
B. Renal cell carcinoma
C. Periodontal disease
D. Osteonecrosis

27 A 73-year-old male who is status post partial glossectomy with segmental mandibulectomy and left radial forearm free flap undergoes a three-phase bone scan. Based on the supplied anterior blood flow, blood pool, delayed planar, and axial SPECT images, what is the most likely diagnosis?

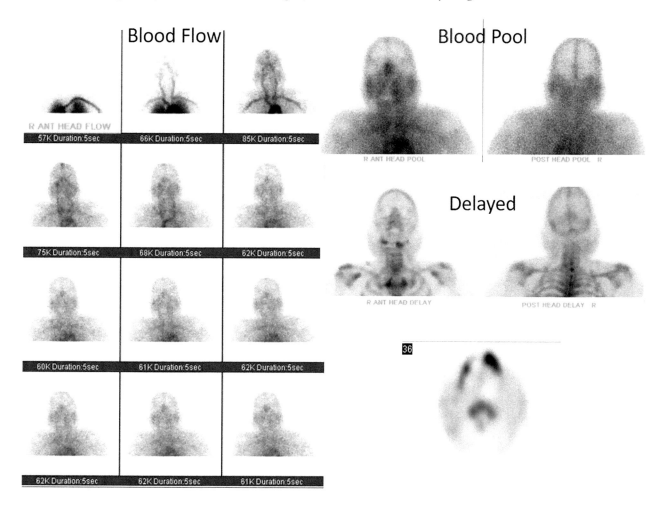

A. Osteonecrosis
B. Osteomyelitis
C. Viable flap
D. Nonviable flap

ANSWERS AND EXPLANATIONS

1 **Answer D.** Excessive aluminum from the generator elution causes colloid formation, which can accumulate in the liver. Causes of diffuse abnormal hepatic activity on bone scan include the following: excessive aluminum in elution from the generator, residual activity from a previous sulfur colloid scan, excessive serum aluminum, hepatic necrosis, hepatic metastases, amyloidosis, and metastatic calcifications.

On the other hand, excessive air in the mixing vial will result in the oxidation of tin from stannous ion (Sn II) to stannous hydroxide (Sn IV). This will cause poor tagging of the radiopharmaceutical and will result in excessive free pertechnetate. Free pertechnetate can also be visualized if the radiopharmaceutical injection is delayed for more than 4 hours after its preparation. Free pertechnetate localizes within the salivary glands, thyroid gland, and stomach and increases the background soft tissue activity. As such, quality control with chromatography should be routinely performed before the injection of the radiopharmaceutical to ensure >95% binding.

References: MacDonald J. Idiopathic hepatic uptake of 99mTc methylene diphosphonate: a case report. *J Nucl Med Technol* 2001;29(1):32–36.

O'Malley JP, Ziessman HA, Thrall JH. *Nuclear medicine: the requisites*, 5th ed. Philadelphia, PA: Saunders, 2020:55, 75–76.

2 **Answer C.** The supplied images demonstrate diffusely increased radiotracer uptake throughout the spine, pelvis, ribs, and the proximal appendicular skeleton with absent visualization of the kidneys. The findings are most compatible with a superscan. Normal physiologic distribution of the radiotracer on the bone scan includes the GU system, and attention to the kidneys should be paid on the bone scan. The kidneys are not visualized on the superscan due to intense uptake within the osseous structures. If these images were windowed down, renal parenchyma would be more evident. Superscan is most commonly secondary to osseous metastatic disease; however, it can also be seen with metabolic disorders such as primary hyperparathyroidism, renal osteodystrophy, myelofibrosis, mastocytosis, and hypervitaminosis D. A patient with renal failure would demonstrate more background soft tissue uptake on 3-hour delayed images secondary to decreased clearance of the radiotracer. An 18- to 24-hour delayed "fourth-phase" scan in patients with renal failure/dialysis may produce a similar appearance and is often referred to as a "beautiful scan." Superscan or beautiful scan associated with primary hyperparathyroidism and renal osteodystrophy (secondary hyperparathyroidism) often demonstrates increased radiotracer uptake within an enlarged mandible, which is referred to as the "Lincoln sign" (see image below) as well as increased uptake within periarticular bones. Hypertrophic osteoarthropathy typically demonstrates increased radiotracer uptake within the periosteum of long bones, which is often referred to as "tram tracking."

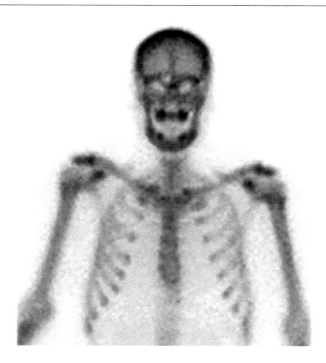

References: Habibian MR. *Nuclear medicine imaging: a teaching file*, 2nd ed. Philadelphia, PA: Lippincott Williams & Wilkins, 2009:326–328.

Mettler FA, Guiberteau MJ. *Essentials of nuclear medicine imaging*, 7th ed. Philadelphia, PA: Saunders, 2019:249.

O'Malley JP, Ziessman HA, Thrall JH. *Nuclear medicine: the requisites*, 5th ed. Philadelphia, PA: Saunders, 2020:77, 90–91.

3 **Answer B.** Delayed anterior and posterior whole-body images demonstrate a large focus of intense radiotracer uptake within the right femoral diaphysis. Multiple small foci of intense radiotracer uptake are seen within the right and left chest, which do not correspond to the locations of the ribs (arrow below). The findings are most compatible with uptake within lung metastasis, typically seen with osteosarcoma. In questionable cases, SPECT-CT may be performed to confirm the location of metastasis in the lungs. Lung metastasis from osteosarcoma demonstrates intense bisphosphonate radiotracer uptake due to the presence of ossification within the metastasis. While the diaphyseal location is typically associated with Ewing sarcoma, lung metastasis from Ewing sarcoma would not be expected to demonstrate intense Tc-99m MDP uptake.

Osteosarcoma commonly arises from the distal femoral metaphysis and demonstrates heterogeneous uptake containing areas of photopenia (see the image from a different patient below). While osteomyelitis may occur in the femoral diaphysis, it will typically demonstrate a well-defined homogeneous increase in radiotracer uptake (see an example case in the pediatrics nuclear medicine chapter). Both osteomyelitis and osteosarcoma would be positive on three-phase bone scintigraphy.

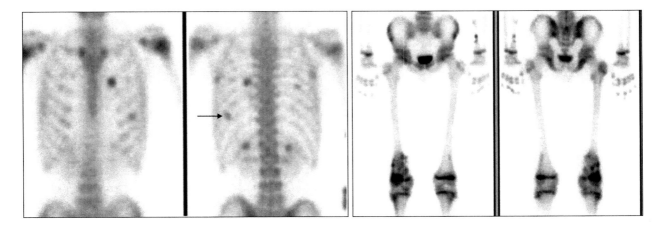

References: Mebarki M, Medjahedi A, Menemani A, et al. Osteosarcoma pulmonary metastasis mimicking abnormal skeletal uptake in bone scan: utility of SPECT/CT. *Clin Nucl Med* 2013;38(10):e392–e394.

Mettler FA, Guiberteau MJ. *Essentials of nuclear medicine imaging*, 7th ed. Philadelphia, PA: Saunders, 2019:253.

O'Malley JP, Ziessman HA, Thrall JH. *Nuclear medicine: the requisites*, 5th ed. Philadelphia, PA: Saunders, 2020:96.

4 **Answer D.** A small round focus of intense uptake (arrow) in the posteromedial aspect of the proximal tibia is surrounded by a more diffuse mild uptake in the proximal tibial metaphysis (arrowheads). The radiograph demonstrates diffuse sclerosis within the proximal tibial metadiaphysis with solid (nonaggressive) periosteal reaction laterally. CT demonstrates a well-defined round low-attenuation nidus (black arrowheads) with a central area of high attenuation/ mineralization (white arrow) within the posteromedial tibial cortex. The combination of these findings is most compatible with an osteoid osteoma. Osteoid osteoma is more common in the femur and tibia (>50%), with less common sites, including the spine, hands, and feet (30%). The least common locations include the skull, scapula, ribs, pelvis, mandible, and patella.

Osteomyelitis would have a more homogenous appearance on bone scintigraphy and lack a hyperintense nidus. Stress fracture would demonstrate linear/ fusiform-shaped, focal intense uptake without the surrounding mild uptake. Bone islands rarely accumulate MDP. Osteosarcoma would appear more diffuse as well and would be expected to have an aggressive periosteal reaction (sunburst appearance) on radiograph and CT. This is the wrong age group for metastatic neuroblastoma. Patients with osteoid osteoma are often adolescents and young adults with the clinical presentation of severe pain that is worse at night.

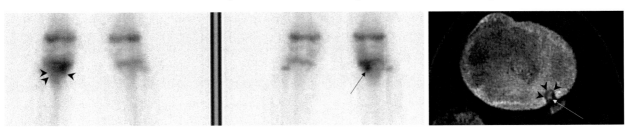

References: Chai JW, Hong SH, Choi JY, et al. Radiologic diagnosis of osteoid osteoma: from simple to challenging findings. *Radiographics* 2010;30(3):737–749.

Mettler FA, Guiberteau MJ. *Essentials of nuclear medicine imaging*, 7th ed. Philadelphia, PA: Saunders, 2019:253–254.

O'Malley JP, Ziessman HA, Thrall JH. *Nuclear medicine: the requisites*, 5th ed. Philadelphia, PA: Saunders, 2020:97.

5 **Answer C.** Anterior and posterior delayed whole-body images demonstrate intense radiotracer uptake within the left hemipelvis involving the left ilium, ischium, and pubic bone in a contiguous fashion. The correlating radiograph demonstrates asymmetric bone expansion, cortical (iliopectineal and ilioischial lines) thickening (arrows below), and coarsened trabeculae. The findings are most compatible with Paget disease. Frequent sites of Paget involvement include pelvis (30% to 75%), spine (30% to 75%), skull (25% to 65%), and proximal long bones (25% to 30%). Less commonly affected sites include the shoulder girdle and forearm. Polyostotic disease (65% to 90%) is more frequent than the monostotic disease (10% to 35%). Pelvic involvement is more often asymmetric than symmetric.

Three phases of Paget's are described. The early resorptive phase is characterized by lysis and thinned cortex. Descriptors such as "blade of grass" and "osteoporosis circumscripta" are seen in this phase. The lytic phase is followed by the mixed phase characterized by coarsening and thickening of trabeculae and cortex. The majority of the cases seen by radiologists are in the mixed phase. The mixed phase later progresses to the final blastic phase at a variable rate. Due to increased blood flow and bone turnover, lytic and mixed phases are typically characterized by intense uptake on bone scintigraphy. The more quiescent late blastic phase may show normal radionuclide uptake. Sarcomatous transformation of Paget's is rare, occurring in approximately 1% of cases, and is seen as focal bone destruction extending through the cortex with an associated soft tissue mass.

Fibrous dysplasia may also demonstrate a similar degree of intense radiopharmaceutical uptake. However, it is typically seen in young patients (75% present by age 30) and can be distinguished from Paget disease based on the pattern of involvement and radiographic findings. While Paget disease involves the end of the bone, fibrous dysplasia typically does not involve the epiphysis. Contiguous involvement of the hemipelvis would be atypical for metastasis. The supplied radiograph also excludes metastasis and osteosarcoma as possibilities.

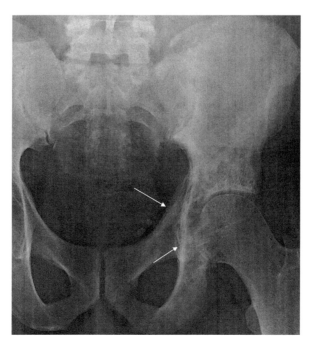

References: Mettler FA, Guiberteau MJ. *Essentials of nuclear medicine imaging*, 7th ed. Philadelphia, PA: Saunders, 2019:272,276.

Smith SE, Murphey MD, Motamedi K, et al. From the archives of the AFIP. *Radiographics* 2002;22(5):1191–1216.

6 **Answer D.** Activity surrounding a cemented prosthesis usually returns to normal within 12 months after surgery. On the other hand, generalized increased activity may be seen for more than 2 years after surgery with a noncemented, porous-coated prosthesis. Persistent activity at the tip of the femoral shaft component and at the trochanter may represent hardware loosening, while a generalized increase in activity around a hip prosthesis, especially the stem, may indicate osteomyelitis. Combined labeled leukocyte–marrow imaging is the radionuclide study of choice for diagnosing prosthetic joint infection. Accuracy of F-18 FDG-PET is lower than that of the combined labeled leukocyte–marrow imaging.

References: Kwee TC, Kwee RM, Alavi A. FDG-PET for diagnosing prosthetic joint infection: systematic review and metaanalysis. *Eur J Nucl Med Mol Imaging* 2008;35(11):2122–2132.

Love C, Marwin SE, Palestro CJ. Nuclear medicine and the infected joint replacement. *Semin Nucl Med* 2009;39(1):66–78.

7 **Answer A.** Supplied anterior and posterior whole-body images demonstrate multiple areas of moderate to severely increased uptake with associated osseous deformities. In a young patient, these findings are characteristic of polyostotic fibrous dysplasia. Fibrous dysplasia (FD) is a benign osseous neoplasm in which the osteoblasts fail to differentiate normally, leading to osteolytic lesions. Frequently, FD occurs in only one bone (monostotic). Typical sites of involvement include the skull, femur, tibia, and humerus. Bone scans are useful in determining the extent of skeletal involvement, especially in polyostotic lesions. Patients with extensive bone disease may present with fractures and deformities of the long bones in early childhood. When these patients suffer femoral involvement, a bowed appearance, referred to as a "shepherd's crook deformity," can be seen. McCune-Albright is a genetic syndrome characterized by cafe au lait spots, polyostotic fibrous dysplasia, and hyperfunctioning endocrinopathies such as hyperthyroidism or precocious puberty. Mazabraud syndrome is a rare combination of fibrous dysplasia and soft tissue myxomas. Fanconi syndrome describes a defect of proximal renal tubules leading to malabsorption of various electrolytes and substances that are usually absorbed by the proximal tubule. WAGR syndrome stands for Wilms tumors, Aniridia, Genital anomalies, and intellectual Retardation. Ollier disease is a skeletal disorder characterized by multiple enchondromas, which are noncancerous (benign) growths of cartilage that develop within the bones.

Reference: Kairemo KJ, Verho S, Dunkel L. Imaging of McCune-Albright syndrome using bone single photon emission computed tomography. *Eur J Pediatr* 1999;158(2):123–126.

8 **Answer C.** Dual-energy x-ray absorptiometry (DEXA) is the technique of choice for the assessment of bone mineral density (BMD). BMD is the average concentration of mineral in a defined section of bone and is measured in grams per square centimeter. A reference database is used to obtain T-score and Z-score. T-score represents the standard deviation by which the patient's BMD differs from the mean BMD of a young adult reference population of the same sex and ethnicity. Z-score represents the standard deviation by which the BMD differs from the mean BMD of a healthy population of the same sex, ethnicity, and age as the person undergoing DEXA. The posteroanterior (PA) spine and total body less head (TBLH) are the most accurate and reproducible skeletal sites for performing BMD in children. The hip (including total hip and proximal femur) is not a reliable site for measurement in growing children due to the fact that there is significant variability in femoral maturation, which results in the lack of reproducibility in the hip region. Vertebral bodies are regarded as the optimal site for monitoring response to treatment. However, when vertebral body BMD is compromised, total hip BMD should be used for comparison as it is the most reproducible measurement of the hip. BMD of the forearm is acquired in the following three scenarios: when two regions from the hip and spine cannot be measured, for patients with hyperparathyroidism, and for patients whose weight exceeds the limit for the table. According to the International Society for Clinical Dosimetry, the distal one-third (33% radius) of the nondominant forearm is the region of choice in the assessment of osteoporosis.

References: Baim S, Binkley N, Bilezikian JP, et al. Official Positions of the International Society for Clinical Densitometry and executive summary of the 2007 ISCD Position Development Conference. *J Clin Densitom* 2008;11(1):75–91.

Baim S, Leonard MB, Bianchi ML, et al. Official Positions of the International Society for Clinical Densitometry and executive summary of the 2007 ISCD Pediatric Position Development Conference. *J Clin Densitom* 2008;11(1):6–21.

Kanis JA; on behalf of the World Health Organization Scientific Group. *Assessment of osteoporosis at the primary health-care level (WHO Collaborating Centre, UK) Technical Report*. University of Sheffield, 2007, 2008.

9 **Answer C.** The delayed whole-body bone scintigraphy demonstrates distinct parallel lines of increased cortical/periosteal uptake in bilateral lower extremities (tibiae and femora). The findings are most compatible with hypertrophic osteoarthropathy. It is most commonly seen with lung cancer. As such, correlation with computed tomography of the chest or chest x-ray should be considered to evaluate for a possible malignancy. Other causes of hypertrophic osteoarthropathy include chest infections, COPD, inflammatory bowel disease, liver disease, and congestive heart failure. Shin splints are usually confined to tibiae and often involve only the posteromedial diaphyseal region. The knee radiograph in this patient demonstrated the characteristic thick wavy periosteal reaction in the distal femur (arrowheads). Chest CT was recommended based on the bone scintigraphy findings, which demonstrated a left upper lobe mass (arrows). The changes seen on bone scintigraphy often resolve after the treatment of the underlying disease.

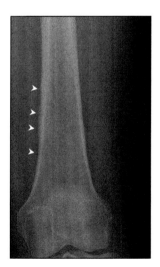 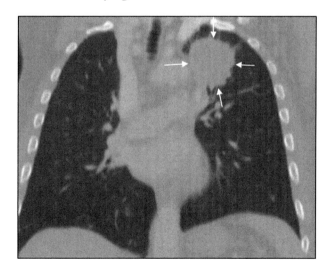

References: Mettler FA, Guiberteau MJ. *Essentials of nuclear medicine imaging*, 7th ed. Philadelphia, PA: Saunders, 2019:276.

O'Malley JP, Ziessman HA, Thrall JH. *Nuclear medicine: the requisites*, 5th ed. Philadelphia, PA: Saunders, 2020:93, 95.

Uchisako H, Suga K, Tanaka N, et al. Bone scintigraphy in growth hormone-secreting pulmonary cancer and hypertrophic osteoarthropathy. *J Nucl Med* 1995;36(5):822–825.

10 **Answer A.** Radium-223 is a bone-seeking, calcium-mimetic alpha-emitting agent with a half-life of 11.4 days that accumulates in areas of increased bone turnover. It is used to treat diffuse painful osseous metastatic disease not responsive to analgesics. The range of the alpha particles (<100 μm) is shorter than 7 mm for Sr-89 or 3.3 mm for Sm-153 beta particles. Also, high-linear energy transfer of alpha radiation results in greater biologic effectiveness than that of beta radiation. Ra-223 is primarily eliminated through feces, and diarrhea is the most common side effect reported with Ra-223 therapy. Of the molecular bone treatment agents available, Ra-223 is the only one that is reported to not only decrease bone pain but increase survival time (4 months). Ra-223 (Xofigo) is currently the only approved agent for the treatment of prostate cancer metastasis.

References: Mettler FA, Guiberteau MJ. *Essentials of nuclear medicine imaging*, 7th ed. Philadelphia, PA: Saunders, 2019:284–285.

O'Malley JP, Ziessman HA, Thrall JH. *Nuclear medicine: the requisites*, 5th ed. Philadelphia, PA: Saunders, 2020:117.

Pandit-Taskar N, Larson SM, Carrasquillo JA. Bone-seeking radiopharmaceuticals for treatment of osseous metastases, part 1: alpha therapy with 223Ra-dichloride. *J Nucl Med* 2014;55(2):268–274.

11 **Answer B.** Xofigo (Radium 223) is used in patients with castrate-resistant prostate cancer and symptomatic bone metastasis without known visceral metastasis. This treatment has been shown to improve life quality by decreasing the pain associated with osseous metastasis and prolonged patient survival. The patients typically receive 1.49 microcurie/kg of Xofigo IV every 4 weeks for a total of 6 cycles. Because of the proximity of the red marrow to the osteogenic cells, patients develop marrow suppression. Nadir in blood counts typically occurs 2 to 3 weeks after the Xofigo administration, and most patients recover approximately 6 to 8 weeks after administration. As such, hematologic evaluation is a prerequisite at baseline and before every dose of Xofigo therapy. Before the first administration of Xofigo, the absolute neutrophil count (ANC) should be $\geq 1.5 \times 10^9$/L, the platelet count $\geq 100 \times 10^9$/L, and hemoglobin ≥ 10 g/dL. Prior to subsequent administrations, the ANC should be $\geq 1 \times 10^9$/L and the platelet count $\geq 50 \times 10^9$/L. The patients should receive blood transfusion for anemia, but a minimum hemoglobin level is not required for the subsequent treatments. There is no PSA requirement before treatments at any time. Xofigo is not recommended for use in combination with abiraterone acetate plus prednisone/prednisolone due to increased risk of fractures and mortality.

References: Mettler FA, Guiberteau MJ. *Essentials of nuclear medicine imaging*, 7th ed. Philadelphia, PA: Saunders, 2019:284–285.

O'Malley JP, Ziessman HA, Thrall JH. *Nuclear medicine: the requisites*, 5th ed. Philadelphia, PA: Saunders, 2020:117.

Pandit-Taskar N, Larson SM, Carrasquillo JA. Bone-seeking radiopharmaceuticals for treatment of osseous metastases, part 1: alpha therapy with 223Ra-dichloride. *J Nucl Med* 2014;55(2):268–274.

Xofigo prescribing information: https://hcp.xofigo-us.com/prescribe-xofigo/overview/

12 **Answer B.** Delayed anterior and posterior whole-body images demonstrate increased radiopharmaceutical uptake in the periarticular regions. There is soft tissue radiopharmaceutical uptake within the thyroid, lungs, stomach, liver, and kidneys. These findings are most compatible with metastatic calcification. Relative photopenia about the left knee is secondary to arthroplasty. Metastatic calcification is calcium deposition caused by abnormal calcium and phosphate metabolism. Increased serum calcium phosphonate product is believed to result in the soft tissue uptake. Thyroid, lungs, heart, stomach, kidneys, and liver are common sites of involvement. It is typically seen in patients with severe hypercalcemia resulting from chronic renal disease, parathyroid tumor, malignancy (i.e., multiple myeloma), and hypervitaminosis D. While free technetium would demonstrate radiopharmaceutical uptake within the thyroid and stomach, it would not be present in the lungs or liver. The findings seen are not typical for hypertrophic osteoarthropathy, metastatic lung cancer, or nephrogenic systemic fibrosis.

References: Imanishi Y, Kishiro M, Miyazaki O, et al. Multiple metastatic calcifications detected by bone scintigraphy and demonstrated by CT. *Clin Nucl Med* 1992;17(2):114–118.

Reitz MD, Vasinrapee P, Mishkin FS. Myocardial, pulmonary, and gastric uptake of technetium-99m MDP in a patient with multiple myeloma and hypercalcemia. *Clin Nucl Med* 1986;11(10):730.

13 **Answer A.** The primary osteoporosis can be divided into postmenopausal osteoporosis (type I) or senile osteoporosis (type II). According to the World Health Organization, postmenopausal women and men 50 years or older are assigned a diagnosis based on T-score. The World Health Organization defines osteoporosis and osteopenia as follows: normal = T-score at or above −1.0 SD; osteopenia or low bone mass = T-score less than −1 and greater than −2.5 SD; and osteoporosis = T-score at or below −2.5 SD. As such, a T-score of −1 is normal.

Z-scores are used in the evaluation of premenopausal women, men younger than 50 years, and children younger than 20 years. In these patients, osteoporosis should not be diagnosed on the basis of densitometric criteria. Instead, a Z-score less than −2 indicates bone mineral density (BMD) below the expected range for age in adults or low density for chronologic age in children.

Although the reference standard for the description of osteoporosis is BMD at the femoral neck, other central sites (i.e., lumbar spine, total hip) can be used for diagnosis in clinical practice. Either hip may be used for DEXA of the proximal femur. Lowest level data of the femoral neck or total hip are used for the diagnosis. BMD measurement of the hip bone (neck or total) is optimal for predicting the risk of hip fracture, whereas BMD measurement of the spine is optimal for monitoring response to treatment.

References: Baim S, Binkley N, Bilezikian JP, et al. Official Positions of the International Society for Clinical Densitometry and executive summary of the 2007 ISCD Position Development Conference. *J Clin Densitom 2008*;11(1):75–91.

Baim S, Leonard MB, Bianchi ML, et al. Official Positions of the International Society for Clinical Densitometry and executive summary of the 2007 ISCD Pediatric Position Development Conference. *J Clin Densitom 2008*;11(1):6–21.

Kanis JA; on behalf of the World Health Organization Scientific Group. *Assessment of osteoporosis at the primary health-care level (WHO Collaborating Centre, UK) Technical Report*. University of Sheffield, 2007, 2008.

Mettler FA, Guiberteau MJ. *Essentials of nuclear medicine imaging*, 7th ed. Philadelphia, PA: Saunders, 2019:281–282.

14 **Answer B.** The anterior and posterior whole-body images demonstrate intense uptake of radiopharmaceutical within the musculature as well as relatively reduced renal uptake. Mild radiopharmaceutical uptake is visualized within the osseous skeleton, suggesting that the correct radiopharmaceutical was injected. These findings are most compatible with severe rhabdomyolysis. Calcium deposition in damaged myocytes is thought to result in radionuclide deposition when combined with phosphate. In rhabdomyolysis, the amount of radiopharmaceutical uptake within the musculature is proportional to the extent of muscle injury. Bone scintigraphy is invariably positive during the acute phase, with the greatest uptake occurring in the first 24 to 48 hours, which gradually resolves over a week. As such, it provides a good way of estimating the extent of involvement and allows for following recovery.

Patients with rhabdomyolysis typically present with myoglobinuria, elevated creatine phosphokinase levels, and renal failure. Patients with nephrogenic systemic fibrosis (end-stage renal disease with exposure to gadolinium-based contrast agents) would demonstrate more heterogeneous muscular uptake accompanied by increased radiopharmaceutical uptake in the skin and superficial soft tissues, which is not seen in this patient. Metastatic calcifications (markedly elevated calcium levels) would have soft tissue uptake in the thyroid, lungs, heart, stomach, liver, and kidneys.

References: Habibian MR. *Nuclear medicine imaging: a teaching file*, 2nd ed. Philadelphia, PA: Lippincott Williams & Wilkins, 2009:395–396.

Mettler FA, Guiberteau MJ. *Essentials of nuclear medicine imaging*, 7th ed. Philadelphia, PA: Saunders, 2019:257.

O'Malley JP, Ziessman HA, Thrall JH. *Nuclear medicine: the requisites*, 5th ed. Philadelphia, PA: Saunders, 2020:107.

15 **Answer B.** The anterior, posterior, and left lateral delayed scintigraphic images of the tibia and fibula demonstrate a moderate-sized, oval focus of mild to moderately increased activity along the anterolateral aspect of the tibia. On CT scan, there is an oval region of ossification within the musculature of the anterolateral shin with mature peripheral calcifications, characteristic of myositis ossificans.

Myositis ossificans, more correctly known as heterotopic ossification, is development of bone in soft tissues such as muscle, tendon, ligaments, or subcutaneous fat. The pathogenesis is felt to be secondary to the metaplasia of pluripotent mesenchymal cells into the osteoblasts. The majority of the cases of focal myositis ossificans/heterotopic bone formation are secondary to direct trauma. Other causes include joint replacement, spinal cord injury, and burn. Postsurgical heterotopic bone formation is commonly visualized around the hip joint. Three-phase bone scintigraphy is the most sensitive modality for the early detection of heterotopic ossification. In acute stages, three-phase bone scintigraphy of heterotopic ossification demonstrates hyperperfusion, increased blood pool, and increased uptake on the delayed images. As the lesion matures, the degree of radiotracer uptake decreases. Heterotopic ossification is differentiated from bone-forming malignancies such as parosteal or periosteal osteosarcoma by the presence of more mature calcifications along its periphery rather than in the center. With osteosarcoma, the bone formation would be more organized and denser centrally and less organized and less dense along the outer edge. Early heterotopic ossification may be intensely FDG avid on PET-CT, and close attention to CT characteristics is paramount in differentiation from tumor recurrence.

References: Habibian MR. *Nuclear medicine imaging: a teaching file*, 2nd ed. Philadelphia, PA: Lippincott Williams & Wilkins, 2009:397–398.

Mettler FA, Guiberteau MJ. *Essentials of nuclear medicine imaging*, 7th ed. Philadelphia, PA: Saunders, 2019:257, 263.

O'Malley JP, Ziessman HA, Thrall JH. *Nuclear medicine: the requisites*, 5th ed. Philadelphia, PA: Saunders, 2020:107, 112.

16 **Answer C.** Anterior, and right and left lateral spot view images of the lower extremities demonstrate irregular linear areas of increased activity tracking along the posteromedial and anterolateral aspects of the tibiae bilaterally. The findings are in keeping with shin splints, also known as medial tibial stress syndrome. Three-phase bone scintigraphy is often used to diagnose and differentiate shin splints from tibial stress fractures. Three-phase bone scintigraphy of shin splints demonstrates normal blood flow and normal blood pool with irregular linear areas of increased activity along the one-third or more of the tibial diaphyseal cortex on the delayed images. On the other hand, tibial stress fractures tend to be more focal and fusiform on the delayed images and show increased activity on the blood flow (hyperemia) and blood pool phases (hyperperfusion). Because both shin splints and stress fractures are secondary to abnormal stress on normal bone, such as that from running, they are often seen concomitantly; the image below shows shin splints (arrowheads) accompanied by a stress fracture (arrow).

Shin splints is a stress-induced periosteal reaction at the insertion of the soleus and tibialis muscles onto the tibia, which commonly occurs from repetitive long-distance running on hard surfaces. Patients with shin splints usually present with pain on the medial aspect of the tibia, which is aggravated while running and relieved with rest. Radiographs are often unrevealing, and bone scans are diagnostic. Conservative treatment with rest, analgesics, and orthotics are usually sufficient in the management of shin splints. The uptake in hypertrophic pulmonary osteoarthropathy (HPOA) is more intense than that in the shin splints and is not confined to the tibiae. Also, HPOA would be seen in an older population than that of shin splints. The appearance of areas of increased activity seen in this case is not typical for that of metastatic disease, which tends to present as a focal area of increased activity.

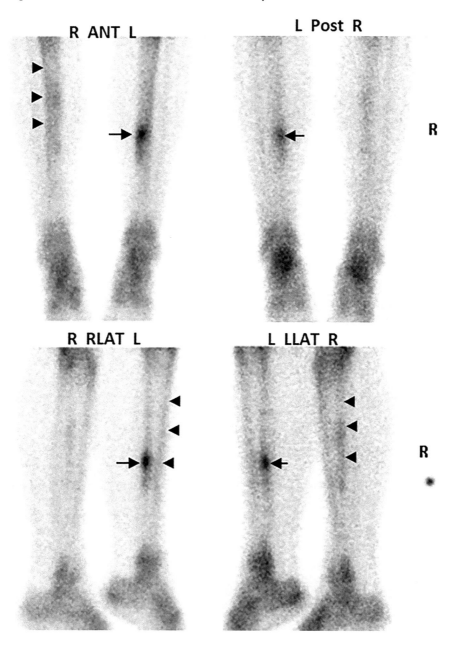

References: Mettler FA, Guiberteau MJ. *Essentials of nuclear medicine imaging*, 7th ed. Philadelphia, PA: Saunders, 2019:265, 285.

O'Malley JP, Ziessman HA, Thrall JH. *Nuclear medicine: the requisites*, 5th ed. Philadelphia, PA: Saunders, 2020:107.

Rupani HD, Holder LE, Espinola DA, et al. Three-phase radionuclide bone imaging in sports medicine. *Radiology* 1985;156(1):187–196.

17 **Answer B.** Delayed anterior, and posterior whole-body scintigraphy images demonstrate asymmetrically increased radiopharmaceutical uptake within an enlarged right breast (arrowheads). The findings are highly suspicious for primary breast malignancy. As such, further correlation with mammography should be considered. Increased activity within the left axilla (black arrow) is likely secondary to the combination of physiologic breast uptake and overlap of radiopharmaceutical uptake within the soft tissues. A subsequent contrast-enhanced CT of this patient demonstrated the presence of a large necrotic mass within the right breast (asterisk). The contour abnormality of the bladder seen on the anterior images was secondary to an enlarged uterus from leiomyomata (#). Differential considerations of increased breast activity on bone scintigraphy include mastitis and trauma.

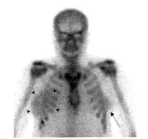 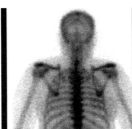 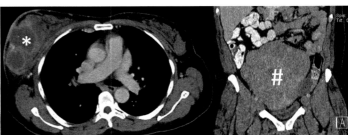

References: Mettler FA, Guiberteau MJ. *Essentials of nuclear medicine imaging*, 7th ed. Philadelphia, PA: Saunders, 2019:257.

O'Malley JP, Ziessman HA, Thrall JH. *Nuclear medicine: the requisites*, 5th ed. Philadelphia, PA: Saunders, 2020:83.

18 **Answer E.** The supplied anterior and posterior delayed whole-body images and spot views of the skull demonstrate increased activity within the skull base and periorbital regions as well as diffusely increased marrow activity within the axial and appendicular skeleton suspicious for bone marrow involvement. A large mass with intense activity is present within the right upper quadrant. The findings are most compatible with neuroblastoma with diffuse marrow involvement. Because they contain microcalcifications, approximately 30% to 50% of primary neuroblastomata demonstrate avidity on bone scintigraphy. The findings seen are not typical of nonaccidental trauma, fibrous dysplasia, or Paget disease. Soft tissue lesions of Wilms tumor and rhabdomyosarcoma are not typically avid on bone scintigraphy.

I-123 metaiodobenzylguanidine (MIBG) scan is more sensitive than bone scintigraphy for the evaluation of neuroblastoma metastasis. The combination of both MIBG and bone scintigraphy gives the highest sensitivity. Since there is no physiologic activity of MIBG in the osseous skeleton, any abnormal osseous uptake should be presumed to be metastatic. The osseous involvement is easier to appreciate on the MIBG scan from the same child shown below. Since early metastasis typically involves physeal and metaphyseal regions, it is difficult to diagnose on bone scan owing to normal intense activity in the growth plates. A subtle increase in metaphyseal activity is often the only clue for marrow involvement on the bone scan.

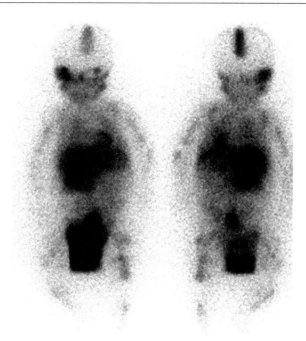

References: Mettler FA, Guiberteau MJ. *Essentials of nuclear medicine imaging*, 7th ed. Philadelphia, PA: Saunders, 2019:251, 260.

O'Malley JP, Ziessman HA, Thrall JH. *Nuclear medicine: the requisites*, 5th ed. Philadelphia, PA: Saunders, 2020:94.

19 Answer B. The anterior and posterior delayed whole-body bone scintigraphy images demonstrate the presence of intense uptake in bilateral sacral alae forming two vertical lines with a joining intense horizontal line of uptake extending across the sacral body. This so-called H pattern or "Honda" sign is characteristic of sacral insufficiency fracture (SIF). However, this pattern of radiopharmaceutical uptake is seen in only 20% to 40% of patients with SIF. Sacral insufficiency fractures are a type of stress fractures that are the result of normal stresses on abnormal bone. SIF is most frequently seen in the setting of osteoporosis. Long-term bisphosphonate use has also been associated with insufficiency fractures. Bone scintigraphy and MR imaging are the most sensitive examinations and can be diagnostic of SIFs in the right clinical settings. Bone scintigraphy has a reported sensitivity of 96% and a positive predictive value of 92% for the detection of SIFs. However, correlation with the patient's presentation is essential as occasionally metastatic disease to the sacrum may mimic insufficiency fractures.

References: Fujii M, Abe K, Hayashi K, et al. Honda sign and variants in patients suspected of having a sacral insufficiency fracture. *Clin Nucl Med* 2005;30(3):165–169.

Mettler FA, Guiberteau MJ. *Essentials of nuclear medicine imaging*, 7th ed. Philadelphia, PA: Saunders, 2019:257, 266.

Ries T. Detection of osteoporotic sacral fractures with radionuclides. *Radiology* 1983;146(3):783–785.

20 Answer D. Samarium-153 EDTMP emits a beta particle with a maximum energy of 0.81 MeV and a 28% abundant gamma emission with a photopeak of 0.103 MeV. This gamma emission allows for imaging, which can be usually done at 6 hours after administration. Strontium-89 is a calcium-mimetic agent that accumulates in the areas of increased bone turnover. Unlike radium-223, it is a beta-emitting agent with a maximum tissue range of 7.2 mm. It is primarily excreted through urine. Like Sr-89, bone marrow toxicity is common with Ra-223 and Sm-153 EDTMP. These agents have been used in patients with metabolically active metastases from breast cancer, prostate cancer, and osteogenic sarcoma.

References: Mettler FA, Guiberteau MJ. *Essentials of nuclear medicine imaging*, 7th ed. Philadelphia, PA: Saunders, 2019:284.

O'Malley JP, Ziessman HA, Thrall JH. *Nuclear medicine: the requisites*, 5th ed. Philadelphia, PA: Saunders, 2020:117.

Pandit-Taskar N, Larson SM, Carrasquillo JA. Bone-seeking radiopharmaceuticals for treatment of osseous metastases, part 1: alpha therapy with 223Ra-dichloride. *J Nucl Med* 2014;55(2):268–274.

21 **Answer D.** The PA lumbar spine and bilateral hip DEXA images demonstrate diffusely increased bone mineral density. Close attention to the images reveals heterogeneously distributed areas of increased bone mineral density, which are highly suspicious for osseous metastasis. As such, correlation with either radiograph or PSA levels should be considered. Other causes of increased bone mineral density include renal osteodystrophy, hypervitaminosis D, lymphoma, and leukemia.

Reference: Lorente-Ramos R, Azpeitia-Armán J, Muñoz-Hernández A, et al. Dual-energy x-ray absorptiometry in the diagnosis of osteoporosis: a practical guide. *Am J Roentgenol* 2011;196(4):897–904.

22 **Answer C.** The radionuclide angiographic images demonstrate markedly increased blood flow through the right anterior and posterior tibial arteries. The blood pool images demonstrate marked hyperperfusion throughout the visualized right lower extremity. On the delayed images, increased activity is seen in periarticular distribution within the right ankle, hindfoot, and midfoot. These findings are classic for complex regional pain syndrome or reflex sympathetic dystrophy. The image below is from a different patient with a left-hand involvement. Scintigraphic findings are variable and depend on the stage of the disease. This classic pattern is seen in <50% of the patients but has the highest diagnostic accuracy. Later in the course of the disease, the blood flow may be normal or decreased in the affected limb. Periarticular increase in uptake on the delayed images is the most sensitive finding (>95%) but has lower specificity as it can be seen with arthritis or infection. Charcot arthropathy would demonstrate regional hyperemia and hyperperfusion, but diffuse involvement, such as in this case, would be atypical. Similarly, diffuse involvement by cellulitis with increased periarticular uptake would be atypical; also, the patient's history is atypical for cellulitis.

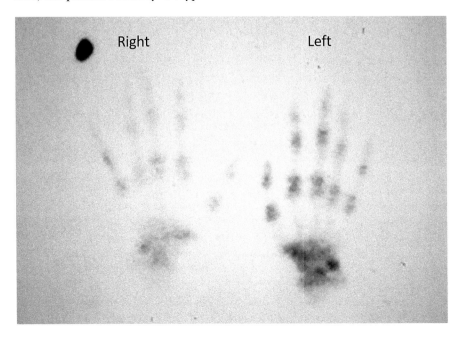

References: Fournier RS, Holder LE. Reflex sympathetic dystrophy: diagnostic controversies. *Semin Nucl Med* 1998;28(1):116–123.

Mettler FA, Guiberteau MJ. *Essentials of nuclear medicine imaging*, 7th ed. Philadelphia, PA: Saunders, 2019:278.

23 **Answer B.** Anterior and posterior delayed whole-body bone images demonstrate enlarged kidneys with diffusely increased uptake within the renal cortex. A small focus of moderate activity in the left upper quadrant above the left kidney on the posterior images corresponds to activity in the atrophic spleen (arrow on the image below). Also, mild heterogeneity of radiotracer is seen in the long bones, related to prior infarcts. Photopenia about the right hip is secondary to prior hip arthroplasty. The constellation of these findings is typically seen with sickle cell anemia. Uptake superior to the left kidney is related to infarcted splenic uptake and not related to adrenal metastasis. The port was used for injection of the radiotracer, explaining the uptake in the associated vascular territory. Port infection alone would not have uptake on a bone scan.

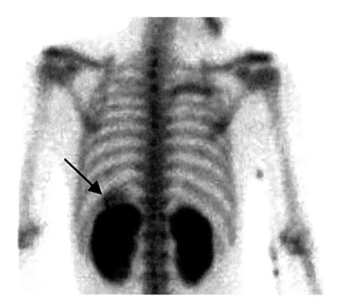

Reference: Cerci SS, Suslu H, Cerci C, et al. Different findings in Tc-99m MDP bone scintigraphy of patients with sickle cell disease: report of three cases. *Ann Nucl Med* 2007;21(5):311–314.

24 **Answer A.** Desirable characteristics of F-18 sodium fluoride (NaF) PET/CT include shorter uptake time (secondary to rapid bone uptake and very rapid blood clearance), better sensitivity, and better specificity. F-18 NaF PET scan is better than Tc-99m MDP in spatial and anatomical resolution. However, F-18 NaF PET is more expensive and delivers more radiation dose to the patient (~7 times compared to that of Tc 99m MDP). NaF PET/CT scans are performed 45 to 60 minutes after the intravenous injection of the agent, while bone scans are typically performed approximately 3 hours postinjection. Compared to the whole-body bone scan, NaF PET scans have increased sensitivity for the detection of lesions within the axial skeleton, while sensitivity to lesions within the extremity is comparable. Both NaF PET scans and planar bone scans demonstrate uptake in degenerative changes and fractures.

References: Mettler FA, Guiberteau MJ. *Essentials of nuclear medicine imaging*, 6th ed. Philadelphia, PA: Saunders, 2012:272,273.

Mettler FA, Guiberteau MJ. *Essentials of nuclear medicine imaging*, 7th ed. Philadelphia, PA: Saunders, 2019:243–244.

O'Malley JP, Ziessman HA, Thrall JH. *Nuclear medicine: the requisites*, 5th ed. Philadelphia, PA: Saunders, 2020:78–80.

Schirrmeister H, et al. Early detection and accurate description of extent of metastatic bone disease in breast cancer with fluoride ion and positron emission tomography. *J Clin Oncol* 1999;17:2381–2389.

Schirrmeister H, et al. Sensitivity in detecting osseous lesions depends on anatomic localization: planar bone scintigraphy versus 18F PET. *J Nucl Med* 1999;40:1623–1629.

Schirrmeister H, et al. Prospective evaluation of the clinical value of planar bone scans, SPECT, and 18F-labeled NaF PET in newly diagnosed lung cancer. *J Nucl Med* 2001;42:1800–1804.

Segall GM. PET/CT with sodium 18F-fluoride for management of patients with prostate cancer. *J Nucl Med* 2014;55(4):531–533.

25 **Answer B.** Anterior and posterior delayed whole-body images demonstrate foci of markedly increased activity including right scapula, left acetabulum, and left femoral head in keeping with prostate cancer metastases. Additionally, there is diffusely increased soft tissue retention of the radiotracer below the thorax with normal soft tissue clearance above that level. This finding is likely secondary to soft tissue edema and decreased tracer clearance from an inferior vena cava (IVC) obstruction. This appearance on bone scan is also referred to as the "Wader sign" as it resembles a pair of fisherman's waders. When present, a CT scan of the abdomen and pelvis should be obtained to ascertain the cause of IVC obstruction. This patient had IVC obstruction secondary to retroperitoneal lymphadenopathy. In superior vena caval obstruction, the distribution would be reversed with increased radiotracer retention in the soft tissues of the head and neck, upper extremities, and thorax. Cellulitis is unlikely to give this pattern of distribution. Rhabdomyolysis presents with increased uptake in the involved skeletal muscles and not in the soft tissues.

References: Chu YK, Hu LH. Waders sign on bone scan: a manifestation of portal hypertension. *Clin Nucl Med* 2012;37(4):385–386.

Rodman DJ, Atkinson LK, Maxwell DD, et al. Bone scan in inferior vena cava obstruction. *Clin Nucl Med* 1990;15(10):740–741.

26 **Answer D.** Anterior and posterior whole-body bone scan images demonstrate intense radiotracer uptake in the body of the mandible, which extends to involve the left mandibular ramus. The extent and degree of abnormal activity are highly suspicious for osteonecrosis of the mandible. Patients who receive bisphosphonate therapy to reduce the risk of pathologic fractures are often at the risk of developing osteonecrosis. Bone scintigraphy is highly sensitive and can detect early cases of osteonecrosis, which can be missed on conventional imaging secondary to the subtle nature of findings in the early stages. The typical appearance of an area of photopenia surrounded by increased activity is a rare finding in cases of jaw osteonecrosis, and diffusely increased activity is more common. Osteonecrosis of the jaw can be seen with dental extraction, after radiation, or with drugs such as steroids and bisphosphonate. While periodontal disease can have increased uptake in the mandible, it tends to be more focal, surrounding the tooth involved, and not diffuse, as shown in this image. Asymmetric uptake in the left pelvicalyceal system is suggestive of left-sided hydronephrosis, which can be related to any obstructive causes such as renal stone (in most of the cases) or underlying obstructive lesion. Further workup should be obtained with a diagnostic CT or ultrasound. There are no areas of reduced radioactivity in the kidneys to suggest a space-occupying mass indicative of renal cell carcinoma. Asymmetrically increased uptake in the left breast is related to the known breast cancer.

References: Dore F, Filippi L, Biasotto M, et al. Bone scintigraphy and SPECT CT of bisphosphonate induced osteonecrosis of the jaw. *J Nucl Med* 2009;50:30–35.

Morag Y, Morag-Hezroni M, Jamadar D, et al. Bisphosphonaterelated osteonecrosis of the jaw: a pictorial review. *RadioGraphics* 2009;29:1971–1986.

27 **Answer D.** Blood flow, blood pool, and delayed images demonstrate an area of absent radiotracer uptake in the mandible, which is better seen on the SPECT image. The finding is in keeping with a nonviable flap. Osteocutaneous flaps are commonly used for the reconstruction of bone defects after oncologic surgery. The success of surgery depends on the viability of the bone flap, and the bone scan is often used to evaluate the viability of the flap. Absent uptake in the flap is suggestive of a nonviable flap, while a viable flap would show uptake on all three phases. Osteomyelitis and osteonecrosis would show increased uptake.

Reference: Srivastava MK, Penumadu P, Kumar D, et al. Role of (99m) Tc-methylene diphosphonate bone scan in the evaluation of the viability of the bone flap in mandibular reconstruction in patients with oromaxillofacial malignancies. *Indian J Nucl Med* 2015;30(3):280–282.

4 Head and Neck

1 Which of the following is true regarding the brain perfusion imaging using HMPAO and ECD?

   A. HMPAO and ECD are lipophilic agents with low first-pass extraction.
   B. The distribution of HMPAO and that of ECD within the brain parenchyma are identical.
   C. Images are usually acquired 30 to 60 minutes after the injection.
   D. Peak brain activity occurs at 15 to 20 minutes after the injection.

2 Which of the following is true regarding the localization of seizure focus using SPECT perfusion and F-18 FDG-PET metabolism imaging?

   A. Interictal studies are more sensitive than ictal studies.
   B. Interictal perfusion SPECT study is superior to interictal PET.
   C. Interictal hypometabolism/hypoperfusion is common with extratemporal epilepsy.
   D. Interictal PET is most helpful in patients with complex partial seizures.

3 Which of the following procedures is most sensitive in diagnosing seizures of extratemporal origin?

   A. Ictal FDG-PET
   B. Interictal FDG-PET
   C. Ictal perfusion SPECT
   D. Interictal perfusion SPECT

4 F-18 FDG hypometabolism in which region helps differentiate dementia with Lewy bodies from Alzheimer disease?

   A. Basal ganglia
   B. Anterior cingulate gyrus
   C. Occipital cortex
   D. Anterior temporal lobes
   E. Frontal lobes

5   The following brain death examination was performed using Tc-99m HMPAO
in a 16-year-old boy who was found to have dilated and fixed pupils after
an ATV accident. Which of the following is the most appropriate conclusion
regarding this examination?

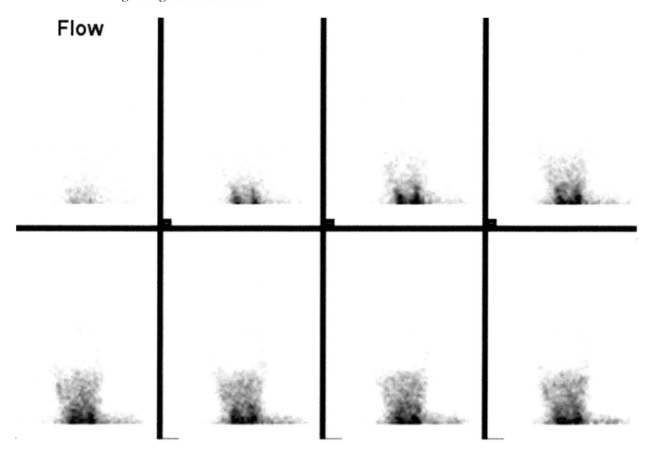

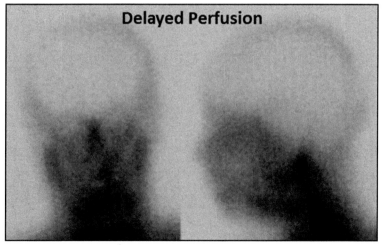

A. The study is nondiagnostic due to inadequate tracer bolus.
B. A conclusion cannot be made without correlation with EEG.
C. Hot nose sign is specific for brain death.
D. Findings are consistent with brain death.
E. Findings are NOT consistent with brain death.

6   The following coronal interictal (A) and ictal (B) Tc-99m HMPAO SPECT-CT images, as well as axial interictal F-18 FDG-PET (C), images are from a patient with a clinical history of intractable complex partial seizures. What is your conclusion?

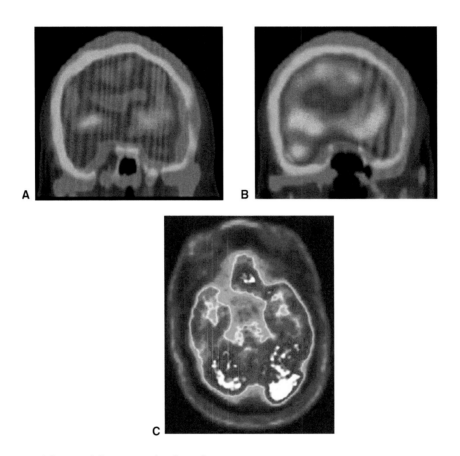

A. Right mesial temporal sclerosis.
B. Left mesial temporal sclerosis.
C. Seizure focus cannot be localized.
D. Right temporal glioblastoma multiforme.
E. Left temporal glioblastoma multiforme.

7 The following F-18 FDG-PET imaging is from a 65-year-old gentleman with progressive cognitive decline and a normal MRI. What is the most likely diagnosis?

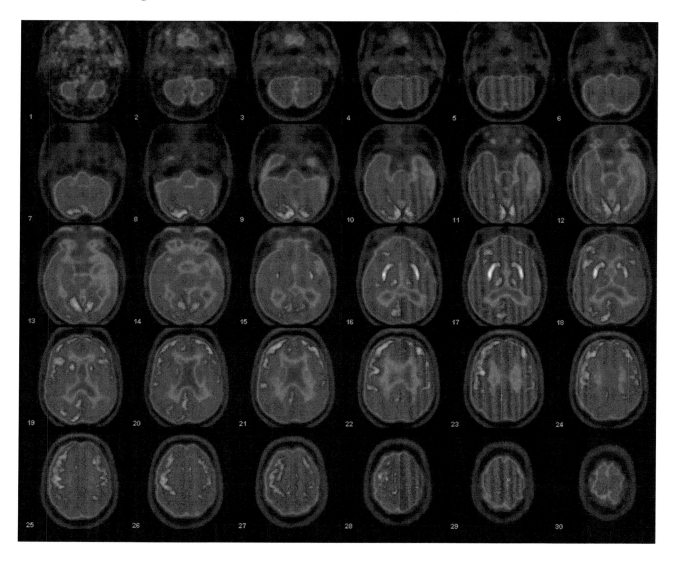

A. Multi-infarct dementia (MID)
B. Alzheimer disease (AD)
C. Frontotemporal dementia (FTD)
D. Dementia with Lewy bodies (DLB)

8 The following F-18 florbetapir axial imaging is from a patient undergoing evaluation of cognitive dysfunction. Which of the following statements is MOST accurate regarding the amyloid imaging of the brain?

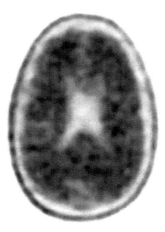

A. A positive Amyvid scan establishes the diagnosis of Alzheimer disease.
B. Amyvid scan can predict the development of dementia and cognitive decline.
C. Amyvid scan can be used for monitoring the treatment response of Alzheimer disease.
D. A negative scan reduces the likelihood of Alzheimer disease.

9a The following examination was performed on a patient with tremors. This radiopharmaceutical is an analog of what naturally occurring substance?

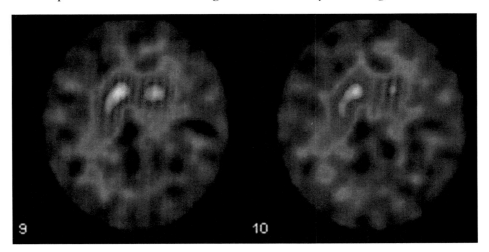

A. Dopamine
B. Cocaine
C. Somatostatin
D. Serotonin

9b If this patient had a clinical history of progressive cognitive decline, what would be the most likely cause of this patient's memory impairment?

A. Huntington chorea
B. Multi-infarct dementia
C. Alzheimer disease
D. Frontotemporal dementia
E. Dementia with Lewy bodies

10 Acetazolamide challenge has been used to evaluate cerebrovascular reserve in patients with chronic cerebrovascular diseases such as moyamoya. What is the mechanism by which acetazolamide assesses the cerebrovascular reserve?

A. Vasodilatation by binding to adenosine receptors
B. Vasodilatation by blocking adenosine uptake by cells
C. Vasodilatation by increasing nitrous oxide concentration
D. Vasodilatation by increasing carbon dioxide concentration
E. Increased cerebral blood flow by increasing the cardiac output

11 The following cisternogram images are from a 60-year-old gentleman who has a history of unsteady gait and memory loss. What is the most likely diagnosis?

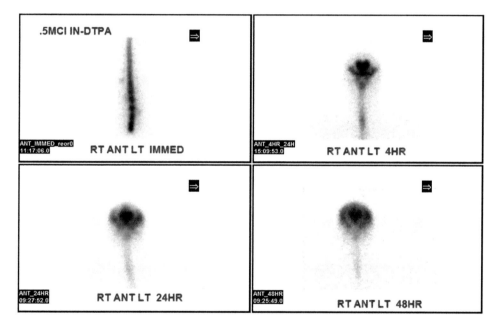

A. Alzheimer disease
B. Normal-pressure hydrocephalus
C. Cerebral atrophy
D. CSF leak

12 Examination with which of the following radiopharmaceuticals would be most helpful in differentiating between Alzheimer disease and frontotemporal dementia?

A. F-18 FDG
B. I-123 ioflupane
C. F-18 florbetapir
D. F-18 flurpiridaz

13 A 60-year-old patient with a history of trauma and positional headaches presents for further evaluation. Based on the supplied planar and SPECT/CT images, what is the most likely diagnosis?

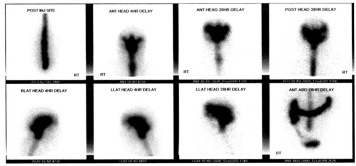

	Right Superior	Right Middle	Right Inferior	Left Superior	Left Middle	Left Inferior
Pledget Wt (wet)	11.379	10.500	10.934	11.113	10.614	10.802
Pledget Wt (dry)	9.602	9.458	9.670	9.602	9.344	9.518
Net Pledget Wt "W"	**1.777**	**1.042**	**1.264**	**1.511**	**1.270**	**1.284**
Pledget Activity (cp5m)	5970	20636	11133	1276322	887661	66542
Bkgrnd Activity (cp5m)	321	321	321	321	321	321
Net Pledget Activity "A"	**5649**	**20315**	**10812**	**1276001**	**887340**	**66221**
Net Pledget Activity						
Net Pledget Weight	3179	19496	8554	844475	698693	51574
Net Pledget Activity						
Plasma Net Activity	0.204	1.251	0.549	54.196	44.840	3.310

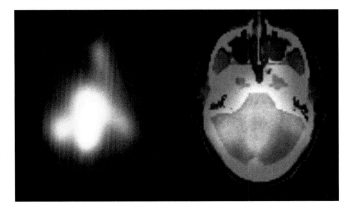

A. CSF leak
B. Normal-pressure hydrocephalus
C. Meningitis
D. Obstructive hydrocephalus
E. Basal cistern arachnoiditis

14 A teenager with mild neurologic impairment complains of worsening headaches. Which of the following radiopharmaceuticals was used to perform this examination?

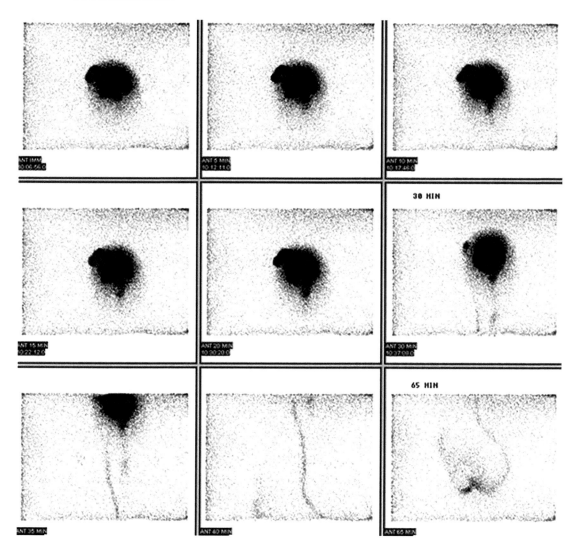

A. Tc-99m pertechnetate
B. Tc-99m HMPAO
C. Tc-99m DTPA
D. Tc-99m sulfur colloid

15 The following coronal F-18 FDG PET image is from an 85-year-old gentleman with a history of stroke. What is the most likely diagnosis?

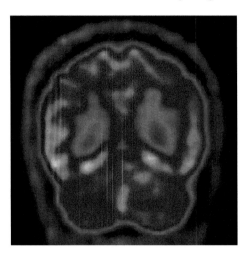

A. Alzheimer dementia
B. Normal-pressure hydrocephalus
C. Pick disease
D. Crossed cerebellar diaschisis

ANSWERS AND EXPLANATIONS

1 **Answer C.** Tc-99m hexamethylpropyleneamine oxime (HMPAO [Ceretec]) and ethyl cysteinate dimer (ECD [Neurolite]) are lipophilic agents with a high first-pass extraction across the blood–brain barrier (see image below for an example of examination with a preserved brain flow and parenchymal perfusion). Peak brain activity occurs within the first few minutes of the injection. Once inside the neuron, both become trapped by metabolic conversion into nondiffusible forms. As such, their distribution on delayed images corresponds to the regional cerebral blood flow at the time of injection. However, in order to allow for an optimal target to background noise ratio, imaging is usually delayed for 30 to 60 minutes for ECD and 30 to 90 minutes for HMPAO after the injection. The distribution of Tc-99m HMPAO differs slightly from that of Tc-99m ECD. HMPAO accumulates more in the frontal lobes, thalami, and cerebellum, while ECD has a high affinity for the parietal and occipital lobes. As such, the same agent should be used for serial examinations, such as those done for seizure evaluation.

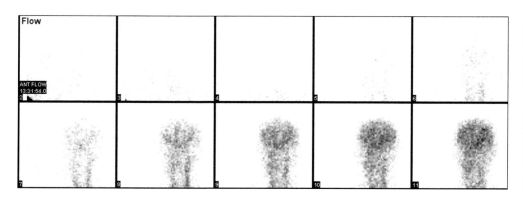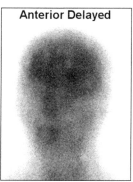

References: Mettler FA, Guiberteau MJ. *Essentials of nuclear medicine imaging*, 7th ed. Philadelphia, PA: Saunders, 2019:62–63.

O'Malley JP, Ziessman HA, Thrall JH. *Nuclear medicine: the requisites*, 5th ed. Philadelphia, PA: Saunders, 2020:364–367.

2 **Answer D.** Ictal perfusion SPECT studies are more sensitive than interictal studies for seizure focus localization. Due to seizure-induced increased blood flow, seizure foci present as areas of increased activity on the ictal perfusion SPECT. On the other hand, blood flow in the region of epileptic foci is either normal or reduced soon after or in between seizures. As such, seizure foci are harder to detect on the interictal SPECT images. In this regard, the interictal F-18 FDG-PET is superior to the interictal SPECT perfusion. Specifically, interictal FDG-PET is very sensitive (80%) in localizing refractory complex partial seizures, which typically originate from the temporal lobe. Interictal SPECT or PET is frequently used to increase the specificity of the findings seen on the ictal study.

References: Mettler FA, Guiberteau MJ. *Essentials of nuclear medicine imaging*, 7th ed. Philadelphia, PA: Saunders, 2019:71–72.

O'Malley JP, Ziessman HA, Thrall JH. *Nuclear medicine: the requisites*, 5th ed. Philadelphia, PA: Saunders, 2020:365–368.

3 **Answer C.** While interictal F-18 FDG is very sensitive (80%) in localizing refractory partial complex seizures originating from the temporal lobe, it is not sensitive in the evaluation of extratemporal seizure focus. Ictal perfusion SPECT with ECD or HMPAO is most sensitive when extratemporal seizure focus is expected. Interictal hypometabolism and hypoperfusion are uncommon with extratemporal epilepsy, and interictal SPECT or PET is not ideal for its evaluation. For ictal studies, the patients are taken off their seizure medications, admitted, and continuously monitored for the onset of a seizure. The radiopharmaceutical is kept at the bedside until the seizure occurs. Once the seizure is identified, the radiotracer is injected during or within 20 seconds after the completion of the seizure.

References: Mettler FA, Guiberteau MJ. *Essentials of nuclear medicine imaging*, 7th ed. Philadelphia, PA: Saunders, 2019:71–72.

O'Malley JP, Ziessman HA, Thrall JH. *Nuclear medicine: the requisites*, 5th ed. Philadelphia, PA: Saunders, 2020:365–368.

4 **Answer C.** Dementia with Lewy bodies (DLB) is the second most common type of primary dementia. The pattern of FDG hypometabolism in DLB may be similar to that in Alzheimer disease (AD). However, DLB shows the involvement of the visual cortex, which is spared in AD. Involvement of the visual cortices in DLB may explain visual hallucinations reported by the patients with DLB.

Reference: Bohnen NI, Djang DSW, Herholz K, et al. Effectiveness and safety of 18F-FDG PET in the evaluation of dementia: a review of the recent literature. *J Nucl Med* 2012;53(1):59–71.

5 **Answer D.** Anterior dynamic images of the brain death examination with Tc-99m HMPAO demonstrates termination of the internal carotid artery flow at the skull base with absent cortical uptake on the delayed anterior and lateral perfusion images. The findings are consistent with absent cerebral perfusion and brain death. A blush of increased activity is seen in the nasal region, which is referred to as the "hot nose" sign. It is felt to be secondary to the diversion of the intracranial blood flow to the external carotid circulation. However, this sign is nonspecific for brain death as it can be seen in internal carotid artery occlusion without brain death. While dynamic flow images can be obtained with both HMPAO and ECD, unlike for Tc-99m DTPA, they are not necessary as the absence of cerebral uptake on delayed images implies absent blood flow. Lack of intracerebral blood flow is diagnostic of brain death, and radionuclide brain death study alone is sufficient for its diagnosis. The brain death study is usually performed in the setting of an equivocal clinical examination and/or EEG. And unlike EEG, it is not affected by drug intoxication or hypothermia. While the lack of intracerebral blood flow can be demonstrated with four-vessel arteriography, radionuclide brain death study is noninvasive, simple, rapid, and specific.

References: Donohoe KJ, Agrawal G, Frey KA, et al. SNM practice guideline for brain death scintigraphy 2.0. *J Nucl Med Technol* 2012;40:198–203.

Mettler FA, Guiberteau MJ. *Essentials of nuclear medicine imaging*, 7th ed. Philadelphia, PA: Saunders, 2019:63–65.

O'Malley JP, Ziessman HA, Thrall JH. *Nuclear medicine: the requisites*, 5th ed. Philadelphia, PA: Saunders, 2020:398–399.

6 **Answer A.** The coronal ictal SPECT-CT image (B) demonstrates increased perfusion to the right temporal lobe compared to the left (arrow). Coronal interictal SPECT-CT (A) and axial F-18 FDG-PET (C) images demonstrate relatively decreased perfusion and metabolism to the right temporal lobe compared to the left, respectively (arrowheads). These findings are most compatible with seizure focus within the right temporal lobe, likely from mesial temporal sclerosis. Glioblastoma multiforme is a high-grade primary brain malignancy that would demonstrate increased perfusion and metabolism.

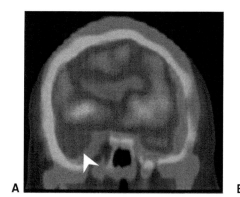 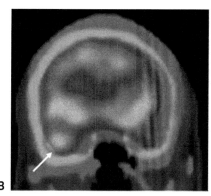 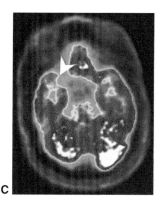

A   B   C

References: Mettler FA, Guiberteau MJ. *Essentials of nuclear medicine imaging*, 7th ed. Philadelphia, PA: Saunders, 2019:71–72.

O'Malley JP, Ziessman HA, Thrall JH. *Nuclear medicine: the requisites*, 5th ed. Philadelphia, PA: Saunders, 2020:393, 396–397.

7 Answer B. The axial F-18 FDG-PET images demonstrate moderate to severe, asymmetric hypometabolism involving bilateral posterior parietal and temporal lobes (left greater than right). This pattern of hypometabolism distribution is typically seen with Alzheimer disease (AD). AD is the most common cause of primary dementia representing 50% to 60% of total cases. The addition of FDG-PET to routine clinical information increases the diagnostic accuracy and physician confidence in diagnosing AD. The added diagnostic value of FDG-PET is similar to the information gleaned during a longitudinal clinical follow-up period of about 4 years. In early AD, there is involvement of the posterior cingulate gyrus and superior posterior parietal cortex, which is often asymmetric. As the disease progresses, there is greater involvement of the temporal lobes and frontal cortices. However, there is sparing of the anterior cingulate (involved in frontotemporal dementia), occipital visual cortex (involved in dementia with Lewy bodies), primary sensory and motor cortices, cerebellum, and basal ganglia.

References: Bohnen NI, Djang DS, Herholz K, et al. Effectiveness and safety of 18F-FDG-PET in the evaluation of dementia: a review of the recent literature. *J Nucl Med* 2012;53(1):59–71.

O'Malley JP, Ziessman HA, Thrall JH. *Nuclear medicine: the requisites*, 5th ed. Philadelphia, PA: Saunders, 2020:371–376.

8 Answer D. A single axial image from F-18 florbetapir (Amyvid) shows diffuse uptake throughout the cortical gray matter, with loss of contrast between the white and the gray matter. The findings are in keeping with the presence of moderate to abundant amyloid plaques. A major limitation of Amyvid is that a positive scan does not establish the diagnosis of Alzheimer disease (AD). While this appearance with moderate to abundant amyloid plaques is seen with Alzheimer disease (AD), corroborative clinical evidence is required to establish the diagnosis of AD as a similar pattern may be seen in patients with other types of neurologic conditions as well as older people with normal cognition. On the other hand, a negative Amyvid PET scan (scan from a different patient below) would make it unlikely that the patient's cognitive impairment would be due to AD. Additionally, the safety and effectiveness of Amyvid have not been established for predicting the development of dementia or other neurologic conditions, determining the severity of dementia, or monitoring responses to therapies.

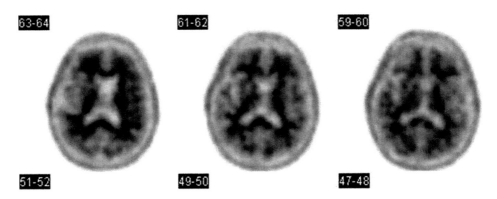

References: Amyvid [package insert]. Indianapolis, IN: Lilly USA, LLC, 2013. (www.amyvid. com)

Johnson KA, Minoshima S, et al. Appropriate use criteria for amyloid PET: a report of the Amyloid Imaging Task Force, the Society of Nuclear Medicine and Molecular Imaging, and the Alzheimer's Association. *J Nucl Med* 2013;54(3):476–490.

9a **Answer B.** I-123 ioflupane is an analog of cocaine. It reversibly binds with high affinity to the dopamine transporter (DaT) protein, a marker for presynaptic terminals in dopaminergic nigrostriatal neurons. In patients with parkinsonian syndromes (idiopathic Parkinson disease, progressive supranuclear palsy, and multiple system atrophy), there is destruction of nigrostriatal neurons leading to decreased uptake of the radiopharmaceutical in the striatum. The decreased uptake initially occurs in the posterior striatum (posterior putamen) and then moves anteriorly (anterior putamen and then caudate nucleus). In the United States, DaTscan is approved as an adjunct to other diagnostic evaluations in differentiating tremor secondary to the parkinsonian syndromes from the essential tremor. A normal DaTscan (see image below) in a patient with movement disorder would suggest essential tremor.

In this case, delayed images acquired after the IV administration of I-123 ioflupane demonstrate absent radiotracer uptake within the left lentiform nucleus (putamen and globus pallidus, aka posterior striatum) with a mild reduction in radiopharmaceutical uptake within the left caudate nucleus. Relatively normal radiopharmaceutical uptake is noted within the right striatum. In this patient with tremor, the findings are most compatible with parkinsonian syndromes. For comparison purposes, a normal DaTscan is shown below.

Stimulants such as cocaine, amphetamines, ephedrine, and methylphenidate severely decrease I-123 ioflupane uptake. Other medications known to interfere with DaTscan include selective serotonin-reuptake inhibitors (SSRI), which bind to DaT with high affinity and may up-regulate or down-regulate its expression. Anti-Parkinson disease medications such as carbidopa or levodopa act on the postsynaptic dopamine receptors and, therefore, do not interfere with DaTscan and may be continued as prescribed.

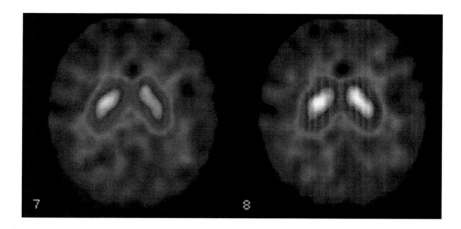

References: Grosset DG, Tatsch K, Oertel WH, et al. Safety analysis of 10 clinical trials and for 13 years after first approval of ioflupane 123I injection (DaTscan). *J Nucl Med* 2014;55(8):1281–1287.

O'Malley JP, Ziessman HA, Thrall JH. *Nuclear medicine: the requisites*, 5th ed. Philadelphia, PA: Saunders, 2020:391–395.

9b   Answer E. Dementia with Lewy bodies (DLB) is usually accompanied by visual hallucinations, fluctuating mental status, and parkinsonism. F-18 FDG-PET in DLB patients demonstrates hypometabolism in the primary visual cortex, which is spared in Alzheimer disease (AD). In cases where the differentiation between AD and DLB is difficult on FDG-PET, DaTscan may help differentiate between the two. Patients with AD and frontotemporal dementia will have a normal DaTscan, while patients with parkinsonian syndromes and DLB will have abnormal DaTscan. It is important to diagnose DLB because patients with DLB may have improved cognition from acetylcholinesterase inhibition, and their movement disorder may benefit from antiparkinsonian therapy. In Huntington chorea, patients have uncontrollable choreiform movements and dementia. Generally, reduced radiotracer uptake is seen in the caudate nucleus on PET or SPECT imaging, followed by atrophy of the basal ganglia seen on the anatomic imaging.

References: Grosset DG, Tatsch K, Oertel WH, et al. Safety analysis of 10 clinical trials and for 13 years after first approval of ioflupane 123I injection (DaTscan). *J Nucl Med* 2014;55(8):1281–1287.

O'Malley JP, Ziessman HA, Thrall JH. *Nuclear medicine: the requisites*, 5th ed. Philadelphia, PA: Saunders, 2020:391–395.

10   Answer D. Acetazolamide (ACZ) penetrates the blood–brain barrier slowly and causes increased carbon dioxide concentration by inhibiting carbonic anhydrase. The resultant carbonic acidosis causes a significant increase in cerebral blood flow (CBF). A standard dose of 1,000 mg intravenously is used for the ACZ challenge test. Peak CBF augmentation occurs at approximately 10 to 15 minutes after intravenous bolus administration with a 30% to 60% increase in CBF achieved in healthy subjects. Systemic blood pressure, heart rate, respiratory rate, arterial CO_2, and arterial pH are unaffected. Adenosine and regadenoson cause vasodilatation by binding to the adenosine receptor, while dipyridamole causes vasodilatation by increasing the adenosine concentration by blocking its uptake by cells. None of these other agents crosses the blood–brain barrier.

References: Rogg J, Rutigliano M, et al. The acetazolamide challenge: imaging techniques and designed to evaluate cerebral blood flow reserve. *AJR Am J Roentgenol* 1989;53:605–612.

Vagal AS, Leach JL, Fernandez-Ulloa M, et al. The acetazolamide challenge: techniques and applications in the evaluation of chronic cerebral ischemia. *AJNR Am J Neuroradiol* 2009;30(5):876–884.

11 **Answer B.** Anterior immediate, 4-hour, 24-hour, and 48-hour images acquired after the intrathecal administration of In-111 DTPA demonstrate the migration of the radiotracer to the skull base at 4 hours. There is a penetration of the radiopharmaceutical into the ventricular system (ventricular reflux) at 4 hours, which persists at 24 and 48 hours. Also, there is delayed migration of the radiotracer over the cerebral convexities with no significant activity over the cerebral convexity at 24 hours. In a patient with the supplied medical history, the findings are most consistent with normal pressure hydrocephalus (NPH). NPH is a form of communicating hydrocephalus in which the opening CSF pressures are normal. It is caused by impaired absorption of the CSF by the arachnoid granulations. The classic clinical triad includes dementia, gait disturbance, and incontinence. Patients with NPH showing ventricular penetration on cisternogram respond better to ventricular shunt placement when compared to those without. Images from a different patient shown below also show delayed migration of the radiotracer over the cerebral convexity without the presence of ventricular penetration, in keeping with NPH.

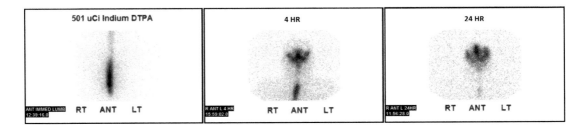

Normal CSF dynamics demonstrate the migration of intrathecally injected radiopharmaceutical into the basal cisterns of the posterior and middle cranial fossae by 1 to 3 hours. It appears in frontal poles and sylvian fissures by 2 to 6 hours, and cerebral convexities by 12 hours. Images from a different patient below show normal CSF flow dynamics with radiopharmaceutical in between the frontal poles and sylvian fissure at 4 hours and over the cerebral convexity at 24 hours.

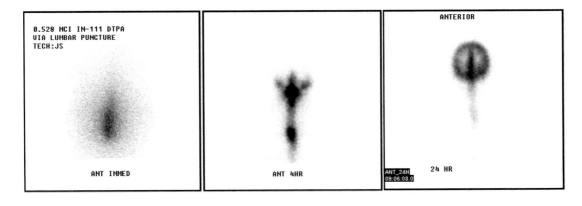

Due to its long half-life of 2.8 days, In-111 DTPA is used in the evaluation of CSF dynamics and slow CSF leaks resulting in otorrhea and rhinorrhea. In cases where high count statistics are necessary and which do not require longer imaging time (i.e., spinal dural leak, CSF shunt evaluation), Tc-99m DTPA can be used instead. DTPA is ideal for CSF imaging as it does not get metabolized or get absorbed across the ependyma. Once at the cerebral convexity, it gets absorbed through the arachnoid villi and rapidly gets cleared by the kidneys.

Reference: Mettler FA, Guiberteau MJ. *Essentials of nuclear medicine imaging*, 6th ed. Philadelphia, PA: Saunders, 2012:91–96.

12 **Answer C.** Because of the prominent involvement of frontal lobes in advanced Alzheimer disease (AD), differentiation of advanced AD from frontotemporal dementia (FTD) is often difficult. The diagnostic accuracy of F-18 FDG-PET in distinguishing AD patients from normal subjects is >90%, but it has poor specificity in differentiating AD from other causes of primary dementia. Beta-amyloid imaging would be most helpful in differentiating AD from FTD as it would be markedly abnormal in AD but normal in FTD. The first FDA-approved and most widely used radiotracer for in vivo identification of beta-amyloid (Aβ) plaques was F-18 florbetapir (Amyvid). Other FDA-approved agents for imaging beta-amyloid include F-18 florbetaben (Neuraceq) and F-18 flutemetamol (Vizamyl). A negative beta-amyloid imaging PET scan would show predominant white matter retention, while a positive scan would display increasing gray matter retention. Amyloid imaging demonstrates the earliest abnormality in AD, even before F-18 FDG-PET is abnormal. However, a positive amyloid PET scan in itself is not definitive for AD; the presence of beta-amyloid in the brain serves to increase the clinical certainty of AD diagnosis. A negative scan indicates few or no amyloid plaques, excluding AD. C-11 Pittsburgh compound B (C-11 PIB), a derivative of a fluorescent amyloid dye (thioflavin T), was the first agent with high affinity and specificity for beta-amyloid plaques used in amyloid imaging. However, the use of C-11 PIB is limited to centers with an on-site cyclotron because of the short 20-minute radioactive half-life of C-11.

References: Mettler FA, Guiberteau MJ. *Essentials of nuclear medicine imaging*, 7th ed. Philadelphia, PA: Saunders, 2019:74–77.

Rowe CC, Villemagne VL. Brain amyloid imaging. *J Nucl Med* 2011;52(11):1733–1740.

Yang L, Rieves D, Ganley C. Brain amyloid imaging—FDA approval of florbetapir F18 injection. *N Engl J Med* 2012;367(10):885–887.

13 **Answer A.** The anterior and lateral cisternogram images acquired after the intrathecal administration of In-111 DTPA show increased radiotracer accumulation within the region of the left nostril, best visualized on the 4-hour left lateral projection (arrow below). This is confirmed by the SPECT/CT images as well as by measuring the activity within the nasal pledgets. The findings are consistent with a CSF leak in the left nostril. Activity within the colon on the 24-hour delayed image is from swallowed nasal secretions containing the radiotracer from the leak. Approximately 80% of CSF rhinorrhea cases are the result of head trauma, with 16% being iatrogenic and the remaining 4% being spontaneous.

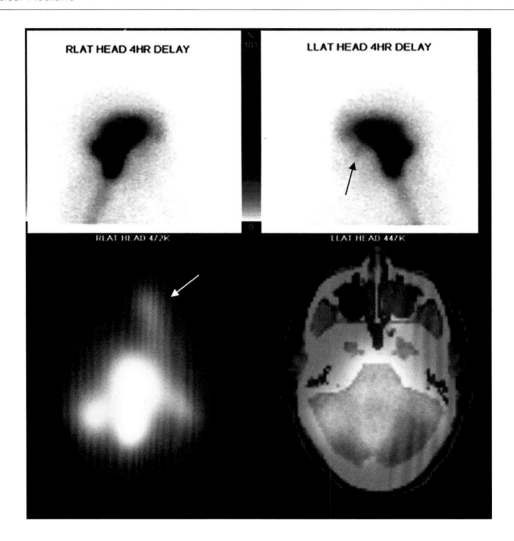

Evaluation of CSF leaks should consist of imaging the site of the leak and measuring differential activity in the pledgets placed deep into each nostril or ear, as per history. Pledgets are placed before the intrathecal injection of the radiotracer and are typically removed 4 hours after the placement and counted in a well counter. Simultaneously, blood serum samples should be obtained and counted. The pledget-to-serum ratio of more than 1.5 is interpreted as evidence of the CSF leak. In our patient, the left nostril ratio is significantly higher than 1.5 at 54 in the superior and 45 in the middle left nostril pledgets. It is important to image for a CSF leak at the time the radiotracer reaches the suspected site of the origin of the leak. Apart from images of the thoracic and lumbar spine, head and neck images should be obtained as leaks generally happen near the basilar cisterns. SPECT/CT images provide better anatomic correlation in cases of major leaks. Any position or activity known by the patient to provoke or aggravate the leak of CSF should be accomplished immediately before or during imaging. A delayed image of the abdomen may be obtained to visualize indirect evidence of a CSF leak from swallowed radiotracer activity within bowel loops, such as in this patient. A higher count study with intrathecal injection of Tc-99m DTPA may be better in cases of CSF leak associated with a suspected tear in the spinal cord dura.

References: Habibian MR. *Nuclear medicine imaging: a teaching file*, 2nd ed. Philadelphia, PA: Lippincott Williams & Wilkins, 2009:176–177.

Mettler FA, Guiberteau MJ. *Essentials of nuclear medicine imaging*, 6th ed. Philadelphia, PA: Saunders, 2012:91–96.

14 **Answer C.** Tc-99m DTPA and In-111 DTPA are the radiopharmaceuticals utilized to evaluate for CSF shunt patency. Tc-99m pertechnetate, Tc-99m sulfur colloid, and Tc-99m HMPAO are not utilized for CSF scintigraphy. In-111-DTPA is the only FDA-approved agent for intrathecal injection. In this examination, Tc-99m DTPA was injected through the reservoir with the distal limb manually occluded to allow the injected tracer to flow into the proximal limb. The images demonstrate prompt flow into the ventricles, followed by spontaneous flow through the distal limb of the shunt catheter into the peritoneal cavity. There is a free distribution of radiopharmaceutical within the peritoneal cavity without pooling of the radiopharmaceutical around the tip of the distal limb. This is a normal CSF shunt evaluation study.

Reference: Mettler FA, Guiberteau MJ. *Essentials of nuclear medicine imaging*, 7th ed. Philadelphia, PA: Saunders, 2019:81–83.

15 **Answer D.** A single coronal PET image demonstrates reduced metabolism in the left cerebral cortex, consistent with a known stroke. There is also a significantly decreased metabolism in the contralateral cerebellum. This finding is consistent with crossed cerebellar diaschisis. Crossed cerebellar diaschisis is defined as a reduction in metabolic activity and blood flow of the cerebellum contralateral to the supratentorial cerebral lesion. Most commonly, the corticopontocerebellar pathway is involved whose origin comes from motor, premotor, parietal association as well as occipital cortices and terminates in the cerebellar gray matter. It can be seen with infarct, supratentorial tumors, epilepsy, or vascular dementia. The cerebellar metabolic and/or perfusion depression is typically asymptomatic. It resolves when occurring with stroke but may persist when associated with brain tumors. It is important to recognize this phenomenon and not to mistake it for a concomitant cerebellar lesion.

References: Flores L, Futami S, Hoshi H, et al. Crossed cerebellar diaschisis: analysis of iodine-123-IMP SPECT imaging. *J Nucl Med* 1995;36(3):399–402.

Mettler FA, Guiberteau MJ. *Essentials of nuclear medicine imaging*, 6th ed. Philadelphia, PA: Saunders, 2012:91–96.

QUESTIONS

1 The following image is from a dual-isotope myocardial perfusion examination. What is the major difference between performing the myocardial perfusion stress imaging with thallium-201 (Tl-201) and technetium-99m (Tc-99m) myocardial perfusion agents?

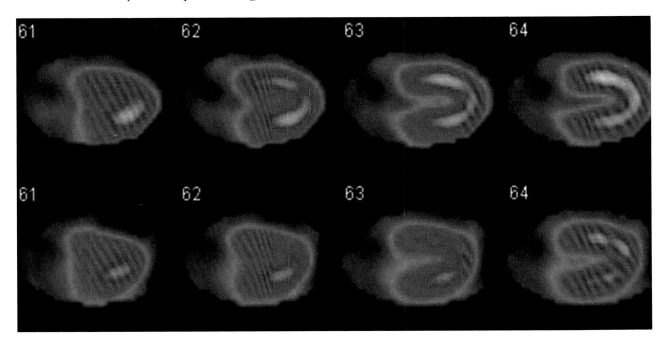

A. A higher dose of thallium-201 is used for imaging.
B. Stress acquisition must begin within 10 minutes of Tl-201 injection.
C. An exercise stress test cannot be performed with Tl-201.
D. A pharmacologic stress test cannot be performed with Tl-201.
E. Imaging is usually begun 30 to 45 minutes after Tl-201 administration.
F. Tl-201 has less soft tissue attenuation.

2 What is the most appropriate dose range for the resting portion of 1-day rest/
stress Tc-99m tetrofosmin SPECT myocardial perfusion imaging?

A. 3 to 5 mCi
B. 8 to 12 mCi
C. 15 to 20 mCi
D. 24 to 36 mCi

3 Which of the following is a correct statement regarding regadenoson
(Lexiscan)?

A. It is a selective A2B receptor agonist.
B. It cannot be used in patients with a history of asthma or COPD.
C. Fixed bolus injection of 400 µg is given over 10 seconds.
D. Atropine is used to treat adverse effects associated with its administration.

4 What is the major difference between the PET myocardial perfusion images
acquired with N-13 ammonia when compared to those acquired with
rubidium-82?

A. Better resolution
B. Larger full width at half maximum
C. No difference
D. Higher energy photon
E. Less signal to noise

5 Which of the following myocardial perfusion agents has the longest half-life?

A. Rb-82
B. F-18 FDG
C. O-15 water
D. N-13 ammonia

6 Which of the following is most commonly associated with an inferior wall
perfusion abnormality?

A. Breast attenuation
B. Diaphragm attenuation
C. Left bundle branch block
D. Left circumflex artery stenosis

7 Name the labeling method where the red blood cells are separated via
centrifugation, washed, incubated with Sn^{2+}, incubated with $99m\text{-}TcO_4^-$, and
reinjected?

A. In vitro
B. In vivo
C. Modified in vivo
D. Modified in vitro

8a A 68-year-old lady underwent rest–stress Tc-99m tetrofosmin myocardial perfusion imaging for chest pain. What is the most likely diagnosis?

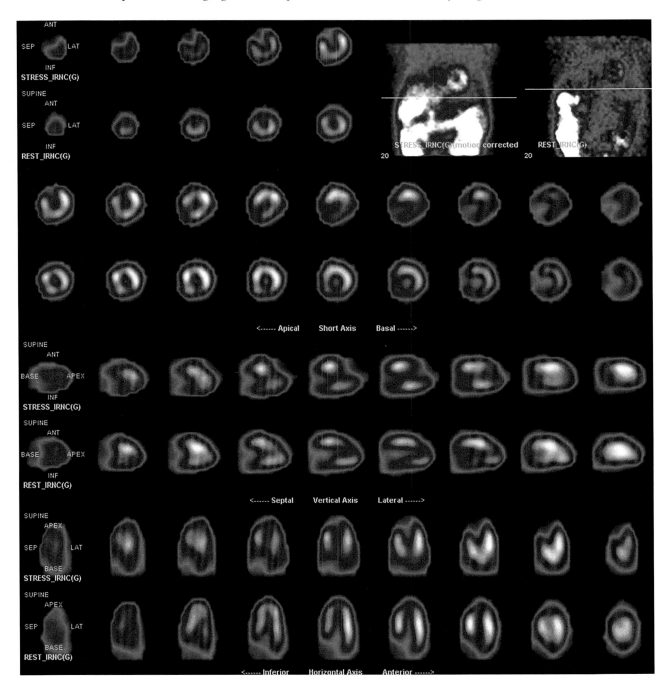

A. Normal
B. Ischemia
C. Infarct
D. Attenuation artifact

8b This territory is supplied by which of the following arteries?

A. Left anterior descending artery (LAD)
B. Left circumflex artery (LCX)
C. Right coronary artery (RCA)
D. Ramus intermedius artery

9 The following patient underwent a regadenoson pharmacologic stress test using Rb-82 rest–stress PET myocardial perfusion imaging. What is the most likely diagnosis?

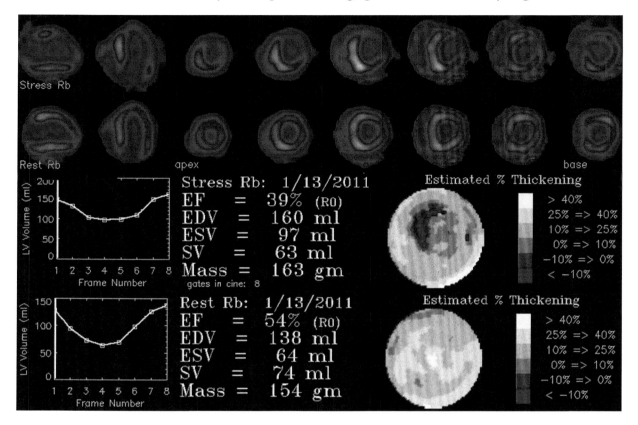

A. Left anterior descending artery disease
B. Left circumflex artery disease
C. Right coronary artery disease
D. Multivessel disease

10a A 63-year-old gentleman with ischemic cardiomyopathy is being evaluated for possible coronary artery bypass grafting with the hope of symptom improvement. Based on the following immediate (top row) and 24-hour delayed (bottom row) short-axis thallium-201 perfusion images, what is the MOST likely diagnosis?

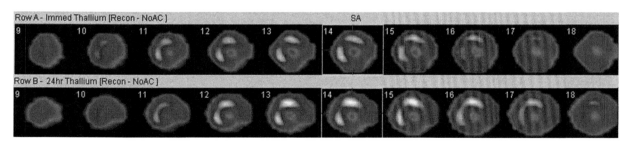

A. Ischemia
B. Attenuation artifact
C. Stunned myocardium
D. Hibernating myocardium
E. Nonviable myocardial infarct

10b What artery supplies this territory?

A. Left anterior descending artery
B. Left circumflex artery
C. Right coronary artery
D. Ramus intermedius artery

11 The patient is a 59-year-old gentleman with ischemic cardiomyopathy and LVEF of 35%. Based on the following resting N-13 ammonia (top row) and F-18 FDG- (bottom row) PET images, what is the most likely diagnosis?

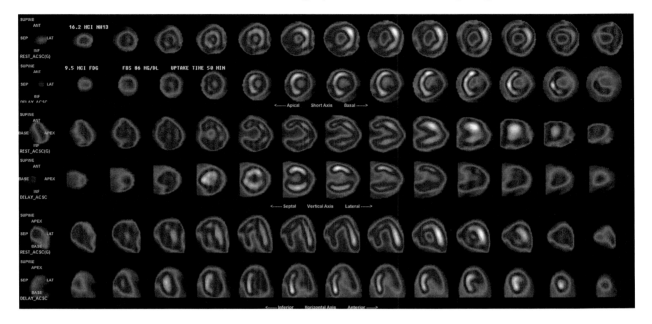

- A. Ischemia
- B. Attenuation artifact
- C. Stunned myocardium
- D. Hibernating myocardium
- E. Nonviable myocardial infarct

12 This patient with decreased LVEF had abnormal patchy enhancement on a prior MRI, which prompted this resting Rb-82 (top) and 18-hour fasting F-18 FDG myocardial PET (bottom) examination. What is the MOST likely explanation for the finding?

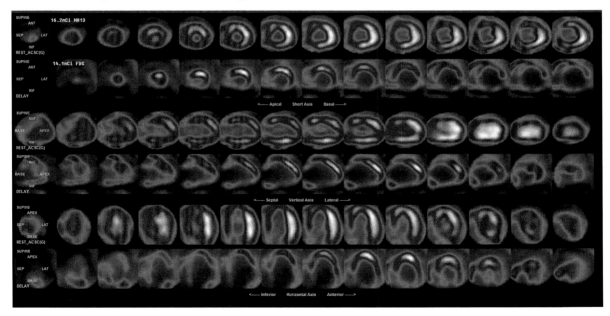

- A. Infarcted nonviable myocardium
- B. Hibernating viable myocardium
- C. Active granulomatous disease
- D. Ischemic myocardium

13 Rest rubidium-82 perfusion (top) and F-18 FDG metabolic (bottom) PET images from a 57-year-old male with a history of hypertension, CHF, and sarcoid are shown below. Based on the supplied images, what is the most appropriate conclusion?

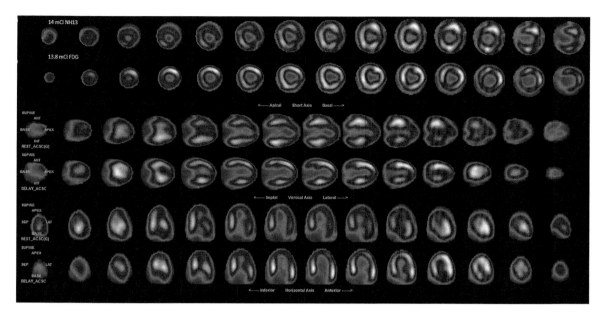

A. Subcutaneous infiltration of dose
B. Dietary noncompliance
C. Diffuse myocardial sarcoidosis
D. Hibernating myocardium

14 The same patient underwent repeat imaging with proper adherence to the dietary instructions. Based on the supplied imaging, which of the following is the most appropriate conclusion regarding cardiac sarcoidosis?

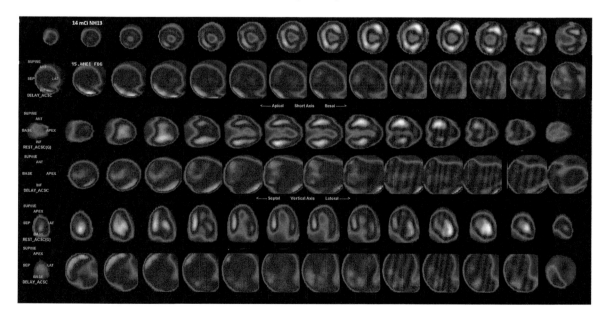

A. Normal study
B. Early-stage sarcoidosis
C. Progressive stage
D. Inconclusive study

15 Based on the Rb-82 resting perfusion (top) and F-18 FDG metabolism (bottom) images as well as reconstructed FDG-PET/CT images from the same dataset in the second figure, what is the most likely diagnosis?

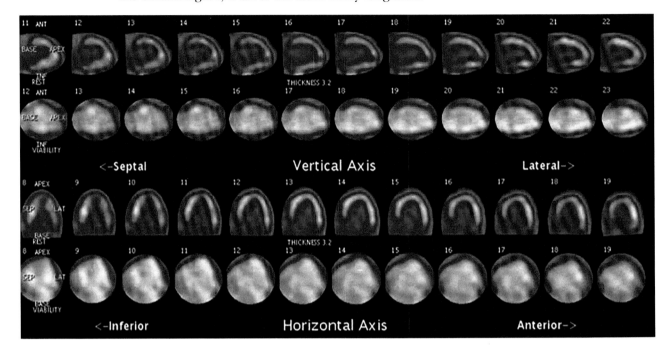

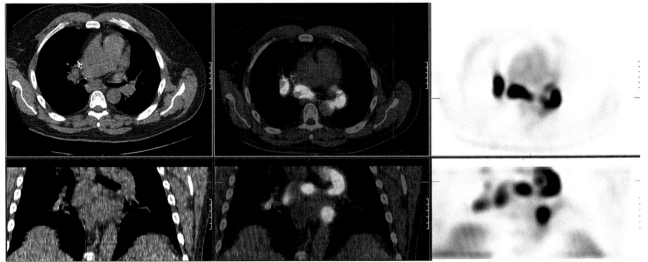

A. Negative cardiac sarcoidosis, positive systemic sarcoidosis
B. Negative cardiac sarcoidosis, negative systemic sarcoidosis
C. Positive cardiac sarcoidosis, positive systemic sarcoidosis
D. Positive cardiac sarcoidosis, negative systemic sarcoidosis

16 A 44-year-old lady was seen in the ED with the complaint of chest pain. The patient underwent a treadmill exercise stress test, during which she achieved her target heart rate. What is the MOST likely explanation for the following findings?

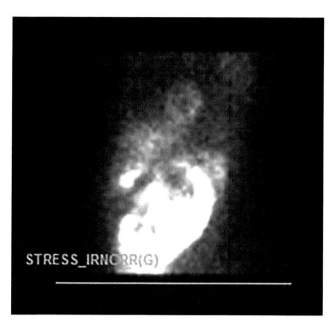

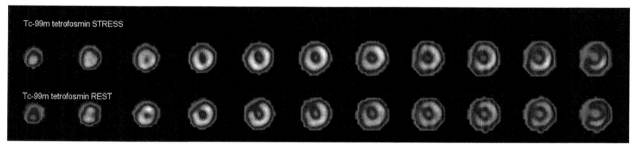

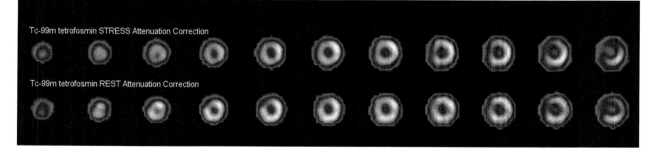

A. Infarct

B. Ischemia

C. Malignancy

D. Motion artifact

E. Gating abnormality

F. Attenuation artifact

G. Hibernating myocardium

17 What is the most likely cause of the artifact demonstrated by the following image?

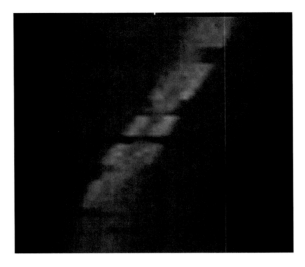

    A. Attenuation
    B. Center of rotation
    C. Patient motion
    D. Abnormal gating
    E. Field nonuniformity

18 A single-frame image below is from a rotating cine of a patient who underwent myocardial perfusion imaging for chest pain. What is the most appropriate next step?

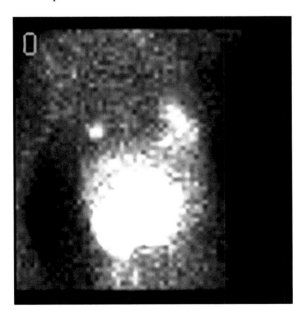

    A. Prone imaging
    B. Repeat supine images with right arm up
    C. HIDA scan
    D. Attenuation correction
    E. Mammogram
    F. CT of the abdomen

19 A 35-year-old with aberrant coronary arteries is being evaluated for demand
ischemia. Based on the following rest–stress myocardial perfusion SPECT
images, what is the most likely cause of the depicted abnormality?

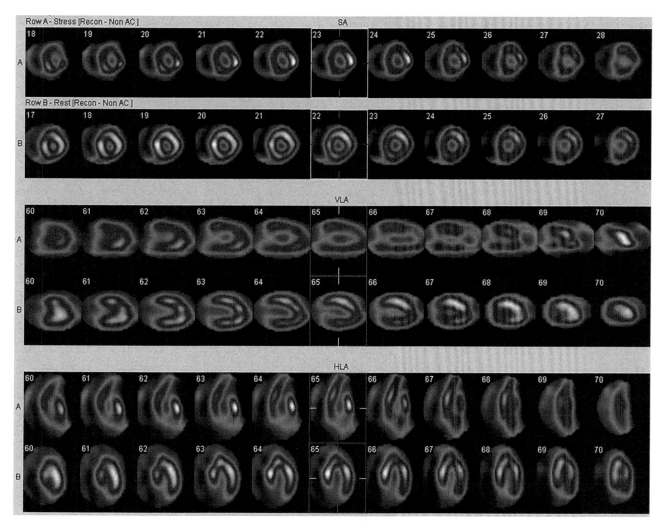

   A. Ischemia
   B. Camera axis error
   C. Attenuation artifact
   D. Patient motion
   E. Field nonuniformity
   F. Dose infiltration

20 Review the single frame from the cine images, sinogram, and the corresponding myocardial perfusion SPECT images. What is the MOST likely cause of the resting perfusion SPECT image degradation?

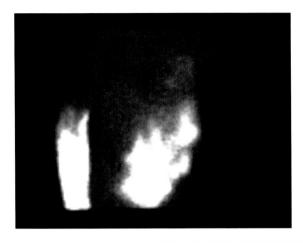

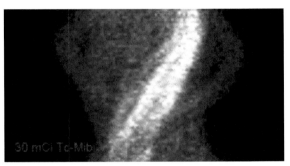

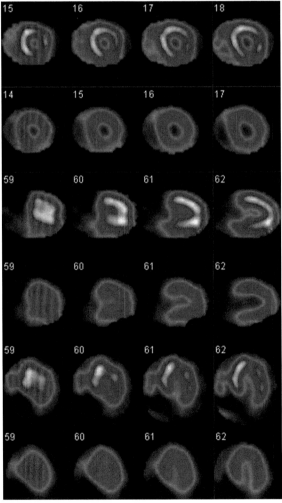

A. Patient motion
B. Attenuation artifact
C. Arterial injection
D. Right forearm malignancy
E. Improper reconstruction

21 A 55-year-old male with known coronary artery disease has a history of persistent chest pains. Based on the supplied PET myocardial perfusion images, what is the most appropriate next step?

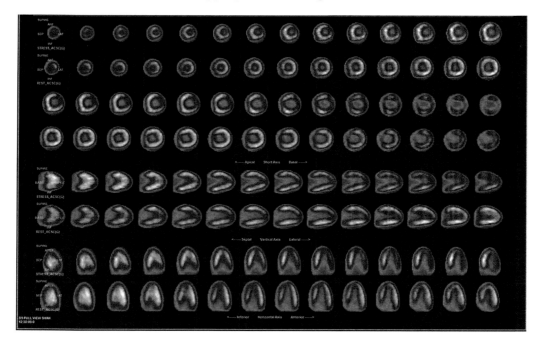

A. Interpret the study as lateral wall ischemia.
B. Review the PET and CT images for misregistration.
C. Interpret the study as hibernating myocardium in the lateral wall.
D. Interpret the study as an infarct in the lateral wall.
E. Interpret the study as a stunned myocardium in the lateral wall.

22 Which of the following statements is most accurate regarding the images provided below?

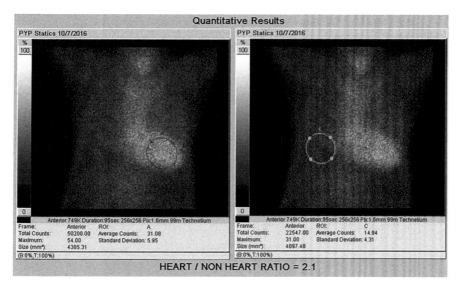

A. The patient is undergoing evaluation of myocardial perfusion.
B. The patient is undergoing an evaluation of amyloid deposits formed from transthyretin.
C. The patient is undergoing evaluation of myocardial ejection fraction.
D. The patient is undergoing evaluation of cardiac sympathetic innervation.

23 The following radionuclide ventriculography (RVG) or gated equilibrium radionuclide angiography (E-RNA) is from a patient who is undergoing evaluation for stem cell transplantation. What conclusion can be made regarding the calculated left ventricular ejection fraction (LVEF)?

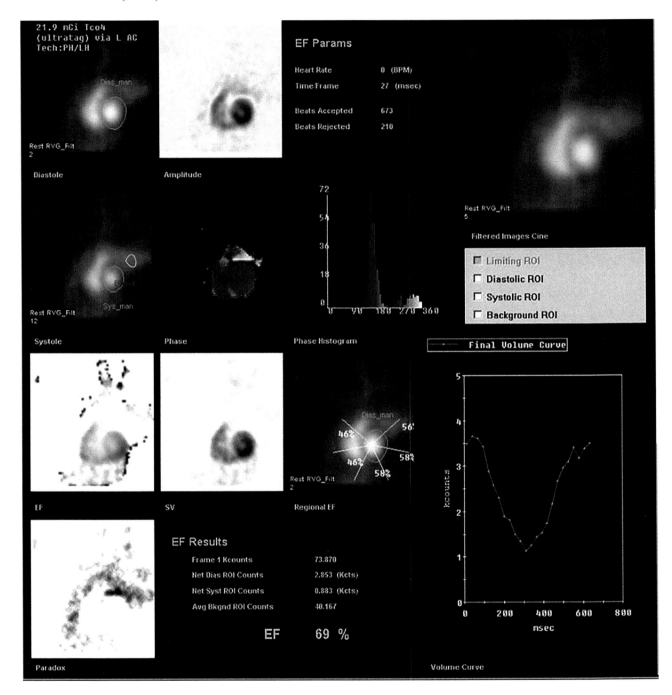

A. LVEF is falsely elevated.
B. LVEF is falsely decreased.
C. LVEF is normal; no further intervention is required.
D. There is evidence of early diastolic failure.
E. There is evidence of right bundle branch block.

ANSWERS AND EXPLANATIONS

1 **Answer B.** Thallium-201 (Tl-201) is a potassium analog, which is transported across the myocardial membrane via the Na^+-K^+ ATPase pump into the myocardial cytosol. It localizes in the myocardium in two phases: initial distribution is mediated by blood flow and cellular extraction by viable myocardium, and delayed redistribution is mediated by the continued dynamic exchange between vascular blood pool and myocardium. It has a very high first-pass extraction rate of approximately 85% compared to about 60% for the Tc-99m–labeled myocardial perfusion imaging agents (sestamibi or tetrofosmin). Unlike Tc-99m–labeled myocardial perfusion imaging agents, Tl-201 quickly undergoes redistribution, which is a dynamic exchange of Tl-201 between the myocardial cytosol and the vascular blood pool. Because of redistribution, poststress images with Tl-201 must be performed quickly after its injection (<10 minutes). Redistribution is also the basis for the use of Tl-201 in the evaluation of myocardial viability with delayed 24-hour imaging. Either exercise or pharmacologic stress protocol can be used with Tl-201. Because of its higher absorbed dose, in part due to its longer half-life of 3 days, the injected dose of the Tl-201 (3 to 4 mCi total) is lower than those of the Tc-99m–labeled myocardial perfusion agents (30 to 45 mCi total). Biliary excretion of Tc-99m–labeled myocardial perfusion agents results in intense activity within the liver. In order to allow clearance from the liver and since these agents do not undergo redistribution, imaging is usually begun 30 to 45 minutes after their administration. In comparison, Tl-201 is excreted slowly and to an equal extent through urine and feces, resulting in less GI scatter. Since Tc-99m photon has higher energy (140 keV) than mercury daughter x-rays from Tl-201 (69 to 81 keV), less soft tissue attenuation would be seen with Tc-99m–labeled agents compared to Tl-201.

Reference: Mettler FA, Guiberteau MJ. *Essentials of nuclear medicine imaging*, 7th ed. Philadelphia, PA: Saunders, 2019:120–123.

2 **Answer B.** Typical rest dose of Tc labeled myocardial perfusion agents for 1-day rest/stress myocardial perfusion study is between 8 and 12 mCi. For 1-day protocol, the rest dose is typically one-third of the stress dose. Some variations may be allowed depending on the length of time between rest and stress injections. If the time between the rest and stress injections is long, a full three times greater dose is not required for the stress injection due to greater decay of activity from the prior resting injection. If the time is short, the stress portion of the study requires a higher dose. With a high rest dose, stress dose will need to be three times higher, which will give patients unnecessary radiation. If a lower dose is used for stress without sufficient time between the two injections, there will be residual activity from the rest study, which can underestimate the amount of ischemia. Newer dedicated cardiac cameras with solid-state detectors and focused cardiac imaging are more efficient and may allow for a lower dose of the radiotracer injection than traditional gamma cameras.

Reference: Henzlova MJ, et al. ASNC Imaging Guidelines for Nuclear Cardiology Procedures: stress protocols and tracers. *J Nucl Cardiol* 2016;23(3):606–639. doi: 10.1007/s12350-015-0387-x.

3 **Answer C.** Regadenoson is the most commonly used pharmacologic stress agent for myocardial perfusion imaging due to its ease of use and favorable side effect profile. It was first approved for clinical use by the FDA in 2009. It is a selective A2A receptor agonist with rapid onset (30 seconds) and vasodilatory effects lasting for approximately 2 to 5 minutes. The recommended IV dose of 400 μg is typically given over 10 to 30 seconds into a peripheral vein. Like adenosine and dipyridamole (Persantine), it induces coronary arteriolar hyperemia approximately 3.5 to 4 times that of the baseline. Unlike adenosine and Persantine, it is a selective adenosine receptor agonist. Since it does not bind to A3 receptors responsible for bronchospasm, severe asthma or COPD are not absolute contraindications to its use. While package insert states that appropriate bronchodilator therapy and resuscitative measures should be available prior to and following Lexiscan administration, we have not encountered serious complications in these patients in our clinical practice. With the exception of seizures, complications or side effects of all of the adenosine agonist agents can be reversed with intravenous administration of aminophylline (50 to 250 mg). Atropine may be used in conjunction with dobutamine or exercise to counteract the effects of beta-adrenergic blocking medications in order to achieve target heart rate and to increase the sensitivity of the myocardial perfusion imaging in certain patient populations.

Receptor Subtype	Effect
A1	AV block
A2A	Coronary arteriolar vasodilation
A2B	Peripheral vasodilation, bronchospasm
A3	Bronchospasm

References: Henzlova MJ, et al. ASNC Imaging Guidelines for Nuclear Cardiology Procedures: stress protocols and tracers. *J Nucl Cardiol* 2016;23(3):606–639. doi: 10.1007/s12350-015-0387-x.

Mettler FA, Guiberteau MJ. *Essentials of nuclear medicine imaging*, 7th ed. Philadelphia, PA: Saunders, 2019:144–146.

4 **Answer A.** N-13 ammonia positron has less energy (1.198 MeV) than the positron emitted by the decay of rubidium-82 (Rb-82, 3.150 MeV). As such, it travels a shorter distance before undergoing annihilation. This decreased range is responsible for the better image resolution (smaller full width at half maximum) of N-13 ammonia myocardial perfusion images compared to that acquired with Rb-82. The energy of photons generated by annihilation is 511 keV for both N-13 ammonia and Rb-82. N-13 ammonia, Rb-82, and F-18 flurpiridaz are the PET radiotracers that can be used to evaluate myocardial perfusion; F-18 FDG is used for the evaluation of myocardial viability. The use of N-13 ammonia (half-life 10 minutes) requires an on-site cyclotron. Rubidium-82 (half-life 76 seconds) is produced by a generator and does not require an on-site cyclotron. F-18 flurpiridaz is a new PET myocardial perfusion radiopharmaceutical in clinical development.

References: Dicarli MF, Liptom MJ. *Cardiac PET and PET/CT imaging*. New York, NY: Springer, 2007:74.

Dilsizian V, Bacharach SL, Beanlands RS, et al. Imaging guidelines for nuclear cardiology procedures: PET myocardial perfusion and metabolism clinical imaging. *J Nucl Cardiol* 2009;16:651. doi: 10.1007/s12350-009-9094-9.

5 **Answer D.** Since currently available PET myocardial perfusion agents have short half-lives, they are best suited for pharmacologic stress. O-15 water, Rb-82, and N-13 ammonia are myocardial perfusion agents with half-lives discussed in the table below. F-18 FDG has a longer half-life, but it evaluates glucose metabolism and not myocardial perfusion. Rb-82 is an analog of potassium. Its extraction in the myocardium is lower at 60% compared to 70% to 80% for N-13 ammonia. F-18 Flurpiridaz is a new PET myocardial perfusion agent in clinical development. It has a longer half-life (110 minutes) and may allow for exercise PET myocardial perfusion imaging evaluation. Also, given that the positron resulting from F-18 annihilation travels the least distance, it also has the highest resolution of the clinically used positron emitters for myocardial perfusion imaging. Please note that because the energy of the Rb-82 positron is the highest, it has a range of 13 to 15 mm in soft tissues before undergoing annihilation. This results in inferior image quality compared to N-13 ammonia or F-18 FDG.

Agent	Mechanism	Production Method	Half-life	Energy (MeV)	Range in Soft Tissue (mm)
O-15	Perfusion	Cyclotron	2 min	1.73	7.3
Rb-82	Perfusion	Generator	75 s	3.15	15
N-13	Perfusion	Cyclotron	10 min	1.09	5.4
F-18 FDG	Glucose metabolism	Cyclotron	110 min	0.635	2.4

References: Mettler FA, Guiberteau MJ. *Essentials of nuclear medicine imaging*, 7th ed. Philadelphia, PA: Saunders, 2019:130–134.

O'Malley JP, Ziessman HA, Thrall JH. *Nuclear medicine: the requisites*, 5th ed. Philadelphia, PA: Saunders, 2020:465–467.

6 **Answer B.** Diaphragm attenuation artifact is typically seen along the mid to basal inferior wall, which is more severe along the base. The use of CT attenuation correction or prone imaging usually results in the resolution of the perfusion defect caused by the diaphragm attenuation artifact. Breast attenuation artifact is commonly seen along the anterior and anteroseptal walls (see below). Left bundle branch–related perfusion abnormalities are commonly seen along the anteroseptal and septal walls (see below). Left circumflex artery disease would be typically seen along the lateral and inferolateral walls.

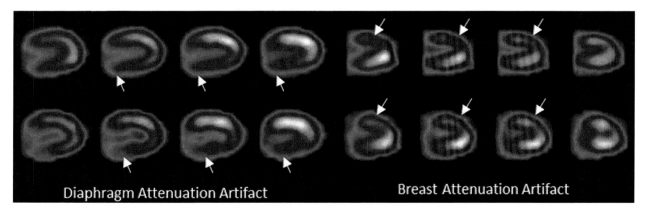
Diaphragm Attenuation Artifact   Breast Attenuation Artifact

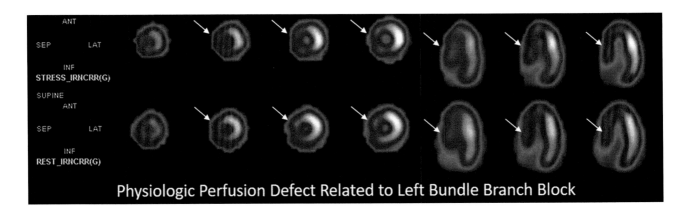

Physiologic Perfusion Defect Related to Left Bundle Branch Block

Reference: O'Malley JP, Ziessman HA, Thrall JH. *Nuclear medicine: the requisites*, 5th ed. Philadelphia, PA: Saunders, 2020:4131–4134.

7 **Answer A.** The described method is in vitro labeling of the red blood cells (RBCs). As the name implies, all steps involved in the labeling of the RBCs with in vitro labeling are performed outside the patient. It has the highest labeling efficiency (>97%) of the three labeling methods. The labeling efficiency of the modified in vivo technique is about 85% to 90%, and in vivo technique is about 75%.

References: Mettler FA, Guiberteau MJ. *Essentials of nuclear medicine imaging*, 7th ed. Philadelphia, PA: Saunders, 2019:166–167.

Saha GB. *Fundamentals of nuclear pharmacy*, 6th ed. New York, NY: Springer, 2010:120–121.

8a **Answer B.** The images demonstrate a large area of severely decreased activity along the anteroseptal wall extending into the apex, which is not present (reversible) on resting images. Findings are most consistent with myocardial ischemia. A myocardial infarct would appear the same on stress and rest perfusion images. Although the breast attenuation artifact would be seen along the anteroseptal wall, it would typically present as a mild to moderate intensity fixed perfusion defect and not as a severe intensity reversible defect. Also, the cine images would show significant attenuation related to the breasts. Diaphragm attenuation artifact would be most prominent along the basal inferior wall.

References: Mettler FA, Guiberteau MJ. *Essentials of nuclear medicine imaging*, 7th ed. Philadelphia, PA: Saunders, 2019:129–134.

O'Malley JP, Ziessman HA, Thrall JH. *Nuclear medicine: the requisites*, 5th ed. Philadelphia, PA: Saunders, 2020:452–455.

8b **Answer A.** Anterior, anteroseptal, and apical walls are typically supplied by the left anterior descending coronary artery (LAD). The left circumflex artery (LCX) typically supplies the lateral and inferolateral walls, while the inferior and inferoseptal walls are usually supplied by the right coronary artery (RCA), as shown in the image below.

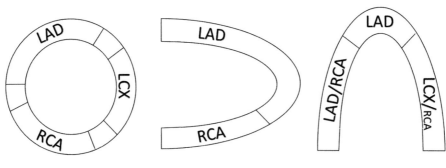

References: Mettler FA, Guiberteau MJ. *Essentials of nuclear medicine imaging*, 7th ed. Philadelphia, PA: Saunders, 2019:130–132.

O'Malley JP, Ziessman HA, Thrall JH. *Nuclear medicine: the requisites*, 5th ed. Philadelphia, PA: Saunders, 2020:444–447.

9 **Answer D.** The rest–stress perfusion images demonstrate a large area of severely decreased activity along the anterior wall extending into the anterolateral and lateral walls. Only a small area of mildly decreased activity is seen along the lateral wall on the rest images. Also, there is evidence of stress-induced dilatation of the left ventricular (LV) cavity and stress-induced reduction of LV ejection fraction (LVEF) from 54% to 39%, both of which suggest multivessel disease.

Because of the short half-lives of current PET radiopharmaceuticals, the patient must undergo the stress perfusion PET imaging during the pharmacologic stress. As such, any reduction in the stress LVEF with PET represents myocardial stunning from significant ischemia with a resultant decrease in myocardial contractility. On the other hand, with Tc-99m tetrofosmin and sestamibi, the patients usually wait 10 to 40 minutes between the injection at peak stress and imaging to allow for clearance from the liver. By this time, the stunned myocardium may have recovered, and stress-induced reduction in the LVEF may have resolved. With these agents, transient ischemic dilatation (TID), dilatation of the LV cavity on stress images compared to the rest images, is thought to be representative of a combination of diffuse subendocardial ischemia and myocardial stunning.

References: Mettler FA, Guiberteau MJ. *Essentials of nuclear medicine imaging*, 7th ed. Philadelphia, PA: Saunders, 2019:137, 156–157.

O'Malley JP, Ziessman HA, Thrall JH. *Nuclear medicine: the requisites*, 5th ed. Philadelphia, PA: Saunders, 2020:465–469.

10a **Answer E.** The immediate images (top row) demonstrate a large-sized area of severely decreased activity along the inferolateral wall, which persists on 24-hour images (bottom row). Findings are consistent with a nonviable myocardial scar. Because of the redistribution phenomenon, Tl-201 would be expected to redistribute from the normal myocardium and localize in the chronically ischemic but viable (hibernating) myocardium on the delayed 6- or 24-hour images when compared to the immediate images. When identified, revascularization of the chronically ischemic but viable myocardium results in significant improvement in the myocardial function. Rest/redistribution Tl-201 myocardial scintigraphy or PET myocardial perfusion/F-18 FDG metabolism study may be used for the evaluation of myocardial viability.

References: Maddahi J, Schelbert H, Brunken R, et al. Role of thallium-201 and PET imaging in evaluation of myocardial viability and management of patients with coronary artery disease and left ventricular dysfunction. *J Nucl Med* 1994;35(4):707–715.

O'Malley JP, Ziessman HA, Thrall JH. *Nuclear medicine: the requisites*, 5th ed. Philadelphia, PA: Saunders, 2020:456–459.

10b **Answer B.** This area is typically supplied by the left circumflex artery, as discussed in explanation 8b.

References: Mettler FA, Guiberteau MJ. *Essentials of nuclear medicine imaging*, 7th ed. Philadelphia, PA: Saunders, 2019:130–132.

O'Malley JP, Ziessman HA, Thrall JH. *Nuclear medicine: the requisites*, 5th ed. Philadelphia, PA: Saunders, 2020:444–447, 456–459.

11 **Answer D.** The resting N-13 ammonia perfusion images demonstrate a large area of severely decreased perfusion along the anterior wall extending into the anteroseptal wall and septum. This defect demonstrates metabolism on the F-18 FDG images. As such, the findings are consistent with a large zone of hibernating myocardium in the LAD and RCA territories. Hibernating myocardium is chronically ischemic but viable myocardium, which should recover function after revascularization.

The patient undergoing F-18 FDG myocardial viability imaging undergoes glucose loading (sometimes with insulin) prior to F-18 FDG administration. This will help switch myocardial metabolism from fatty acids to glucose and increase the amount of F-18 FDG taken up in the heart. F-18 FDG-PET viability images should always be interpreted in conjunction with perfusion images. The perfusion defect is the only area that should be evaluated on the metabolic viability images as the normally perfused myocardium may utilize fatty acids and may not demonstrate significant FDG uptake. Hibernating myocardium will preferentially use glucose over free fatty acids and will demonstrate an area of increased FDG uptake. If this area corresponds to the area of resting perfusion abnormality, then it represents a hibernating myocardium. If the defect is present on both perfusion and metabolism images, then it likely represents a nonviable myocardial scar, and the patient will not benefit from revascularization.

References: Maddahi J, Schelbert H, Brunken R, et al. Role of thallium-201 and PET imaging in evaluation of myocardial viability and management of patients with coronary artery disease and left ventricular dysfunction. *J Nucl Med* 1994;35(4):707–715.

O'Malley JP, Ziessman HA, Thrall JH. *Nuclear medicine: the requisites*, 5th ed. Philadelphia, PA: Saunders, 2020:454–455.

12 **Answer C.** Acquired resting N-13 ammonia perfusion (top) and delayed fasting F-18 FDG metabolism images demonstrate a moderate to large-sized area of increased glucose metabolism in the anterior wall extending into the anterolateral and anteroseptal walls (arrows below). Also, increased FDG metabolism is visualized in the mid to basal aspect of the right ventricle (arrowheads in the image below). Mildly decreased perfusion is noted in the anterior and septal walls. The findings are in keeping with cardiac sarcoidosis, likely in the peak active phase.

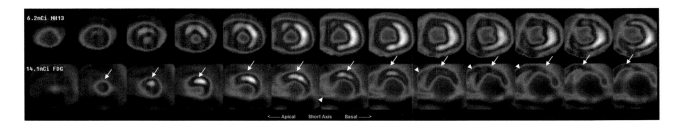

In contrast to the F-18 FDG myocardial viability study in which the patient undergoes glucose loading prior to F-18 FDG administration, F-18 FDG-PET is performed after prolonged fasting if the patient is undergoing evaluation of active granulomatous disease such as sarcoidosis. Active granulomatous disease would demonstrate increased FDG uptake on 18-hour fasting images, while normal myocardium would have switched to fatty acid metabolism after prolonged fasting. The sensitivity and specificity of F-18 FDG-PET for cardiac sarcoidosis are reported to be 89% and 78%, respectively. FDG-PET and delayed contrast-enhanced MRI often play a complementary role in the early identification of cardiac sarcoidosis. The following figure from Skali et al. best summarizes the findings seen with various stages of sarcoidosis on F-18 FDG-PET imaging.

STAGES	Perfusion/FDG Patterns	
	Perfusion Defect	FDG-Uptake
Normal	None	No/ Low
Early	None	FDG uptake high
Progressive	Mild	
Peak active	Moderate	
Progressive myocardial.impairment	Severe	
Fibrosis	Severe	Low

References: Skali H, Schulman AR, Dorbala S. 18F-FDG PET/CT for the assessment of myocardial sarcoidosis. *Curr Cardiol Rep* 2013;15(4):352.

Youssef G, Leung E, Mylonas I, et al. The use of 18F-FDG PET in the diagnosis of cardiac sarcoidosis: a systematic review and metaanalysis including the Ontario experience. *J Nucl Med* 2012;53(2):241–248.

13 **Answer B.** Rest Rb-82 perfusion images demonstrate a small zone of severely decreased activity in distal inferolateral wall. F-18 FDG images demonstrate diffuse F-18 FDG uptake throughout the myocardium with the exception of a small zone of mildly decreased activity along the distal inferolateral wall, similar to the area of reduced resting perfusion seen on N-13 ammonia. Diffuse myocardial uptake is atypical for cardiac sarcoidosis. Questions regarding dietary noncompliance must be raised when diffuse homogeneous myocardial uptake of F-18 FDG is observed in patients undergoing evaluation of cardiac sarcoidosis with F-18 FDG-PET. Generally, focal, focal on diffuse, or multifocal uptake is seen with cardiac sarcoidosis.

Normal myocytes can utilize either glucose or fatty acids for metabolism. In the fasting state, free fatty acids account for 90% of the metabolic demands of normal myocytes. However, this shifts to utilization of glucose in the postprandial state and with a high-carbohydrate diet. Dietary modifications with a high-fat, high-protein, and low-carbohydrate diet have been shown to reduce physiologic glucose uptake by the myocytes. Recent studies suggest that fasting for more than 18 hours further suppresses physiologic myocardial glucose uptake and is preferable for patients undergoing evaluation of cardiac sarcoidosis with F-18 FDG-PET. IV unfractionated heparin activates lipoprotein and hepatic lipases, which ultimately causes increase in plasma free fatty acid levels, and reduces glucose consumption of normal myocytes. Combining low-carbohydrate diet for two meals followed by extended fasting and use of IV unfractionated heparin prior to F-18 FDG administration have shown to result in significant reduction in physiologic myocyte uptake; optimizing the visualization abnormal F-18 FDG uptake by inflammatory granulomatous changes in patients with active cardiac sarcoidosis.

References: Skali H, Schulman AR, Dorbala S. 18F-FDG PET/CT for the assessment of myocardial sarcoidosis. *Curr Cardiol Rep* 2013;15(4):352.

Youssef G, Leung E, Mylonas I, et al. The use of 18F-FDG PET in the diagnosis of cardiac sarcoidosis: a systematic review and metaanalysis, including the Ontario experience. *J Nucl Med* 2012;53(2):241–248.

14 Answer A. Repeat imaging with F-18 FDG shows uptake in the blood pool, but no discrete F-18 FDG uptake is seen in the myocardium. As such, there is no evidence of active sarcoidosis. This can be further confirmed by looking at acquired images in the axial plan, like a study done for malignancy evaluation. As seen in the MIP and axial fused images below, the activity in the region of the heart is in the blood pool and not in the myocardium. Intense metabolic activity is seen within the mediastinal lymph nodes from granulomatous involvement. Therefore, in this patient, the initial diffuse myocardial uptake was likely secondary to dietary noncompliance. Because the normal myocardium can utilize both fatty acids and glucose for metabolism, suppression of normal myocardial glucose uptake is paramount in order to visualize F-18 FDG uptake in the myocardium resulting from lymphocytic infiltration in active cardiac sarcoidosis.

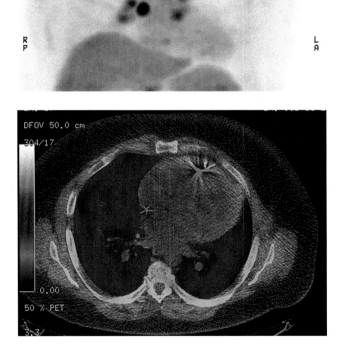

Reference: Skali H, Schulman AR, Dorbala S. 18F-FDG PET/CT for the assessment of myocardial sarcoidosis. *Curr Cardiol Rep* 2013;15:352.

15 Answer A. The supplied images show normal N-13 ammonia resting perfusion (top). No significant myocardial uptake is seen on the F-18 FDG metabolism (bottom). Findings indicate no evidence of active cardiac sarcoidosis. The supplied F-18 FDG processed cardiac images show activity in the blood pool, which appears prominent due to windowing.

Reviewing the F-18 FDG images processed in the axial and coronal planes from the same dataset show intense FDG uptake in bilateral hilar and subcarinal lymph nodes. Note the absent myocardial uptake and mild blood pool activity. Findings indicate active sarcoid involvement in these lymph nodes without the involvement of myocardium. Since activated lymphocytes show intense FDG metabolism, in addition to the evaluation of cardiac sarcoidosis, FDG-PET can be used to evaluate pulmonary and systemic sarcoidosis. FDG PET can also be used to evaluate response to treatment in both cardiac and systemic sarcoidosis.

References: Skali H, Schulman AR, Dorbala S. 18F-FDG PET/CT for the assessment of myocardial sarcoidosis. *Curr Cardiol Rep* 2013;15(4):352.

Youssef G, Leung E, Mylonas I, et al. The use of 18F-FDG PET in the diagnosis of cardiac sarcoidosis: a systematic review and metaanalysis including the Ontario experience. *J Nucl Med* 2012;53(2):241–248.

16 **Answer F.** The poststress images show a small-sized, mild intensity perfusion defect along the distal anteroseptal wall, which appears worse on the rest images and which resolves with the attenuation correction. The findings are consistent with the breast attenuation artifact. A single frame from the raw data demonstrates severe attenuation by the left breast (arrowheads). In the absence of attenuation correction, one could differentiate a myocardial infarct from an attenuation artifact by the presence of normal systolic wall thickening and normal wall motion. Another way to differentiate this artifact from a true defect would be to obtain images with the patient in the prone position. The resultant shift in the breast position may be enough to resolve the attenuation artifact. The breast attenuation artifact usually results in a perfusion defect along the anterior wall, but depending on body habitus, the lateral wall, septum, and apex can be affected as well. On the other hand, the diaphragmatic attenuation artifact is usually most pronounced along the mid to basal inferior wall and is more common in men compared to women.

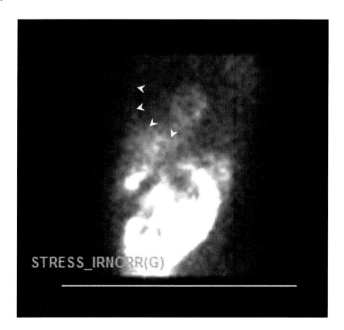

Reference: Burrell S, MacDonald A. Artifacts and pitfalls in myocardial perfusion imaging. *J Nucl Med Technol* 2006;34(4):193–211.

17 **Answer C.** This sinogram demonstrates an artifact related to patient motion. It is generated by stacking a single line of pixels at the level of the heart from the 60 raw projection images on top of each other. The most superior line of pixels is usually from the most posterior projection, 135-degree left posterior oblique (LPO), with the most inferior one from the most anterior projection, 45-degree right anterior oblique (RAO). A normal sinogram would show a smooth continuous contour progressing from the right side of the image to the left (see image below) as the heart moves from the relative right side of the frame to the left as the camera moves from the LPO to RAO projection. Disruption of the smooth contour as seen in this case would suggest the presence of significant patient motion. If the rotating cine images generated from the raw data cannot be viewed, a sinogram can serve as a quick quality control for the patient motion artifact.

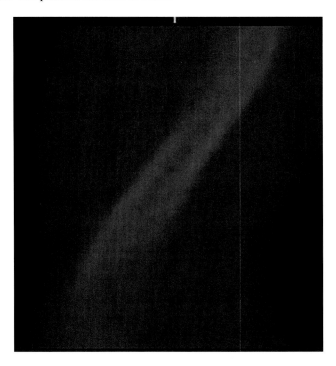

References: Burrell S, MacDonald A. Artifacts and pitfalls in myocardial perfusion imaging. *J Nucl Med Technol* 2006;34(4):193–211.

Case JA, Bateman TM. Taking the perfect nuclear image: quality control, acquisition, and processing techniques for cardiac SPECT, PET, and hybrid imaging. *J Nucl Cardiol* 2013;20(5):891–907.

18 **Answer E.** A moderate-sized focus of intense extracardiac uptake is seen within the right breast, highly suspicious for breast cancer. Both Tc-99m sestamibi (Cardiolite) and tetrofosmin (Myoview) are lipophilic cations that localize in/adjacent to the mitochondria because of their negative transmembrane potential. Since malignancies have a high mitochondrial content, these agents localize into malignancies in high concentration. Therefore, a mammogram would be the next appropriate step to evaluate for breast cancer. It is important to review the cine images for any extracardiac foci of abnormal uptake for unsuspected malignancies such as breast cancer, lung cancer, or lymphoma.

References: Mettler FA, Guiberteau MJ. *Essentials of nuclear medicine imaging*, 7th ed. Philadelphia, PA: Saunders, 2019:130–134.

O'Malley JP, Ziessman HA, Thrall JH. *Nuclear medicine: the requisites*, 5th ed. Philadelphia, PA: Saunders, 2020:454–455.

19 **Answer D.** The poststress perfusion images demonstrate the presence of a large area of decreased activity along the distal anterior, lateral, and inferolateral walls, which is best seen on the horizontal long axis (arrow). There is a "tail" of activity extending from the left ventricular myocardium (arrowheads in the images below), which is often referred to as the "hurricane sign." This finding is typical for patient motion. Vertical (craniocaudal) motion is more common than the horizontal patient motion. While this example represents one of the most severe motion artifacts, the artifact related to patient motion is usually more subtle and can often be confused with areas of ischemia. Their recognition is crucial in the accurate interpretation of myocardial perfusion imaging as a false-positive study would lead to unnecessary cardiac catheterization. As such, routine evaluation of either cine images or sinogram should be performed to ensure that the motion artifact is not present prior to the interpretation of the perfusion images. While software motion correction can be attempted for small degrees of vertical motion, motion correction algorithms cannot correct horizontal or significant vertical patient motion. In such instances, images should be reacquired.

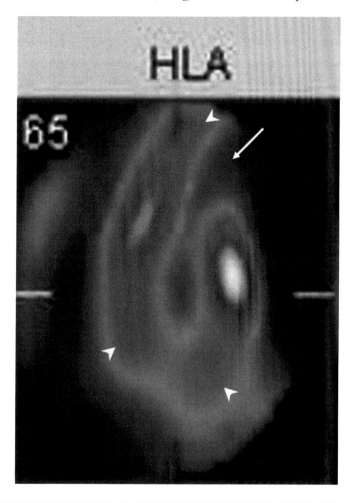

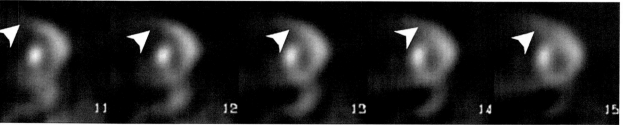

References: Burrell S, MacDonald A. Artifacts and pitfalls in myocardial perfusion imaging. *J Nucl Med Technol* 2006;34(4):193–211.

Case JA, Bateman TM. Taking the perfect nuclear image: quality control, acquisition, and processing techniques for cardiac SPECT, PET, and hybrid imaging. *J Nucl Cardiol* 2013;20(5):891–907.

20 **Answer C.** A single frame from the cine image demonstrates markedly increased activity in the right forearm, which extends distally throughout the forearm; this is compatible with an arterial injection. This would result in a marked decrease in the amount of radiotracer delivered to the myocardium. As such, the study would be nondiagnostic. A normal sinogram excludes patient motion. An attenuation artifact would result in focal, regional perfusion defects. The appearance and distribution are typical for that of an arterial injection. While malignancy would have increased Tc-99m sestamibi or tetrofosmin uptake, the activity would be more focal rather than diffuse, as in this case.

Reference: Burrell S, MacDonald A. Artifacts and pitfalls in myocardial perfusion imaging. *J Nucl Med Technol* 2006;34(4):193–211.

21 **Answer B.** A moderate-sized area of severely decreased activity is present along the anterolateral wall on stress images that is not present on the rest images. This is a typical location of an artifact related to attenuation correction. One of the common artifacts caused by the CT attenuation correction with SPECT–CT or PET–CT myocardial perfusion studies is the false reduction in the activity along the lateral or anterolateral wall. This happens when a portion of the SPECT or PET images project over the adjacent lower attenuation lung or pericardial fat instead of the heart/myocardium on CT scan acquired for attenuation correction (arrow on the image below). Negative attenuation of the lung/fat results in the incorrect application of a lower attenuation correction factor resulting in falsely decreased counts in that region. In order to avoid such artifacts, technologists should always check for proper coregistration of CT and SPECT or PET data when the study is processed. This artifact was responsible for this false-positive study. Once it was recognized and corrective actions were taken, the resulting images showed no significant perfusion defect (image below).

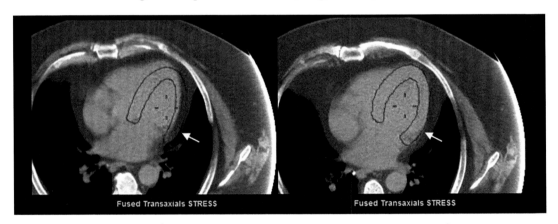

Original   Corrected

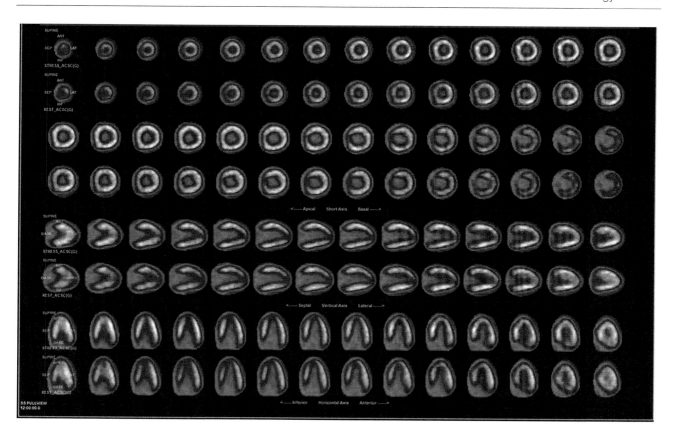

References: Loghin C, Sdringola S, Gould KL. Common artifacts in PET myocardial perfusion images due to attenuation–emission misregistration: clinical significance, causes, and solutions. *J Nucl Med* 2004;45(6):1029–1039.

Mettler FA, Guiberteau MJ. *Essentials of nuclear medicine imaging*, 7th ed. Philadelphia, PA: Saunders, 2019:156–157.

22 Answer B. Anterior images acquired 1 hour after the IV administration of Tc-99m pyrophosphate (PYP) show markedly increased radiotracer uptake diffusely throughout the myocardium. The uptake in the myocardium is significantly greater than that in the adjacent ribs (grade 3), and the heart to contralateral mediastinum ratio is 2.1 (>1.5 abnormal). In the right clinical settings, the findings are most consistent with transthyretin (TTR) amyloidosis. Tc-99m PYP scan is done for the evaluation of TTR-related cardiac amyloidosis. Cardiac sympathetic innervation would be evaluated by the I-123 MIBG scan. Myocardial ejection fraction could be evaluated by in vivo tagging of RBCs by PYP, but gated LAO projection would be utilized for that purpose. Tc-99m tetrofosmin or sestamibi are utilized for myocardial perfusion imaging.

Amyloidosis is characterized by the extracellular deposition of misfolded proteins resulting in the formation of amyloid fibrils. Light chain amyloidosis (AL) is caused by plasma cell dyscrasia while transthyretin amyloidosis (ATTR) is caused by deposition of misfolded transport thyroid retinol made by the liver. Differentiation between AL and ATTR is important as they have different prognosis and therapy. AL carries a poor prognosis and requires chemotherapy/oncology consultation. In contrast, ATTR tends to have a protracted clinical course and can be treated with newer agents such as Tafamidis (transthyretin stabilizer).

Tc-99m PYP was historically utilized for bone scans. Subsequently, it was found to have utility in the evaluation of acute myocardial infarct imaging.

Its most recent utility is in the diagnosis of amyloidosis related to transthyretin deposition (ATTR). PYP binds to the deposited ATTR amyloid fibrils in the myocardium and can be visualized using planar and SPECT imaging at 1 hour. Delayed, 3-hour imaging can be performed in patients with poor renal function and persistent blood pool activity. SPECT images are helpful in distinguishing physiologic blood pool activity from activity in the myocardium. Interpretation is done by visual analysis where the myocardial PYP uptake is compared to that within the rib. The Perugini grading system for semiquantitation is shown in the table below. Also, quantitative analysis is done by drawing a circular region of interest (ROI) over the heart (H) and contralateral lung (CL). Mean H/CL lung ratio of >1.5 at 1 hour is classified as suspicious, while ratio ≤1 is classified as negative for ATTR. The ratio between 1 and 1.5 is equivocal and requires correlation with visual grading and SPECT imaging. Of note, since up to 20% of AL patients can have a positive PYP scan (typically grade 1 or 2), correlation with serum light chains and serum/urine immunofixation is required for accurate interpretation/clinical diagnosis. Also, some mutational forms of ATTR can be falsely negative on PYP imaging. In the setting of high clinical suspicion, correlation with endomyocardial biopsy should be considered.

Grade	Myocardial Tc-99m PYP Uptake	Diagnosis
Grade 0	No myocardial uptake	Not suggestive of ATTR
Grade 1	Myocardial uptake < ribs	Equivocal for ATTR
Grade 2	Myocardial uptake = ribs	Strongly suggestive of ATTR
Grade 3	Myocardial uptake > ribs	Positive for ATTR

References: *ASNC Practice Point-99mTechnetium Pyrophosphate Imaging 2016 guidelines.*

O'Malley JP, Ziessman HA, Thrall JH. *Nuclear medicine: the requisites*, 5th ed. Philadelphia, PA: Saunders, 2020:463.

23 **Answer A.** Improper placement of regions of interest (ROI) is one of the common sources of error for left ventricular ejection fraction (LVEF) calculation by the radionuclide ventriculography (RVG). As such, proper placement of ROIs should always be confirmed. In this case, the background ROI was placed over blood pool activity. The left ventricular ejection fraction (LVEF) is calculated by the following formula: LVEF = (end-diastolic counts − end-systolic counts)/(end-diastolic counts − background counts). Subtraction of the (falsely) increased background counts from the denominator would result in falsely elevated LVEF when the background is erroneously placed over a high activity area (vascular blood pool or spleen). Other causes of a false increase in LVEF include too small systolic ROI and inclusion of the left atrium in the diastolic ROI. Causes of falsely decreased LVEF include too large systolic ROI, single ROI for the systole and diastole frames, and too small diastolic ROI.

References: Mettler FA, Guiberteau MJ. *Essentials of nuclear medicine imaging*, 7th ed. Philadelphia, PA: Saunders, 2019:160, 166–170.

O'Malley JP, Ziessman HA, Thrall JH. *Nuclear medicine: the requisites*, 5th ed. Philadelphia, PA: Saunders, 2020:475–476.

QUESTIONS

1 What radiopharmaceutical was most commonly used for this procedure?

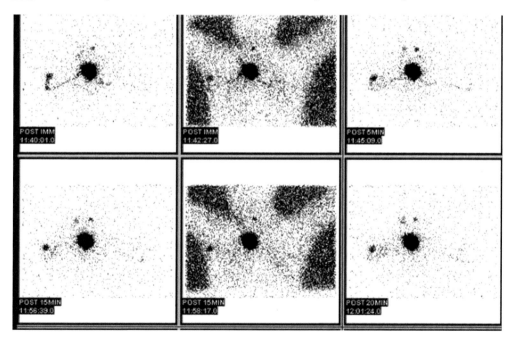

A. Tc-99m sulfur colloid
B. Tc-99m DTPA
C. Tc-99m MAA
D. Tc-99m DMSA

2 In order to expedite the migration as well as to optimize the retention within the lymph nodes, Tc-99m sulfur colloid utilized for lymphoscintigraphy is filtered. What is the typical size of these filtered particles?

A. 100 to 220 nm
B. 10 to 22 nm
C. 100 to 220 μm
D. 10 to 22 μm

3 Which of the following mechanisms is responsible for the localization of filtered Tc-99m sulfur colloid in the sentinel lymph node?

A. Receptor binding of the radiolabeled colloid particles to the metastatic cells
B. Receptor binding of the radiolabeled colloid particles to the macrophages
C. Phagocytosis of the radiolabeled colloid particles by the macrophages
D. Phagocytosis of the radiolabeled colloid particles by the metastatic cells

4 Which of the following characteristics constitutes a lymph node as the sentinel lymph node on the lymphoscintigraphy?

A. Lymph node visualized closest to the tumor
B. Largest visualized lymph node
C. Most intense visualized lymph node
D. First visualized lymph node

5 Which of the following injection sites would be expected to have the most likelihood of internal mammary lymph node visualization?

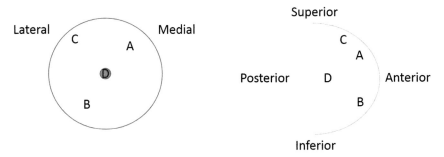

6 The following images are from a bilateral upper extremity lymphangiogram. What is the most likely side and level of the lymphatic obstruction?

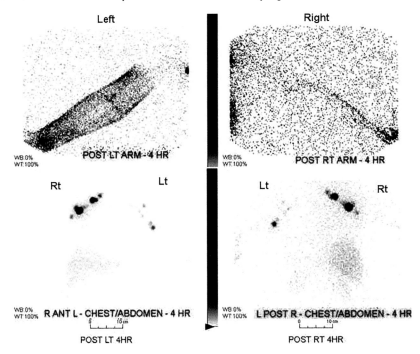

A. Right forearm
B. Left forearm
C. Right upper arm
D. Left upper arm
E. No evidence of obstruction

7 Which of the following is correct regarding the lymphoscintigraphy of the breast?

A. The injection should take place 24 to 48 hours prior to the planned lymph node dissection.

B. Ultrasound guidance is recommended for superficial breast lesions.

C. Lymph nodes visualized in the first 60 minutes of imaging are considered sentinel lymph nodes.

D. A periareolar injection is recommended for lesions in the upper outer quadrant.

8 How was the following image obtained?

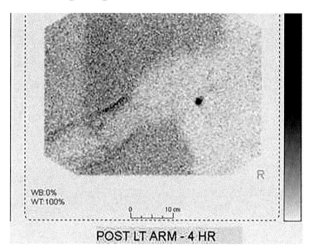

POST LT ARM – 4 HR

A. Cobalt-57 sheet source

B. Cadmium-zinc telluride detector

C. Flat-panel x-ray detector

D. Tungsten x-ray tube

9 The following images were acquired after the intrahepatic injection of Tc-99m MAA. Which of the following would be the best recommendation regarding the planned Yttrium-90 SIR-Spheres treatment?

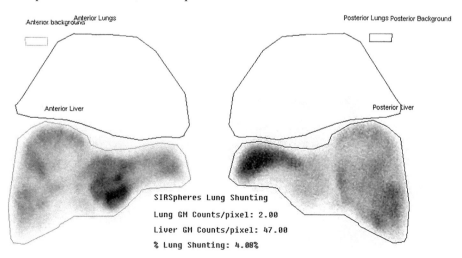

A. No reduction of Y-90 SIR-Spheres dosage necessary

B. Reduction of Y-90 SIR-Spheres dosage by 20%

C. Reduction of Y-90 SIR-Spheres dosage by 40%

D. Reduction of Y-90 SIR-Spheres dosage by 100%

10 Quantitative analysis of anterior and posterior Tc MAA images after the right hepatic intra-arterial injection is provided. What is the MOST correct statement regarding the Y-90 TheraSpheres treatment in this patient?

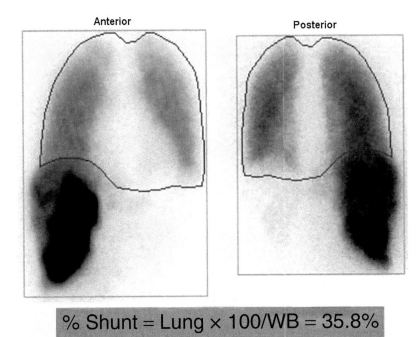

$$\% \text{ Shunt} = \text{Lung} \times 100/\text{WB} = 35.8\%$$

A. No dose adjustment is necessary.
B. Increase the dose.
C. Reduce the dose.
D. Do not treat the patient.

11 What is the most appropriate conclusion based on the supplied planar and SPECT/CT Ga-67 images in this patient with fever of unknown origin?

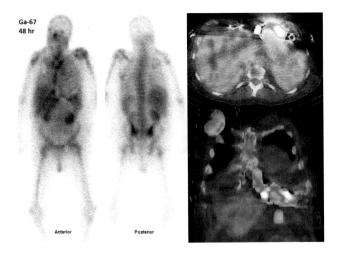

A. No source for the patient's fever is identified.
B. Infected left ventricular assist device pump.
C. Infectious colitis.
D. Attenuation artifact.

12 Which of the following radiotracers would be ideal for the evaluation of abdominal infection?

A. Gallium-67

B. Tc-99m HMPAO–labeled WBC scan

C. In-111 oxine–labeled leukocyte scan

D. Thallium-201

13 In which of the following instances is Ga-67 scintigraphy preferred over In-111 oxine–labeled leukocytes scan?

A. Suspected hip prosthesis infection

B. Suspected intra-abdominal abscess

C. Suspected Crohn disease

D. Suspected vertebral osteomyelitis

14 An 89-year-old male with a history of right femoral vein stent undergoes the following examination for the evaluation of persistent bacteremia. What is the most likely diagnosis?

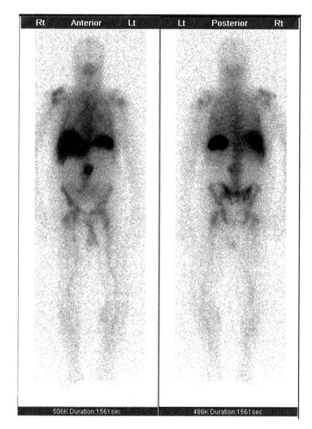
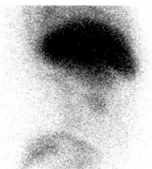

A. Colon cancer

B. Vertebral osteomyelitis

C. Stent infection

D. Mycotic aneurysm

15 The following scan was acquired on a 33-year-old patient who has diarrhea and abdominal discomfort. What is the most likely diagnosis?

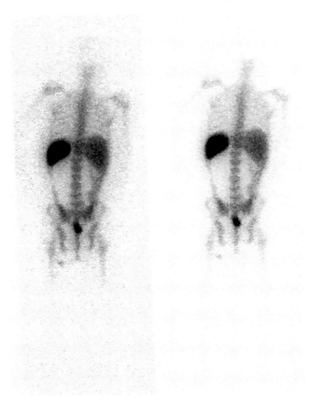

A. Crohn disease
B. Sacral metastasis
C. Splenic lymphoma
D. Colloid shift

16 In truncal melanoma, which basin has the highest chances of harboring the sentinel lymph node?

A. Axillary
B. Inguinal
C. Occipital
D. Truncal

17 Which of the following is most likely to reduce false-negative finding when used in conjunction with lymphoscintigraphy, and is usually combined by many surgeons with the use of the intraoperative gamma probe?

A. Intraoperative ultrasound
B. F-18 FDG PET-CT
C. Blue dye injection
D. Palpation of lymph nodes

18 Which of the following is responsible for the accumulation of Tc-99m tilmanocept (Lymphoseek) in the sentinel lymph node?

A. Receptor-based binding to the metastatic cells
B. Receptor-based binding to the macrophages
C. Phagocytosis by the macrophages
D. Active transport by Na-K ATPase pump into the cytosol
E. Binding of the radiotracer to the mitochondria

19 What is the advantage of Tc-99m tilmanocept (Lymphoseek) compared to Tc-99m sulfur colloid?

A. Higher distal lymph node uptake
B. Faster injection site clearance
C. Appearance of more lymph nodes
D. Lower proximal lymph node uptake

20 What is the required minimum time interval between the injection of Tc-99m tilmanocept (Lymphoseek) and initiation of the intraoperative lymphatic mapping?

A. 15 minutes
B. 30 minutes
C. 45 minutes
D. 60 minutes

ANSWERS AND EXPLANATIONS

1 **Answer A.** In the United States, filtered Tc-99m sulfur colloid (particle size 100 to 200 nm) is most commonly used for sentinel lymph node (SLN) localization by lymphoscintigraphy. Tc-99m nanocolloidal albumin (particle size 5 to 100 nm) is preferred in most of Europe, while Tc-99m antimony trisulfide (particle size 3 to 30 nm) is preferred in Australia and Canada. Tc-99m tilmanocept (Lymphoseek) is an alternative to radiocolloid, which was approved by the FDA in 2014. It targets dextran–mannose receptors on the surface of macrophages. Its use is gaining traction.

This case illustrates why imaging is important (particularly for trunk melanoma lesions) because cancers may drain to a nodal pattern that is different from what would be clinically expected. If the SLN is positive for the disease, this triggers a full nodal dissection of that basin. If the SLN is negative for the disease, this prevents additional nodal dissection and reduces the associated morbidity such as extremity swelling from poor lymphatic drainage.

References: Giammarile F, Alazraki N, Aarsvold JN, et al. The EANM and SNMMI practice guideline for lymphoscintigraphy and sentinel node localization in breast cancer. *Eur J Nucl Med Mol Imaging* 2013;40(12):1932–1947.

Mettler FA, Guiberteau MJ. *Essentials of nuclear medicine imaging*, 7th ed. Philadelphia, PA: Saunders, 2019:322–324.

2 **Answer A.** The sulfur colloid (SC) particles in standard preparations are too large for the purposes of sentinel lymph node (SLN) lymphoscintigraphy. Particles >400 nm in size may not migrate to the regional lymph nodes at all. Particles that are too small may migrate too quickly through the entire nodal basin, making the identification of a single sentinel lymph node difficult. Unfiltered Tc-99m SC is composed of particles ranging from 15 to 5,000 nm, with an average size of 305 to 340 nm. For SLN scintigraphy, the SC is usually filtered using a 0.22-µm filter, which results in the suspension of colloid particles ranging in size between 100 and 220 nm. This results in a more uniform mixture of smaller particles, which makes it more conducive to lymphatic drainage.

References: Mettler FA, Guiberteau MJ. *Essentials of nuclear medicine imaging*, 7th ed. Philadelphia, PA: Saunders, 2019:322–324.

Newman EA, Newman LA. Lymphatic mapping techniques and sentinel lymph node biopsy in breast cancer. *Surg Clin North Am* 2007;87(2):353–364, viii.

3 **Answer C.** Tc-99m sulfur colloid (SC) gets phagocytized by the macrophages. The reticuloendothelial system is responsible for removing large particles such as colloid and immune complexes from healthy persons' circulation. It is composed of monocytes in the blood, Kupffer cells in the liver, and macrophages in connective tissue, lymphoid organs, bone marrow, and lungs. As such, when injected intravenously, Tc-99m SC localizes in the Kupffer cells in the liver and macrophages in the spleen and bone marrow. When injected intradermally, filtered sulfur colloid travels through the lymphatic channel and gets phagocytized by the macrophages residing in the draining lymph node.

Reference: Mettler FA, Guiberteau MJ. *Essentials of nuclear medicine imaging*, 7th ed. Philadelphia, PA: Saunders, 2019:322–324.

4 **Answer D.** According to Morton's original definition, the sentinel lymph node is "the first lymph node that receives afferent lymphatic drainage from a primary tumor." Sentinel lymph nodes (SLN) are regional nodes that are directly connected to the primary tumor by lymphatic channels. Early dynamic images frequently demonstrate a channel leading to the SLN, which is the first lymph node to be visualized in a nodal drainage basin. The major criteria for identifying SLNs are the time of appearance and occasionally visualization of the connecting lymphatic channels. SLN need not be the hottest, the closest, or the largest lymph nodes visualized. As one or more lymph nodes may be connected to the tumor by the lymphatic channels, multiple SLNs may be seen. In such a case, all should be surgically removed and tested for metastatic disease. SLN biopsy is now the gold standard for lymph node staging in breast cancer and melanoma. SLN resection reduces morbidity and has similar mortality rates compared to more invasive lymph node dissections.

References: Chakera AH, Hesse B, Burak Z, et al. EANM-EORTC general recommendations for sentinel node diagnostics in melanoma. *Eur J Nucl Med Mol Imaging* 2009;36(10):1713–1742.

Nieweg OE, Tanis PJ, Kroon BB. The definition of a sentinel node. *Ann Surg Oncol* 2001;8:538–541.

5 **Answer D.** While one would surmise that the ideal injection site to visualize internal mammary nodes would be superficial skin injection medial to the midclavicular line (A), it has been shown that internal mammary node identification is better with deep peritumoral injections. A recent anatomical study on breast lymphatics found that separate lymphatic networks exist in the ventral and dorsal parts of the breast with the former draining to the axilla and latter to the internal mammary chain. Important advantages of the deep injections include improved detection of the extra-axillary sentinel lymph nodes and the possibility of using larger injection volumes. A major advantage of superficial injections (subdermal, periareolar, intradermal, or subareolar) is that they are easy to perform; however, they are often more painful than peritumoral injections. A combination of both techniques may improve sentinel lymph node detection and decrease false-negative findings.

References: Hindie E, Groheux D, Espie M, et al. [Sentinel node biopsy in breast cancer]. *Bull Cancer* 2009;96(6):713–725.

Shimazu K, Tamaki Y, Taguchi T, et al. Lymphoscintigraphic visualization of internal mammary nodes with subtumoral injection of radiocolloid in patients with breast cancer. *Ann Surg* 2003;237(3):390–398.

Suami H, Pan WR, Mann GB, et al. The lymphatic anatomy of the breast and its implications for sentinel lymph node biopsy: a human cadaver study. *Ann Surg Oncol* 2008;15(3):863–871.

6 **Answer D.** The patient was injected between the webs of the fingers in order to visualize the lymphatic drainage. The supplied images demonstrate subcutaneous activity tracking along the left upper extremity, which stops at the mid-upper arm. In contrast, normal lymphatic drainage via lymphatic channels is visualized on the right. Lymph node visualization is present but decreased within the left axilla when compared to the right. The combination of these findings suggests partial left-sided lymphatic obstruction. With complete obstruction, the left axillary lymph nodes would not be visualized at all, and superficial activity would be seen throughout the left arm. Typical indications for lymphatic drainage evaluation by lymphoscintigraphy include lymphedema, chyluria, chylothorax, and chyloperitoneum. The most common secondary causes of abnormal lymphatic drainage are prior surgery, cancer, infection, and radiation.

References: Mettler FA, Guiberteau MJ. *Essentials of nuclear medicine imaging*, 7th ed. Philadelphia, PA: Saunders, 2019:324.

Moshiri M, Katz DS, Boris M, et al. Using lymphoscintigraphy to evaluate suspected lymphedema of the extremities. *Am J Roentgenol* 2002;178(2):405–412.

O'Malley JP, Ziessman HA, Thrall JH. *Nuclear medicine: the requisites*, 5th ed. Philadelphia, PA: Saunders, 2020:353–358.

Yuan Z, Chen L, Luo Q, et al. The role of radionuclide lymphoscintigraphy in extremity lymphedema. *Ann Nucl Med* 2006;20(5):341–344.

7 **Answer D.** In some centers, all patients get periareolar injections; however, periareolar injections are specifically recommended for lesions located within the upper outer quadrant near the area of the axilla. Injection in the periareolar area in these patients helps differentiate the sentinel lymph node (SLN) from activity in the primary lesion if the injection was around the primary lesion close to the axilla. Injections should take place no more than 18 hours prior to planned SLN resection as intraoperative gamma detection is used to confirm the presence of radioactivity within the lymph nodes. While ultrasound guidance is recommended for deep lesions of the breast, subdermal and intradermal injections without guidance are usually sufficient for more superficial lesions. The first lymph nodes detected within a nodal drainage basin on imaging are considered to be the sentinel lymph node(s). While other lymph nodes may also be marked for potential resection, care should be taken to clearly document the SLN. Lymphoscintigraphy detects the SLN in 90% to 98% of cases.

References: Mettler FA, Guiberteau MJ. *Essentials of nuclear medicine imaging*, 7th ed. Philadelphia, PA: Saunders, 2019:322–324.

O'Malley JP, Ziessman HA, Thrall JH. *Nuclear medicine: the requisites*, 5th ed. Philadelphia, PA: Saunders, 2020:353–358.

8 **Answer A.** This is a transmission image acquired using a cobalt-57 sheet source to help provide better anatomical localization. The sheet source is placed behind the patient. The radiation from the sheet gets attenuated by the soft tissues and does not reach the detector. The remaining radiation reaches the detector creating an outline of the patient's body. Sheet sources are a simple and cheap method to enhance the localization of lesions without contributing significant radiation dose to the patient. An x-ray tube can be used when acquiring SPECT/CT images but not in the transmission image that is shown.

References: Mettler FA, Guiberteau MJ. *Essentials of nuclear medicine imaging*, 7th ed. Philadelphia, PA: Saunders, 2019:322–324.

Moshiri M, Katz DS, Boris M, et al. Using lymphoscintigraphy to evaluate suspected lymphedema of the extremities. *Am J Roentgenol* 2002;178(2):405–412.

O'Malley JP, Ziessman HA, Thrall JH. *Nuclear medicine: the requisites*, 5th ed. Philadelphia, PA: Saunders, 2020:220–229.

Yuan Z, Chen L, Luo Q, et al. The role of radionuclide lymphoscintigraphy in extremity lymphedema. *Ann Nucl Med* 2006;20(5):341–344.

9 **Answer A.** The anterior and posterior images acquired after the intra-arterial injection of Tc-99m MAA demonstrate no significant activity within the lungs to indicate arteriovenous shunting. Calculated activity from regions of interest drawn around the lungs and liver demonstrate approximately 4% pulmonary shunting. This is well below the 10% threshold at which dose reduction would be considered with SIR-Spheres. As such, no reduction of Y-90 SIR-Spheres dose is necessary.

Y-90-labeled TheraSpheres and SIR-Spheres are used in the palliative treatment of liver tumors and metastases to selectively deliver a high dose of internal radiation using an intra-arterial infusion. Y-90 is a pure β-emitter with a half-life of 64 hours.

Intra-arterial Tc-99m MAA is used to document the vascular distribution and assess for arteriovenous shunting to nontarget organs as well as lungs prior to the administration of Y-90 microsphere therapy. If significant gastrointestinal activity is seen, embolization of the supplying vessels is indicated prior to Y-90 therapy.

If pulmonary shunting is present, the therapeutic dose may be decreased to prevent radiation pneumonitis. With SIR-Spheres, the activity should be adjusted according to the percentage of lung shunting as shown in the table below.

Percentage of Lung Shunting	Amount of SIR Sphere Reduction (% Total)
<10%	None
10%–15%	Reduce by 20%
15%–20%	Reduce by 40%
>20%	SIR-Spheres are contraindicated.

References: Mettler FA, Guiberteau MJ. *Essentials of nuclear medicine imaging*, 7th ed. Philadelphia, PA: Saunders, 2019:325–327.

O'Malley JP, Ziessman HA, Thrall JH. *Nuclear medicine: the requisites*, 5th ed. Philadelphia, PA: Saunders, 2020:212–213.

Uliel L, Royal HD, Darcy MD, et al. From the angio suite to the gamma-camera: vascular mapping and 99mTc-MAA hepatic perfusion imaging before liver radioembolization—a comprehensive pictorial review. *J Nucl Med* 2012;53(11):1736–1747.

10 **Answer D.** Intra-arterial Tc-99m MAA is used to document the vascular distribution and assess arteriovenous shunting to nontarget organs and lungs prior to the administration of Y-90 microsphere therapy. If significant gastrointestinal activity is seen, the embolization of the supplying vessels is indicated prior to Y-90 therapy.

If pulmonary shunting is present, the therapeutic dose may be decreased to prevent radiation pneumonitis. With TheraSpheres, the upper limit of injected activity shunted to the lung (percentage of shunting to the lungs times the planned therapy activity) is 16.5 mCi (610.5 mBq). As such, in a patient with 35.8% pulmonary shunting, the therapy is contraindicated as it would result in radiation-induced pneumonitis.

References: Mettler FA, Guiberteau MJ. *Essentials of nuclear medicine imaging*, 7th ed. Philadelphia, PA: Saunders, 2019:325–327.

O'Malley JP, Ziessman HA, Thrall JH. *Nuclear medicine: the requisites*, 5th ed. Philadelphia, PA: Saunders, 2020:212–213.

Uliel L, Royal HD, Darcy MD, et al. From the angio suite to the gamma-camera: vascular mapping and 99mTc-MAA hepatic perfusion imaging before liver radioembolization—a comprehensive pictorial review. *J Nucl Med* 2012;53(11):1736–1747.

11 **Answer B.** The 48-hour delayed anterior and posterior images as well as axial and coronal SPECT/CT images acquired after the intravenous administration of gallium-67 demonstrate the presence of a focal area of intense activity surrounding the patient's left ventricular assist device (LVAD) pump. The findings are abnormal and likely represent hardware infection in this patient with a history of fever of unknown origin. In general, there should not be any abnormal accumulation of Ga-67 around the hardware on 48-hour delayed images. Because of increased attenuation from metallic portions of the LVAD, falsely increased activity can be seen on SPECT/CT images from the overcorrection of attenuation. As such, the correlation should be made with non–attenuation corrected and/or planar images. In this patient, the planar images demonstrate abnormal activity in the left upper quadrant anteriorly (arrows). Without the SPECT/CT images, it would be easy to confuse this activity as physiologic bowel uptake. However, SPECT/CT images accurately localize this activity surrounding the hardware, confirming hardware infection and excluding infectious colitis.

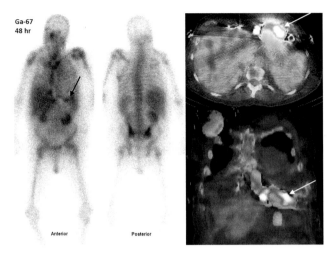

References: Mettler FA, Guiberteau MJ. *Essentials of nuclear medicine imaging*, 7th ed. Philadelphia, PA: Saunders, 2019:268–272.

O'Malley JP, Ziessman HA, Thrall JH. *Nuclear medicine: the requisites*, 5th ed. Philadelphia, PA: Saunders, 2020:111–114.

12 Answer C. In-111-labeled leukocytes are preferred for the evaluation of abdominal infection because they lack normal physiologic bowel activity associated with Ga-67 and Tc-99m HMPAO-labeled leukocyte scan. Also, the presence of significant hepatic and splenic activity with Ga-67 may hamper the detection of infections in the upper abdomen. When present, In-111-labeled leukocyte activity in the gastrointestinal tract is nonspecific and may indicate etiologies including Crohn disease, ulcerative colitis, pseudomembranous colitis, diverticulitis, or ischemia. Also, false-positive results may occur due to swallowing of leukocytes in patients with respiratory tract infections, sinusitis, endotracheal or nasopharyngeal tubes, or gastrointestinal bleeding. Tl-201 has no role in infection imaging. In current clinical practice, a CT of the abdomen and pelvis is usually the initial ordered and preferred imaging modality for suspected intra-abdominal infections/inflammation.

Reference: O'Malley JP, Ziessman HA, Thrall JH. *Nuclear medicine: the requisites*, 5th ed. Philadelphia, PA: Saunders, 2020:409–440.

13 Answer D. In-111 oxine-labeled leukocyte scan is less sensitive than Ga-67 in the evaluation of vertebral osteomyelitis. This may be secondary to regional hypoperfusion in the setting of vertebral osteomyelitis with resultant decrease in the uptake. When used with bone imaging, gallium scan provides increased sensitivity for the diagnosis of vertebral osteomyelitis. In-111 oxine–labeled leukocyte scan is preferred over gallium scan in the evaluation of intra-abdominal infectious or inflammatory processes because of interference from normal physiologic activity within the bowel seen on Ga-67 scans. Combination of In-111 oxine–labeled leukocyte scan and Tc-99m sulfur colloid marrow scan is preferred in the diagnosis of suspected hip or knee prosthesis infection.

Reference: O'Malley JP, Ziessman HA, Thrall JH. *Nuclear medicine: the requisites*, 5th ed. Philadelphia, PA: Saunders, 2020:418–426.

14 **Answer D.** Anterior and posterior whole-body images and right lateral spot view image demonstrate physiologic distribution of the radiopharmaceutical in the liver, spleen, and bone marrow. The images appear coarse, suggesting that this is a polyenergetic medium-energy radiopharmaceutical. These images are from an In-111–oxine labeled leukocyte (In-111 WBC) scan. A large focus of intense activity is seen in the lower abdomen left to the midline, which is more intense on the anterior image compared to the posterior image and localizes anterior to the spine on the lateral projection. The findings are highly suspicious of a mycotic aneurysm in this patient with a history of bacteremia. Since intra-abdominal abscess can present similarly and SPECT-CT could not be obtained, correlation with CT scan was suggested. CT image (below) demonstrates an abdominal aortic aneurysm with surrounding soft tissue stranding in keeping with the suspected mycotic aneurysm.

Because mycotic aneurysm carries a poor prognosis, early diagnosis is crucial. While Crohn disease would be positive on the In-111 WBC scan, the distribution would be more diffuse, and the uptake would be lower than seen in this case. Since the abnormality is not in the expected location of the femoral vein, stent infection is less likely as well. In-111 WBC is not a sensitive modality for the evaluation of vertebral osteomyelitis; Osteomyelitis tends to present as an area of photopenia and not increased activity on In-111 WBC scan. Ga-67 or F-18 FDG is preferred for the evaluation of vertebral osteomyelitis. Unlike Ga-67, a major advantage of the In-111 WBC scan in the evaluation of the abdomen is the lack of normal physiologic intra-abdominal activity. False positives with In-111 WBC scan in the abdomen include accessory splenic tissue, pseudoaneurysm, and a noninfected hematoma. Intraluminal intestinal activity resulting from swallowed or shedding cells that occur with esophagitis, pharyngitis, and sinusitis may also appear on In-111 WBC scan.

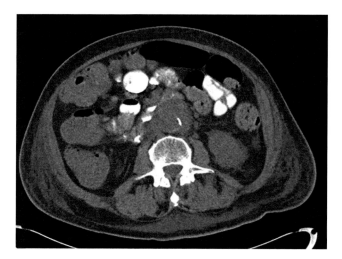

Reference: O'Malley JP, Ziessman HA, Thrall JH. *Nuclear medicine: the requisites*, 5th ed. Philadelphia, PA: Saunders, 2020:413–415.

15 **Answer A.** This is an In-111 oxine–labeled WBC scan with physiologic distribution in the spleen, liver, and bone marrow. Mild diffuse activity is seen in the colon. This is typically seen with infectious or inflammatory colitis such as *Clostridium difficile* colitis, Crohn disease, or ulcerative colitis. A small focus of intense activity overlying the region of the sacrum is from a rectal fissure. Sacral metastasis and lymphoma would not show up on an In-111 WBC scan. The colloid shift is seen on the Tc-99m sulfur colloid scan. It is typically associated with chronic liver dysfunction resulting in the shift of the colloid from the liver to spleen, making the spleen the most intense organ rather than the liver.

Reference: Mettler FA, Guiberteau MJ. *Essentials of nuclear medicine imaging*, 7th ed. Philadelphia, PA: Saunders, 2019:363–368.

16 **Answer A.** The most common drainage pathway in truncal melanoma is to the axillary basin (~90%). Approximately 50% of the truncal melanomas of the upper back may drain to a contralateral basin. About one-third of lesions on the back will drain to multiple basins. As such, performing lymphoscintigraphy in truncal melanoma is imperative. Since the migration to unanticipated drainage pathways may take longer time, delayed imaging at 2 to 4 hours may be useful. If more than one lymph node is visualized in the basin on the delayed imaging, the early or dynamic imaging can be used to determine the identity of the first draining (sentinel) lymph node.

Reference: Mettler FA, Guiberteau MJ. *Essentials of nuclear medicine imaging*, 7th ed. Philadelphia, PA: Saunders, 2019:323.

17 **Answer C.** In sentinel lymph node excision, many surgeons use information obtained by vital blue dye (VBD) injection along with radioactivity to increase sensitivity as well as reduce false negatives. According to the American Society of Clinical Oncology (ASCO), using radioisotope and blue dye during the sentinel lymph node biopsy could achieve a much higher SLN identification rate (>90%) and a relatively low false-negative rate (<5% to 10%) than either tracer alone. This is compared to approximately 83% for the blue dye alone and 89% for the radiocolloid alone according to one widely cited meta-analysis.

References: Kim T, Agboola O, Giuliano A, et al. Lymphatic mapping and sentinel lymph node sampling in early-stage breast cancer: a meta-analysis. *Cancer* 2006;106:4–16.

Lyman GH, Giuliano AE, Somerfield MR, et al. American Society of Clinical Oncology guideline recommendations for sentinel lymph node biopsy in early-stage breast cancer. *J Clin Oncol* 2005;23:7703–7720.

Mettler FA, Guiberteau MJ. *Essentials of nuclear medicine imaging*, 7th ed. Philadelphia, PA: Saunders, 2019:324.

18 **Answer B.** Tc-99m diethylenetriaminepentaacetic acid (DTPA)-mannosyl-dextran (Tc-99m Tilmanocept) was approved by the FDA on October 15, 2014 for lymphatic mapping in solid tumors. Tilmanocept (Lymphoseek) is a macromolecule with an average diameter of 7 nm, consisting of multiple units of DTPA and mannose covalently attached to the dextran backbone. The mannose acts as a ligand for the CD206 receptor, and the DTPA serves as the binding site for Tc-99m. The CD206 receptor protein is found on the surface of macrophages and dendritic cells, which are found in high concentration in lymph nodes.

References: Mettler FA, Guiberteau MJ. *Essentials of nuclear medicine imaging*, 7th ed. Philadelphia, PA: Saunders, 2019:322–323.

O'Malley JP, Ziessman HA, Thrall JH. *Nuclear medicine: the requisites*, 5th ed. Philadelphia, PA: Saunders, 2020:354–355.

19 **Answer B.** The advantages of tilmanocept over radiocolloids include rapid clearance of the injection site, high sentinel lymph node (SNL) extraction, and low distal node accumulation. Because the average diameter of 7mm for Tc-99m tilmanocept is smaller than the average size of the filtered Tc-99m SC particles of 100 to 200 nm, it has faster injection site clearance. Specific and high-affinity binding of mannose to the CD206 receptors on macrophages and dendritic cells results in high sentinel lymph node extraction and lower distal node accumulation.

Baker et al. found that fewer SLNs were removed from patients mapped with Tc-99m tilmanocept plus VBD than patients receiving filtered Tc-99m SC plus VBD. Also, a larger proportion of removed nodes were found to be positive (1.7 times greater) with Tc-99m tilmanocept compared to Tc-99m SC. In two nonrandomized phase III trials, Tc-99m tilmanocept identified more SLNs in more patients than did VBD.

References: Baker JL, Pu M, Tokin CA, et al. Comparison of Tc-99m Tilmanocept and filtered Tc-99m sulfur colloid for identification of SLNs in breast cancer patients. *Ann Surg Oncol* 2015;22:40–45.

Sondak VK, King DW, Zager JS, et al. Combined analysis of phase III trials evaluating [^{99}mTc] tilmanocept and vital blue dye for identification of sentinel lymph nodes in clinically node-negative cutaneous melanoma. *Ann Surg Oncol* 2013;20(2):680–688.

Wallace AM, Han LK, Povoski SP, et al. Comparative evaluation of [^{99}mTc] Tilmanocept and vital blue dye for identification of sentinel lymph nodes in clinically node-negative cutaneous melanoma. *Ann Surg Oncol* 2013;20:2590–2599.

20 **Answer A.** In clinical studies, Tc-99m tilmanocept (Lymphoseek) was detectable in lymph nodes within 10 minutes and up to 30 hours. It is recommended that lymphatic mapping with Tc-99m tilmanocept (Lymphoseek) be conducted no earlier than 15 minutes and up to 15 hours postinjection.

References: Mettler FA, Guiberteau MJ. *Essentials of nuclear medicine imaging*, 7th ed. Philadelphia, PA: Saunders, 2019:322–323.

O'Malley JP, Ziessman HA, Thrall JH. *Nuclear medicine: the requisites*, 5th ed. Philadelphia, PA: Saunders, 2020:354–355.

7 Pulmonary System

1 Which one of the following sentences is true regarding the acquisition of perfusion images using Tc-99m MAA?

   A. Rapid tight bolus injection is preferred over slower injection.
   B. The perfusion scan should be performed before the ventilation scan.
   C. Tc-99m MAA should be administered with the patient in the supine position.
   D. Central venous catheter injection is preferred over peripheral venous injection.
   E. Clinically significant pulmonary emboli can result if the blood is drawn into the syringe prior to the Tc-99m MAA injection.

2 Ventilation images can be acquired with an aerosol such as Tc-99m DTPA or a gas such as Xe-133. Which of the following is an advantage of Tc-99m DTPA compared to Xe-133?

   A. DTPA is more sensitive in the evaluation of airway disease.
   B. DTPA does not interfere with subsequent MAA perfusion images.
   C. DTPA has a short biologic half-life with lower radiation exposure to the patient.
   D. DTPA has better photon flux and allows for the acquisition of multiple projections.

3 In which of the following instances can a normal MAA particle dose be administered to the patient?

   A. Pregnancy
   B. Right-to-left shunt
   C. Pediatric population
   D. Pulmonary hypertension
   E. Saddle pulmonary embolus

4 What radiopharmaceuticals were likely used to perform the following ventilation–perfusion study?

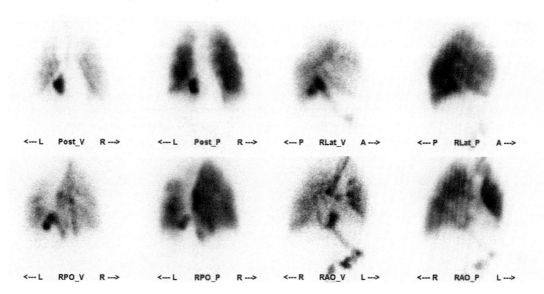

A. Xenon-133 and Tc-99m MAA
B. Tc-99m DTPA and Tc-99m MAA
C. Xenon-133 and Tc-99m DTPA
D. Tc-99m sulfur colloid and Tc-99m DTPA
E. Krypton-81m and Tc-99m DTPA

5 Based on the following imaging, what is the most appropriate next step?

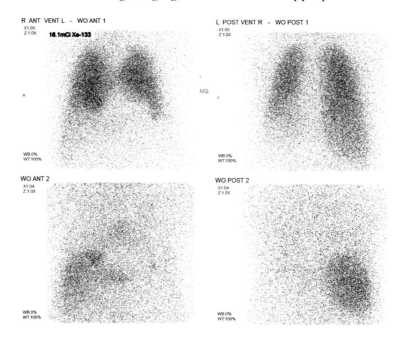

A. Radioiodine treatment
B. FDG-PET/CT
C. Liver function tests
D. Pulmonary function tests
E. CT chest
F. CT abdomen

6 A 36-year-old female in the first trimester of pregnancy presents to the emergency department with chest pain. Which of the following is true regarding the CT pulmonary angiogram (CTPA) compared to the ventilation–perfusion scan (V/Q) in this patient?

A. CTPA has lower specificity.
B. CTPA has lower fetal radiation exposure.
C. CTPA has lower maternal breast radiation exposure.
D. CTPA has lower maternal total body radiation exposure.

7 What is the most appropriate next step based on the following perfusion scintigraphy findings?

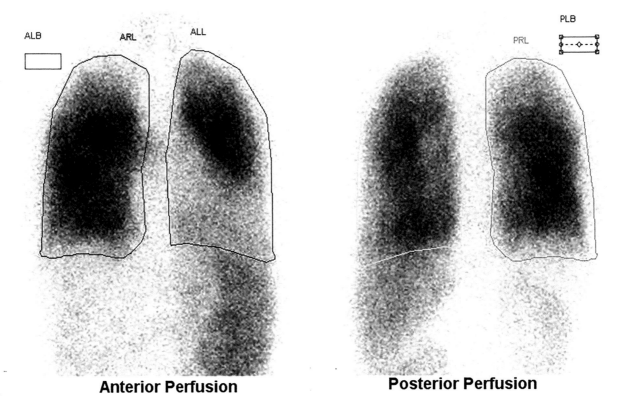

Anterior Perfusion　　　　**Posterior Perfusion**

A. Cardiac MRI
B. CT angiography
C. Planar images of the brain
D. Contrast echocardiography

8 What degree of FDG uptake is typically associated with a pulmonary hamartoma?

A. Less than that of the mediastinum
B. Greater than mediastinum but less than liver
C. Greater than liver but less than bladder
D. Greater than bladder

9 A 63-year-old lady presents with shortness of breath. Given the following images, what is your interpretation based on the modified PIOPED II criteria?

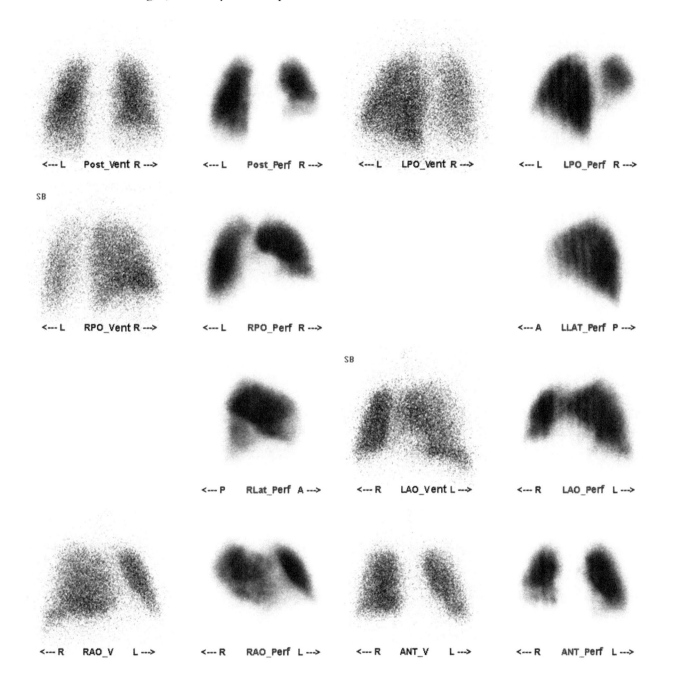

A. Very low probability
B. Low probability
C. Nondiagnostic
D. High probability

10 According to the modified PIOPED II criteria, what is the probability of pulmonary embolism in this patient?

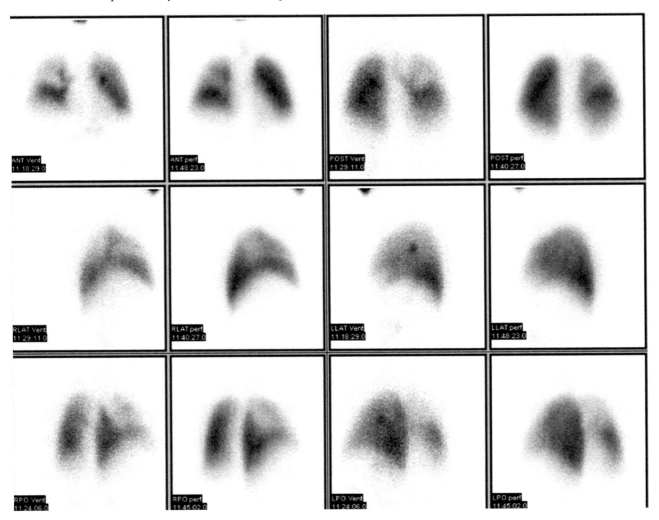

A. Very low probability
B. Low probability
C. Nondiagnostic
D. High probability

11 Diffuse lung uptake 1 hour after the injection of Indium-111–labeled white blood cells is secondary to which of the following?

A. Pneumonia
B. Radiation pneumonitis
C. Pleural effusion
D. Physiologic
E. Chemotherapy

12 A 78-year-old male with a past medical history of smoking presents with the complaint of shortness of breath and palpitations. The ED physician was concerned for pulmonary embolism and requested a V/Q scan. What is the most likely interpretation using the modified PIOPED II criteria?

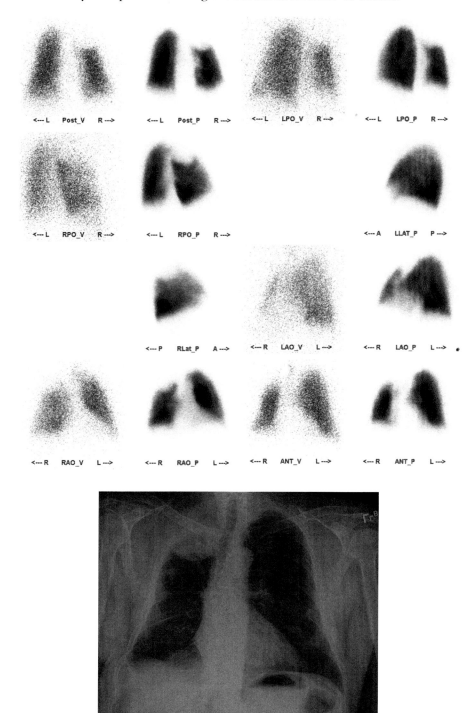

A. Very low probability
B. Low probability
C. Nondiagnostic
D. High probability

13 A 44-year-old female presents with shortness of breath. You are given the following images. What is the most important thing to review prior to the interpretation of this examination?

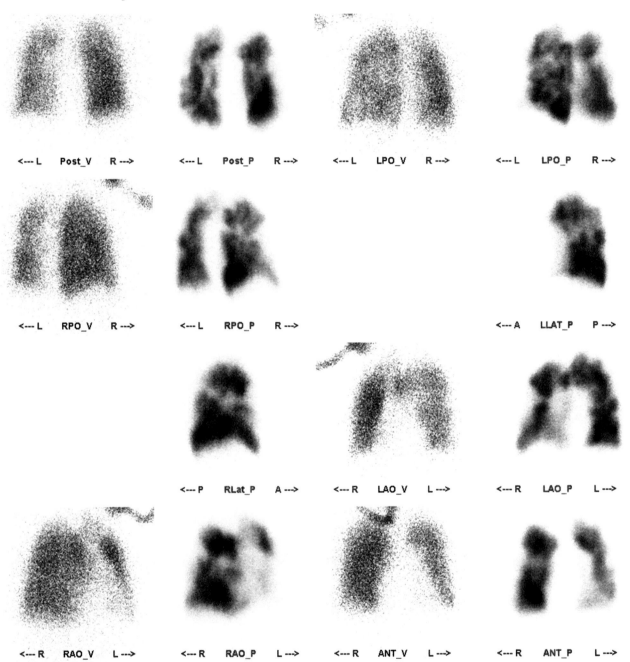

A. Chest x-ray
B. Venous Doppler
C. Prior V/Q scan
D. Prior chest CT

14 A 67-year-old gentleman with coronary artery bypass grafting 2 days ago presents with new-onset shortness of breath and tachycardia. Because of these symptoms, a V/Q scan was performed. What is your interpretation based on the provided images?

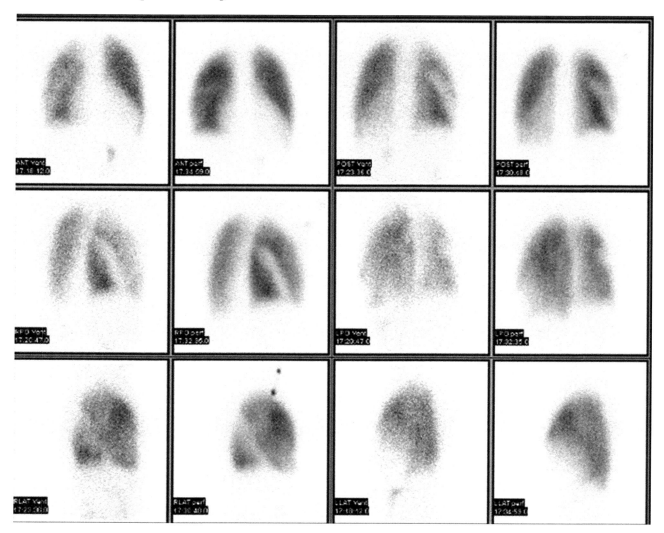

    A. Very low probability for PE
    B. Low probability for PE
    C. Nondiagnostic for PE
    D. High probability for PE

15 What is the most likely cause of bilateral diffuse intense lung uptake on a delayed whole-body bone scintigraphy?

    A. Malignant pleural effusion
    B. Pulmonary alveolar microlithiasis
    C. Pulmonary radiation
    D. Pulmonary osteosarcoma metastasis

16 Based on the provided V/Q scan and chest x-ray, which of the following is the most likely diagnosis?

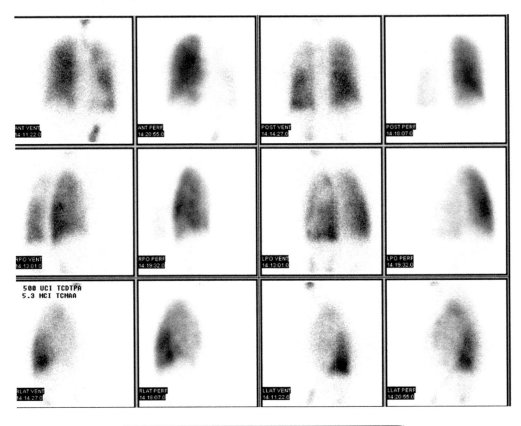

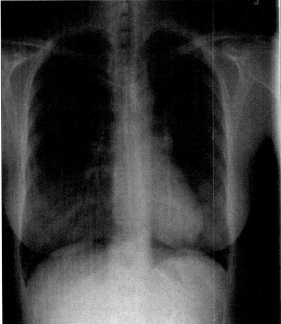

A. Swyer-James syndrome
B. Pulmonary embolus
C. Pulmonary atresia
D. Pneumonectomy
E. Lung cancer

17 A 75-year-old smoker presents with shortness of breath. Based on the images provided, how would you interpret this examination using the modified PIOPED II criteria?

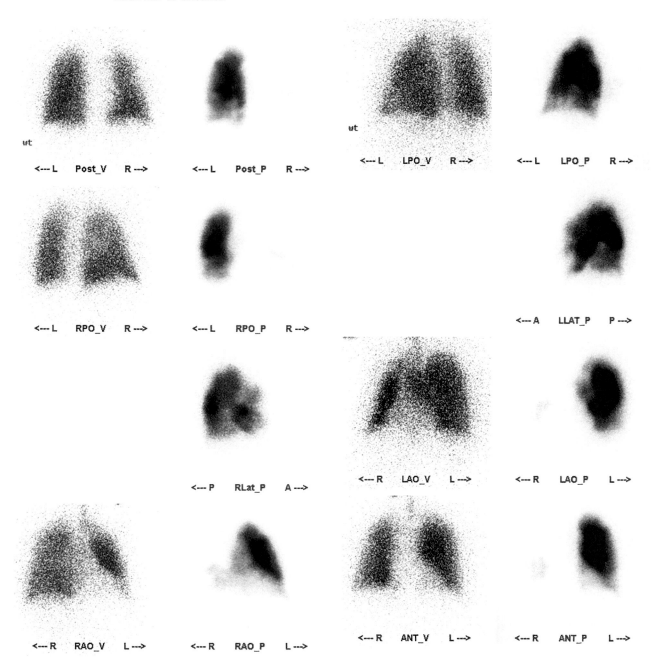

A. Very low probability.
B. Low probability.
C. Nondiagnostic.
D. High probability.
E. The patient does not have a PE but should be evaluated for a hilar mass.

18 An 82-year-old female with history of renal cell carcinoma undergoes the following scan to evaluate for a possible left below-the-knee amputation osteomyelitis. What is the most likely cause of the abnormal activity in the chest?

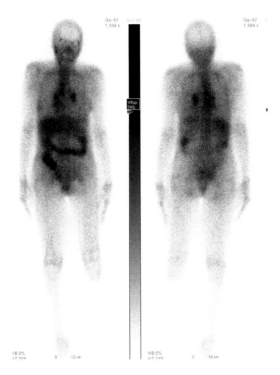

A. Lymphoma
B. Metastasis
C. Pulmonary abscesses
D. Granulomatous disease

19 The following Ga-67 scan is from a 34-year-old gentleman with a history of HIV and cough. Which of the following is the LEAST likely diagnosis?

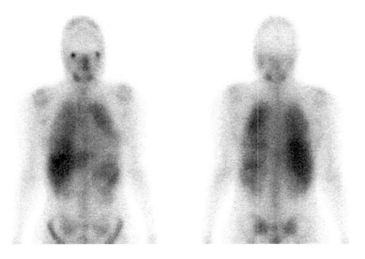

A. *Pneumocystis jiroveci* pneumonia
B. Kaposi sarcoma
C. Radiation pneumonitis
D. Pulmonary drug toxicity
E. *Mycobacterium avium-intracellulare*

20 A patient with severe emphysema and a FEV1 of 2 L needs to undergo a right pneumonectomy for a right upper lobe lung cancer. Based on the perfusion images provided, what would you advise?

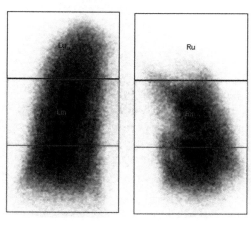
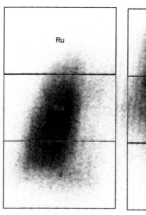
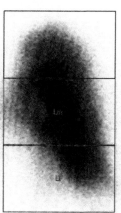

	Posterior Kct			Geometric Mean Kct				Anterior Kct			
	Left		Right		Left Lung		Right Lung		Right		Left	
	%	Kct	%	Kct	%	Kct	%	Kct	%	Kct	%	Kct
Upper Zone:	13.5	97.09	2.7	19.82	14.8	105.52	2.7	19.55	2.7	19.28	16.2	114.68
Middle Zone:	27.8	200.26	20.4	147.44	31.0	220.04	19.8	140.92	19.0	134.69	34.2	241.78
Lower Zone:	19.4	139.58	16.2	116.92	17.7	125.57	14.0	99.26	11.9	84.27	16.0	112.96
Total Lung:	60.6	436.93	39.4	284.17	63.5	451.13	36.5	259.72	33.7	238.24	66.3	469.42

A. The patient can safely undergo right pneumonectomy.
B. The patient cannot safely undergo right pneumonectomy.
C. Study is incomplete as ventilation images were not done.
D. Findings are inconclusive/indeterminate.

21 What is the most likely etiology for the following findings?

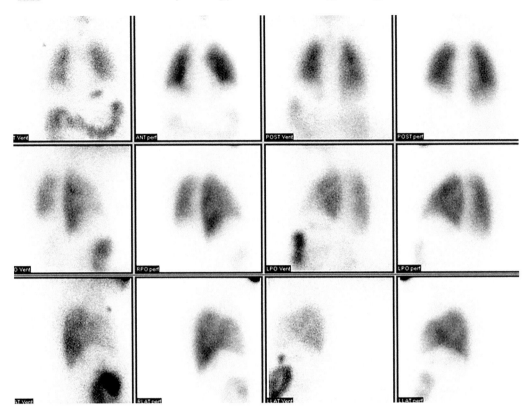

A. Poor tagging
B. GI bleed
C. Prior examination
D. Metastatic calcifications

22 The following examination was performed after oral administration of the radiopharmaceutical. What is the most likely indication for performing this study?

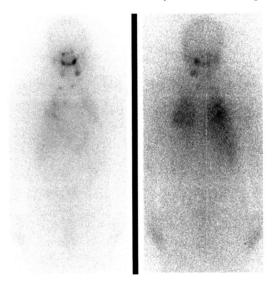

A. Elevated WBC count
B. Shortness of breath in a patient with AIDS
C. Increasing CEA levels
D. Increasing thyroglobulin levels

ANSWERS AND EXPLANATIONS

1 **Answer C.** Because of the gradient created by gravity, the lung bases receive about three times the amount of blood flow compared to the apex when the patient is in the upright position. In order to minimize this gravity-induced physiologic perfusion gradient, Tc-99m MAA should be injected with the patient in the supine position. Also, to allow proper mixing with blood and to prolong the bolus, peripheral vein injection is preferred and injection through the central venous catheter should be avoided. The injection should be slow over more than four respiratory cycles and have large enough volume to assist in homogeneous pulmonary distribution. Labeled blood clots formed by blood drawn into the syringe may result in focal hot spots on the perfusion scan (see arrows in image below); however, they are clinically insignificant. Since both DTPA and MAA are labeled with Tc-99m, sequential ventilation/perfusion images require a smaller dose of the first imaging agent to prevent interference with the second. Because it is difficult to deliver high doses of aerosolized DTPA to the lungs and since better count statistics are preferred for the perfusion imaging, the ventilation portion of the imaging is usually performed first. Because of the low photopeak and short biologic half-life, Xe-133 ventilation is also performed before the perfusion component of the study.

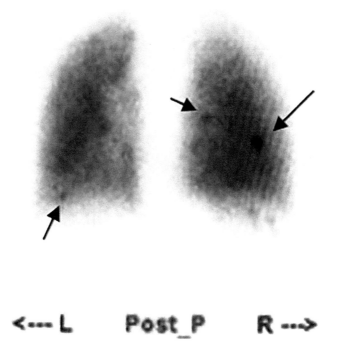

References: Mettler FA, Guiberteau MJ. *Essentials of nuclear medicine imaging*, 7th ed. Philadelphia, PA: Saunders, 2019:177–179.

O'Malley JP, Ziessman HA, Thrall JH. *Nuclear medicine: the requisites*, 5th ed. Philadelphia, PA: Saunders, 2020:128–132.

2 **Answer D.** Advantages of Tc-99m DTPA include the ability to acquire multiple projections, ready availability, and ideal photon energy resulting in better imaging. Disadvantages include interference with subsequent perfusion images from crosstalk as well as central clumping of the radiopharmaceutical in the setting of poor respiratory effort or increased air turbulence (i.e., COPD or asthma).

Advantages of Xe-133 compared to Tc-99m DTPA include superior sensitivity to detect COPD and lack of interference with the subsequent perfusion images owing to its short biologic half-life as well as low photopeak of 81 keV. Disadvantages include higher soft tissue attenuation due to low photon energy, inability to acquire multiple protections (with a single dose) or SPECT images due to rapid washout, and requirement of the special exhaust system, traps, and negative air pressure rooms.

References: Mettler FA, Guiberteau MJ. *Essentials of nuclear medicine imaging*, 7th ed. Philadelphia, PA: Saunders, 2019:177–179, 197.

O'Malley JP, Ziessman HA, Thrall JH. *Nuclear medicine: the requisites*, 5th ed. Philadelphia, PA: Saunders, 2020:128–132.

3 **Answer E.** Usually, 200,000 to 500,000 particles of MAA are administered to the patient undergoing a ventilation–perfusion study for the evaluation of pulmonary embolism. In children, this number is decreased to 10,000 for the neonates and 50,000 to 150,000 for children <5 years of age. Also, reduction in the particle dose (100,000 to 150,000) should be considered in patients with pulmonary hypertension, right-to-left shunt, and pregnancy. Saddle pulmonary embolus is not an indication for the reduction in the particle dose.

References: Mettler FA, Guiberteau MJ. *Essentials of nuclear medicine imaging*, 7th ed. Philadelphia, PA: Saunders, 2019:177.

O'Malley JP, Ziessman HA, Thrall JH. *Nuclear medicine: the requisites*, 5th ed. Philadelphia, PA: Saunders, 2020:128.

4 **Answer B.** The acquired ventilation images demonstrate a large focus of intense activity within the posterior upper abdomen toward the left of the midline in what appears to be the stomach (arrows); activity is also visualized in the proximal small bowel. Findings are secondary to swallowed aerosol particles. The deposition of the radiopharmaceutical is also identified within the trachea and central airways (arrowheads). These findings are seen with the Tc-99m DTPA ventilation scan. Tc-99m DTPA is aerosolized using nebulizer into small particles. Because of its particulate nature, unlike ventilation performed with a gas such as Xe-133, central accumulation of DTPA may occur in patients unable to cooperate with deep breathing or in patients who have increased central airway flow turbulence from COPD or asthma. Also, the ingestion of the noninhaled particles from the oral cavity may result in activity within the esophagus and stomach. This patient had a hiatal hernia (arrows in the chest x-ray below) explaining the activity in the posterior mediastinum. Tc-99m MAA is currently the only agent used for lung perfusion imaging. Because the majority of the particles (60% to 80%) range in size from 10 to 30 μm, it is appropriate for the blockage of pulmonary capillaries, which measure approximately 10 μm in diameter. Since perfusion portion of the study is acquired after the ventilation, shine through of activity in stomach and central airways from the ventilation study is often seen on the perfusion images (as is the case with this patient).

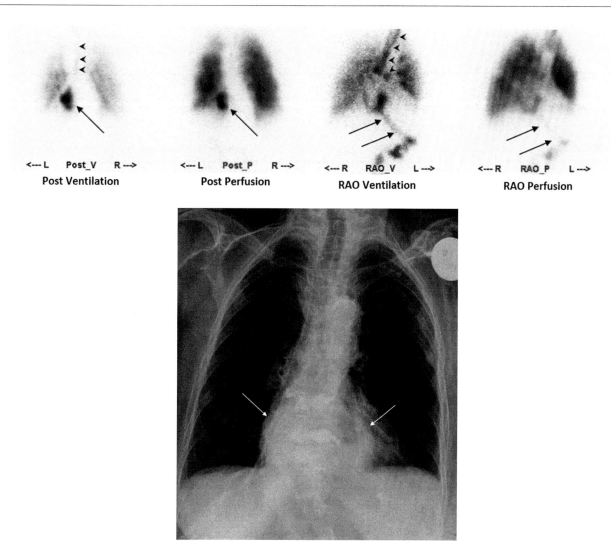

<--- L   Post_V   R --->
Post Ventilation

<--- L   Post_P   R --->
Post Perfusion

<--- R   RAO_V   L --->
RAO Ventilation

<--- R   RAO_P   L --->
RAO Perfusion

References: Mettler FA, Guiberteau MJ. *Essentials of nuclear medicine imaging*, 7th ed. Philadelphia, PA: Saunders, 2019:179–181.

O'Malley JP, Ziessman HA, Thrall JH. *Nuclear medicine: the requisites*, 5th ed. Philadelphia, PA: Saunders, 2020:132–135.

5 **Answer C.** The sequential anterior and posterior Xe-133 images demonstrate retention of Xe-133 within the right upper quadrant (arrow). This is typically seen in patients with fatty infiltration due to the retention of fat-soluble Xe-133 in the liver parenchyma. Liver function tests would be the most appropriate next step in this case, and the other choices would not be appropriate. Retained Xe-133 uptake within the lungs on washout images is associated with air trapping from small airways disease. However, careful inspection of the images demonstrates that the retained radiopharmaceutical is in the liver and not in the lung parenchyma. When present, this finding should not be mistaken for trapping of Xe-133 in the right lower lung.

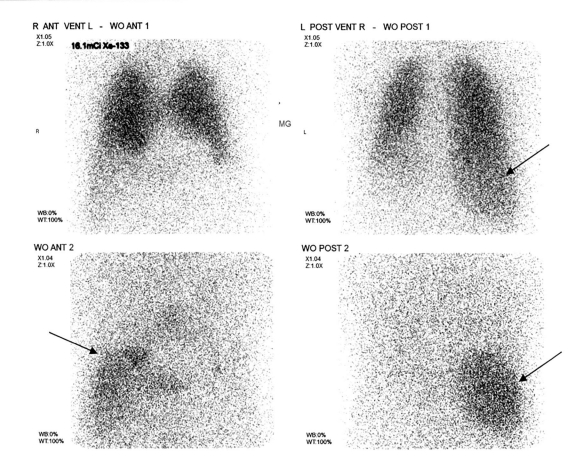

References: Conn HL Jr. Equilibrium distribution of radioxenon in tissue: xenon-hemoglobin association curve. *J Appl Physiol* 1961;16:1065–1070.

Mettler FA, Guiberteau MJ. *Essentials of nuclear medicine imaging*, 7th ed. Philadelphia, PA: Saunders, 2019:179–181, 182.

O'Malley JP, Ziessman HA, Thrall JH. *Nuclear medicine: the requisites*, 5th ed. Philadelphia, PA: Saunders, 2020:135,138.

6 **Answer B.** Even though CT pulmonary angiogram (CTPA) may be the initial test of choice to diagnose pulmonary embolism, the maternal radiation dose is higher with CTPA (3 to 5 mSv) compared to the V/Q scan (2 mSv or less). Admittedly the maternal total body radiation dose is highly variable given the wide variety of CT scanners and protocols currently available. While CT scans with newer detector technology can reduce maternal dose further, CTPA delivers higher radiation to the breast tissue compared to the V/Q scan, increasing the risk of breast cancer. On the other hand, even with reduced dose (1 to 2 mCi of Tc-99m MAA), the fetal dose from the V/Q scan may be higher than that from the CTPA. According to the PIOPED II trial, the V/Q scan and pulmonary CT angiogram performed about equally in the diagnosis of pulmonary embolism. However, the specificity of CTPA for pulmonary emboli detection is greater than that of the V/Q scan. Other weaknesses of the V/Q scan include longer examination time and lack of ready availability as the preparation of radiopharmaceutical requires extra time.

References: Mettler FA, Guiberteau MJ. *Essentials of nuclear medicine imaging*, 7th ed. Philadelphia, PA: Saunders, 2019:209–211.

O'Malley JP, Ziessman HA, Thrall JH. *Nuclear medicine: the requisites*, 5th ed. Philadelphia, PA: Saunders, 2020:142–145.

7 **Answer C.** Anterior and posterior Tc-99m MAA perfusion images demonstrate activity within the spleen (arrows) and kidneys (arrowheads). Activity is not visualized within the stomach (as would be expected with free pertechnetate). As such, findings represent right-to-left shunt, which should be confirmed with planar images of the brain. Visualization of activity within the brain would indicate a right-to-left shunt. Since Tc-99m pertechnetate cannot cross the blood–brain barrier, absence of radiotracer uptake within the brain would confirm free pertechnetate.

Activity within the kidneys and thyroid may be seen due to either free pertechnetate or right-to-left cardiac shunt. When seen, planar images of the brain should be acquired to differentiate between the two.

The right to left shunt may be assessed by Tc-99m MAA perfusion imaging. It can be intracardiac (patent foramen ovale, atrial septal defect, or anomalous pulmonary venous return) or extracardiac (pulmonary arteriovenous malformation or hepatopulmonary syndrome). The shunt fraction is calculated as follows: Percentage of R-L shunt = [(total body geometric mean count − total lung geometric mean count)/total body geometric mean count] ×100.

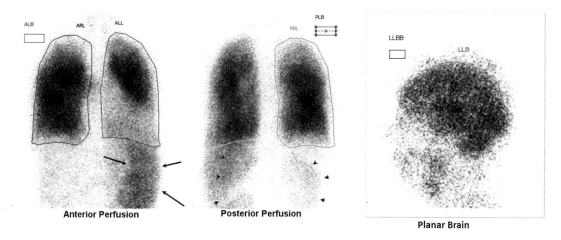

Anterior Perfusion   Posterior Perfusion

Planar Brain

References: Chokkappan K, Kannivelu A, Srinivasan S, et al. Review of diagnostic uses of shunt fraction quantification with technetium-99m acroaggregated albumin perfusion scan as illustrated by a case of Osler–Weber–Rendu syndrome *Ann Thorac Med* 2016;11(2):155–160. PMID: 27168866.

Mettler FA, Guiberteau MJ. *Essentials of nuclear medicine imaging*, 7th ed. Philadelphia, PA: Saunders, 2019:177–178.

O'Malley JP, Ziessman HA, Thrall JH. *Nuclear medicine: the requisites*, 5th ed. Philadelphia, PA: Saunders, 2020:134.

8 **Answer A.** Pulmonary hamartomas generally have no significant uptake (less than the mediastinum) on the F-18 FDG-PET imaging. If a lung nodule has a CT appearance that is benign but demonstrates increased metabolic activity, malignancy should be suspected. False-positive causes of FDG-PET imaging include infectious or granulomatous processes. Also, since well-differentiated adenocarcinoma with lepidic pattern and carcinoid may demonstrate no significant FDG activity, correlation with prior imaging, follow-up imaging, or biopsy should be considered for lesions with a low level of F-18 FDG uptake. If the nodule demonstrates characteristic popcorn-like calcifications within it, then hamartoma is likely and further workup would be unnecessary.

References: Bury T, Dowlati A, Paulus P, et al. Evaluation of the solitary pulmonary nodule by positron emission tomography imaging. *Eur Respir J* 1996;9(3):410–414.

Chang JM, Lee HJ, Goo JM, et al. False-positive and false-negative FDG-PET scans in various thoracic diseases. *Korean J Radiol* 2006;7(1):57–69.

Mettler FA, Guiberteau MJ. *Essentials of nuclear medicine imaging*, 7th ed. Philadelphia, PA: Saunders, 2019:345.

9   **Answer D.** There is a large multisegmental mismatched perfusion defect involving the entire right lower lobe (arrowheads in the first image below). Since there are ≥2 (superior and four basilar segments of the right lower lobe) large (>75% of the lung segment), segmental (wedge-shaped, extending to pleura), mismatched perfusion defects, the findings are compatible with a high probability (85% to 90%) of pulmonary embolism. Occasionally, large defects such as this are misinterpreted when multiple adjacent segments are involved; close attention and correlation with a ventilation scan should help prevent this mistake. A more typical appearance of a high-probability ventilation–perfusion scan is shown in the second image below, which demonstrates multiple, large, wedge-shaped, mismatched segmental perfusion defects in the right and left lungs.

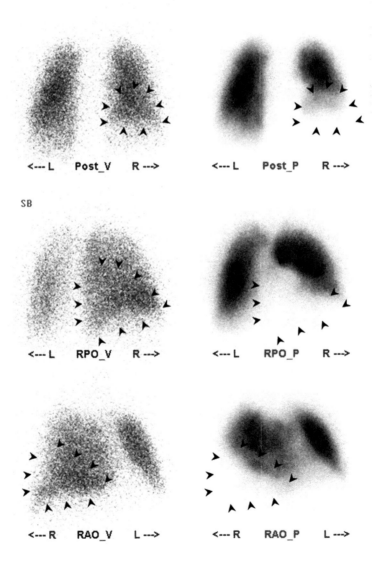

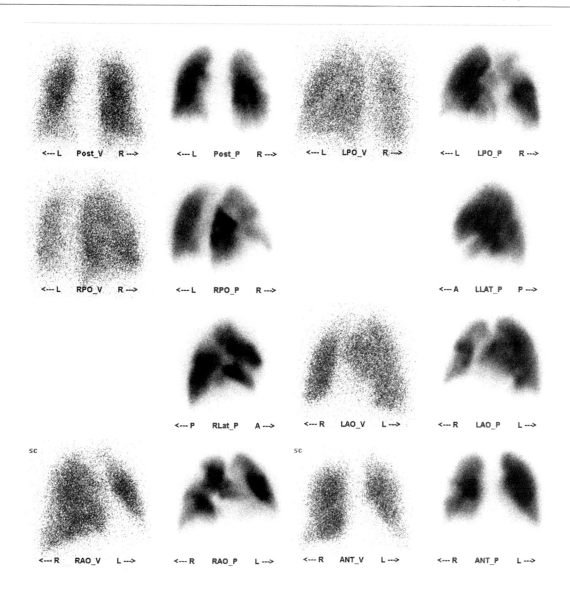

Modified PIOPED II Criteria*	
High probability	≥2 large mismatched segmental defects
Very low probability	Nonsegmental defects
	Stripe sign
	1–3 small segmental defects
	Single triple-matched defect in the upper lung
	Perfusion defect smaller than corresponding radiograph abnormality
Normal	Normal perfusion. No defects

*If the perfusion does not fall into one of these categories, then it is nondiagnostic and requires further workup.

References: Mettler FA, Guiberteau MJ. *Essentials of nuclear medicine imaging*, 7th ed. Philadelphia, PA: Saunders, 2019:190–197.

O'Malley JP, Ziessman HA, Thrall JH. *Nuclear medicine: the requisites*, 5th ed. Philadelphia, PA: Saunders, 2020:135–142.

10 **Answer A.** The ventilation and perfusion images demonstrate the presence of a large, nonsegmental, matched perfusion defect involving the right upper lobe. Perfusion is present at the periphery of this defect (arrows); this is known as the stripe sign and represents a very low probability (<10%) of pulmonary embolus. A nonsegmental perfusion defect does not correspond to the bronchopulmonary anatomic segment and is generally not wedge shaped. It may be caused by pulmonary abnormalities such as emphysema/bullae (most common), atelectasis, neoplasm, pneumonia, hemorrhage, or edema. Extrapulmonary abnormalities resulting in nonsegmental perfusion defects include normal variance or pathology of hilar or mediastinal structures and alterations in diaphragmatic contour. According to modified PIOPED II criteria, the category of very low probability includes the following: nonsegmental perfusion defect, a perfusion defect with a stripe sign, one to three small segmental defects, single triple-matched defect in the upper or middle lung zone, and a perfusion defect smaller than the corresponding chest radiograph abnormality. If a V/Q scan does not fall into a high probability, a very low probability, or a normal category, then it should be assigned a nondiagnostic category requiring further workup.

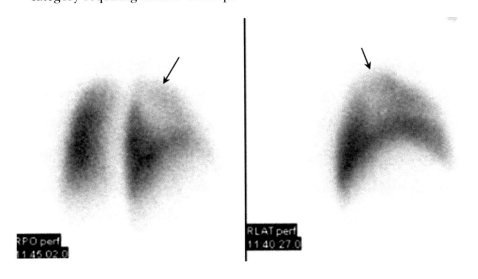

References: Mettler FA, Guiberteau MJ. *Essentials of nuclear medicine imaging*, 7th ed. Philadelphia, PA: Saunders, 2019:190–197.

O'Malley JP, Ziessman HA, Thrall JH. *Nuclear medicine: the requisites*, 5th ed. Philadelphia, PA: Saunders, 2020:135–142.

11 **Answer D.** On early images after intravenous administration of In-111–labeled WBC scan, diffuse physiologic lung activity is visualized. However, this activity should reduce over the course of 4 hours after the injection, reducing to the background. Persistent lung uptake can be secondary to damaged WBCs during the labeling process. Pneumonia, pneumonitis, and chemotherapy can all be associated with increased pulmonary uptake of tagged WBCs, but it would be present on delayed images. Benign pleural effusion would result in no significant abnormality.

References: Love C, Opoku-Agyemang P, Tomas MB. Pulmonary activity on labeled leukocyte images: physiologic, pathologic, and imaging correlation. *Radiographics* 2002;22(6):1385–1393.

Mettler FA, Guiberteau MJ. *Essentials of nuclear medicine imaging*, 7th ed. Philadelphia, PA: Saunders, 2019:364.

12 Answer A. The ventilation and perfusion images demonstrate a large matched perfusion defect involving the right lung apex, which corresponds to a mass-like density on the chest radiograph (arrows). Findings are consistent with a triple-matched upper lobe perfusion defect, which is considered to be a very low probability (<10%) of PE by the modified PIOPED II criteria. In this case, the perfusion defect is secondary to the right apical lung cancer. On the other hand, a triple-matched perfusion defect within the lower lungs would be considered nondiagnostic secondary to an increased prevalence of PE in the lower lobes. In this case, some would advocate an approach stating that there is no evidence of pulmonary embolus and the perfusion defect corresponds to the pulmonary malignancy.

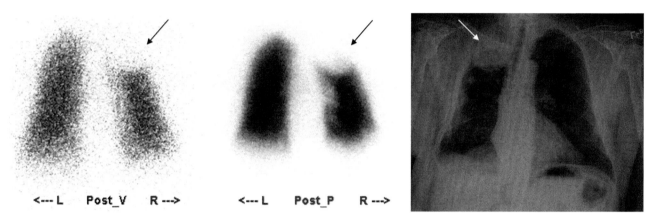

References: Mettler FA, Guiberteau MJ. *Essentials of nuclear medicine imaging*, 7th ed. Philadelphia, PA: Saunders, 2019:190–197.

O'Malley JP, Ziessman HA, Thrall JH. *Nuclear medicine: the requisites*, 5th ed. Philadelphia, PA: Saunders, 2020:135–142.

13 Answer C. The perfusion images demonstrate multiple, large, bilateral, mismatched, segmental defects consistent with a high probability of pulmonary embolism. Incomplete resolution of prior pulmonary emboli is one of the most common causes of mismatched perfusion defects. As such, any prior ventilation/perfusion scan should be reviewed prior to rendering the diagnosis of an acute PE. While it is true that V/Q scans should be interpreted with a recent chest x-ray (at a minimum within the past 48 hours and preferably within 24 hours), a chest x-ray is unlikely to change your interpretation in this case with normal ventilation. This patient had a prior V/Q scan, which was identical in appearance making acute PE less likely. One should closely look for new mismatched defects in these patients, which would indicate new pulmonary emboli. Patients with a high burden of pulmonary emboli and elderly patients are less likely to return to normal after the treatment of PE. In these patients, perfusion lung imaging is preferred over CTPA to follow the course of the disease. A 3-month follow-up study should be considered to serve as a baseline for future reference since perfusion defects persisting at 3 months are less likely to resolve.

References: Mettler FA, Guiberteau MJ. *Essentials of nuclear medicine imaging*, 7th ed. Philadelphia, PA: Saunders, 2019:197–201.

O'Malley JP, Ziessman HA, Thrall JH. *Nuclear medicine: the requisites*, 5th ed. Philadelphia, PA: Saunders, 2020:138.

14 Answer A. A curvilinear-matched perfusion and ventilation defect is seen within the right lung that tracks along the expected course of the major fissure. This finding is known as the "fissure sign" and is commonly seen in the presence of pleural effusion. The corresponding radiograph below demonstrates the blunting of the right costophrenic angle and fluid within the right major fissure. Since this would qualify as a nonsegmental perfusion defect, it would be placed in the category of a very low probability for pulmonary embolus by the modified PIOPED II criteria.

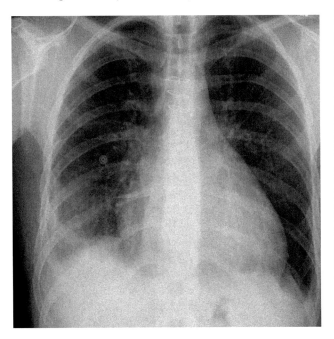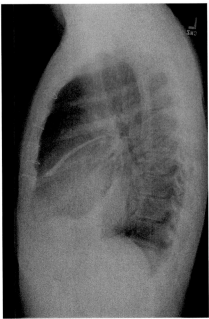

References: Mettler FA, Guiberteau MJ. *Essentials of nuclear medicine imaging*, 7th ed. Philadelphia, PA: Saunders, 2019:190–197.

O'Malley JP, Ziessman HA, Thrall JH. *Nuclear medicine: the requisites*, 5th ed. Philadelphia, PA: Saunders, 2020:135–142.

15 **Answer B.** Diffuse bilateral lung uptake can be seen with pulmonary alveolar microlithiasis. It is a rare disease of unknown etiology, which is characterized by the presence of calcific concretions in the alveolar spaces and development/deposition of intra-alveolar microliths. Diffuse pulmonary metastatic calcification from renal failure and hypercalcemia would also present with similar diffuse lung uptake on bone scan. Malignant pleural effusion may demonstrate a unilateral mild-to-moderate increase in activity, which is seen best on the posterior projection images. Pulmonary radiation–induced fibrosis would demonstrate a regional increase in activity while pulmonary osteosarcoma metastasis would demonstrate focal areas of increase in activity.

References: Rosenthal DI, Chandler HL, Azizi F, et al. Uptake of bone imaging agents by diffuse pulmonary metastatic calcification. *AJR Am J Roentgenol* 1977;129(5):871–874.

Shah TC, Talwar A, Shah RD, et al. Pulmonary alveolar microlithiasis: radiographic and scintigraphic correlation. *Clin Nucl Med* 2007;32(3):249–251.

16 **Answer C.** The perfusion images demonstrate unilateral absence of perfusion to the entire left lung. Normal homogeneous perfusion is noted within the right lung without presence of any segmental perfusion defects. The ventilation portion of the study demonstrates patchy areas of nonsegmental ventilation defects in the left upper lung zone; however, there is a significant mismatch between the perfusion and ventilation. The chest radiograph demonstrates hypoplastic left lung with lack of pulmonary vascularity on the left. This is a case of pulmonary atresia secondary to the congenital absence of the left main pulmonary artery. Associated findings include atretic pulmonary valve with underdeveloped pulmonary artery. There is typically volume loss to the affected side on the chest x-ray. Reticular vessels from bronchial artery collateral circulation may be seen along with the rib notching from the prominence of the intercostal arteries.

The differential considerations for absent or decreased perfusion to one lung can be remembered by pneumonic SAFE POEM: Swyer-James syndrome, pulmonary Agenesis/hypoplasia, mediastinal Fibrosis, pleural Effusion, Pneumonectomy, Obstruction by tumor, pulmonary Embolus, and Mucous plug. Both mucous plug and Swyer-James syndrome would present with matched ventilation–perfusion defect in the affected lung. A large pleural effusion will demonstrate more severe perfusion abnormality in the posterior projection due to layering in supine patients. Also, pleural effusion and pneumonectomy would be evident on the chest radiograph. Similarly, large enough lung neoplasm to cause compression of the pulmonary vasculature should be evident on the chest radiograph. When secondary to pulmonary embolus, unilateral lack of perfusion to one lung is usually accompanied by segmental mismatched perfusion defects on the contralateral side.

References: Mettler FA, Guiberteau MJ. *Essentials of nuclear medicine imaging*, 7th ed. Philadelphia, PA: Saunders, 2019:201–207.

O'Malley JP, Ziessman HA, Thrall JH. *Nuclear medicine: the requisites*, 5th ed. Philadelphia, PA: Saunders, 2020:139.

17 **Answer D.** There is near complete absence of perfusion to the right lung. Also, multiple large, segmental, mismatched perfusion defects are present within the left lung (arrowheads). The ventilation is normal. Combination of these findings is most compatible with a high probability of pulmonary embolus. While a whole lung mismatched perfusion defect is not commonly secondary to a PE, additional mismatched perfusion defects within the left lung make this case a high probability for pulmonary embolism. The corresponding CTPA below shows a saddle embolus with near occlusion of the right pulmonary artery and smaller embolus within the left pulmonary artery.

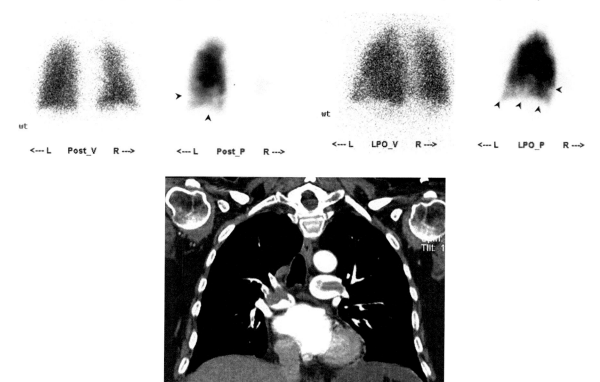

References: Mettler FA, Guiberteau MJ. *Essentials of nuclear medicine imaging*, 7th ed. Philadelphia, PA: Saunders, 2019:201–207.

O'Malley JP, Ziessman HA, Thrall JH. *Nuclear medicine: the requisites*, 5th ed. Philadelphia, PA: Saunders, 2020:139.

18 **Answer D.** Anterior and posterior planar images of the Ga-67 scan demonstrate the presence of physiologic radiopharmaceutical uptake within the liver, spleen, and bowel. Pharmaceutical uptake is noted within bilateral hila and right mediastinum (arrowheads) in a configuration also known as the "lambda sign." While physiologic uptake can be seen in the lacrimal and salivary glands, it appears more intense than is expected. Intense activity in the lacrimal and salivary glands is known as the "panda sign." The patient's head is slightly rotated to the left; as such, the left parotid gland is not visualized. The combination of these findings is typically associated with sarcoidosis. Differential considerations of hilar and mediastinal lymphadenopathy include lymphoma or mycobacterial infectious disease, especially in immunocompromised patients. Lymphoma would be expected to present with a larger mediastinal mass or additional nodal chain involvement. The chest findings are not localized to the lungs, and therefore pulmonary abscess is incorrect.

Half-life of Ga-67 is 3.2 days with principle gamma photons of 93 keV (40%), 184 keV (24%), 296 keV (22%), and 388 keV (7%). The primary route of elimination is through the kidneys in the first 24 hours with intestinal mucosa becoming the major route of elimination after that. The liver has the most intense physiologic activity. Physiologic activity in the spleen, salivary glands, lacrimal glands, and axial skeleton should be less intense than that in the liver. Physiologic activity is seen in the renal collecting system in the first 24 hours and bowel after that. Ga-67 scans were routinely performed to evaluate response to treatment in patients with malignancies such as lymphoma before the advent of F-18 FDG-PET.

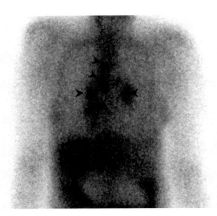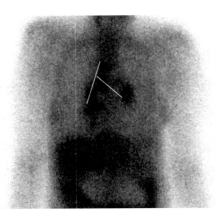

References: Beaumont D, Herry JY, et al. Gallium-67 in the evaluation of sarcoidosis: correlations with serum angiotensin-converting enzyme and bronchoalveolar lavage. *Thorax* 1982;37(1):11–18.

Mettler FA, Guiberteau MJ. *Essentials of nuclear medicine imaging*, 7th ed. Philadelphia, PA: Saunders, 2019:318–321, 370–373.

O'Malley JP, Ziessman HA, Thrall JH. *Nuclear medicine: the requisites*, 5th ed. Philadelphia, PA: Saunders, 2020:434–436.

19 **Answer B.** Diffuse pulmonary uptake of Ga-67 in a patient with known HIV is typically seen with *Pneumocystis jiroveci* pneumonia (PJP), formerly known as *Pneumocystis carinii* pneumonia (PCP). Ga-67 scans have reported sensitivity and negative predictive value of >90% in the diagnosis of PJP. In patients with PJP, Ga-67 scan findings typically precede radiographic changes by days or weeks, allowing for earlier diagnosis and treatment. Kaposi sarcoma does not demonstrate increased lung uptake on Ga-67, but it is Tl-201 avid. Since gallium is a nonspecific infectious/inflammatory agent, radiation pneumonitis, *Mycobacterium avium-intracellulare* infection, and pulmonary drug toxicity will demonstrate increased Ga-67 uptake. Notice intense lacrimal gland activity in this patient, which can be seen in patients with AIDS.

References: Habibian MR. *Nuclear medicine imaging: a teaching file*, 2nd ed. Philadelphia, PA: Lippincott Williams & Wilkins, 2009:85–86.

Mettler FA, Guiberteau MJ. *Essentials of nuclear medicine imaging*, 7th ed. Philadelphia, PA: Saunders, 2019:370–371.

O'Malley JP, Ziessman HA, Thrall JH. *Nuclear medicine: the requisites*, 5th ed. Philadelphia, PA: Saunders, 2020:434.

20 **Answer A.** The purpose of the preoperative pulmonary function test and perfusion scan is to identify those patients who are at an increased risk of having respiratory failure after pneumonectomy. It is particularly important in patients with preoperative FEV1 of <2 L in patients undergoing pneumonectomy or <1.5 L in the case of a lobectomy. Postresection forced expiratory volume in the first second (FEV1) of >1 L is associated with low surgical mortality and acceptable quality of life after surgery. The loss of pulmonary function after pneumonectomy or lobectomy can be accurately predicted by the quantitative Tc-99m pulmonary perfusion scan, and its accuracy is not augmented by the ventilation study. As such, ventilation is not necessary. The postoperative residual function is calculated using the following formula: Postoperative residual function = Preoperative FEV1 × % of perfusion in the remaining lung.

If pneumonectomy is contemplated, right-to-left lung differential function is commonly performed by calculating the geometric mean from the regions of interest drawn around the right and left lung in the anterior and posterior views. If lobectomy is contemplated, posterior oblique views would allow better separation of upper and lower lobes and can be used instead to calculate the percent of total perfusion to the specific lobe. If the predicted FEV1 is <1 L, the patient should not be considered for pneumonectomy until further tests, such as unilateral balloon occlusion of the pulmonary artery, would suggest otherwise. In this example, the postoperative FEV1 in the remaining left lung would be 2 L × 0.635 = 1.27 L. As such, this patient would qualify for a right pneumonectomy.

References: O'Malley JP, Ziessman HA, Thrall JH. *Nuclear medicine: the requisites*, 5th ed. Philadelphia, PA: Saunders, 2020:145, 150.

Wernly JA, DeMeester TR, Kirchner PT, et al. Clinical value of quantitative ventilation-perfusion lung scans in the surgical management of bronchogenic carcinoma. *J Thorac Cardiovasc Surg* 1980;80(4):535–543.

21 **Answer C.** Ventilation and perfusion images acquired after inhalation of aerosolized Tc-99m DTPA and IV administration of Tc-99m MAA respectively demonstrate a large amount of activity in the transverse colon. This activity is more intense on the ventilation images compared to the perfusion images due to higher count influx from lungs related to higher dose on the perfusion images, which are acquired after the ventilation images. A small amount of activity is visualized in the stomach due to swallowed radiotracer during the ventilation portion of the examination. The activity within the colon is likely secondary to a prior examination. In this case, the patient had a Tc-99m tetrofosmin injection for myocardial perfusion imaging done about 30 hours before the V/Q scan. Poor tagging of Tc-labeled agents would result in increased amount of free Tc-99m pertechnetate, which would localize to thyroid gland, salivary glands, and stomach. A GI bleed would not be present on ventilation images. Also, since most of the MAA particles measure 10 to 80 microns in size, they are trapped by the pulmonary capillaries, which are <10 μm in diameter. As such, in the absence of a large right-to-left shunt and the presence of a large GI bleed, colonic activity from GI bleed would not be expected. Metastatic calcifications do not present with increased activity in the colon.

Reference: Mettler FA, Guiberteau MJ. *Essentials of nuclear medicine imaging*, 7th ed. Philadelphia, PA: Saunders, 2019:177.

22 **Answer D.** The anterior and posterior whole-body images demonstrate physiologic activity within the oral cavity and bowel. Small-sized foci of moderate to intense activity are noted within bilateral neck. Also, diffusely increased activity is identified throughout the lungs. Physiologic activity within the liver is noted in the right upper quadrant. This is a posttherapy radioiodine scan with diffuse lung uptake secondary to diffuse military pattern of thyroid metastasis within the lungs. The patients with high-risk, well-differentiated thyroid carcinoma are treated with radioiodine and subsequently followed with serial serum thyroglobulin levels and/or whole-body radioiodine study acquired after the oral administration of I-123 or I-131. One of the early signs of disease recurrence in these patients is elevating serum thyroglobulin levels.

Reference: Mettler FA, Guiberteau MJ. *Essentials of nuclear medicine imaging*, 7th ed. Philadelphia, PA: Saunders, 2019:106–108.

8 Gastrointestinal System

1 Based on the consensus recommendations, what constitutes the solid-phase gastric emptying study standardized meal?

A. 4 oz egg whites, 2 slices white bread, 30 g strawberry jam, 120 mL water
B. 4 oz egg whites, 2 slices white bread, 30 g peanut butter, 120 mL water
C. 4 oz egg whites, 2 slices white bread, 15 g strawberry jam, 120 mL water
D. 4 oz egg whites, 2 slices white bread, 15 g peanut butter, 120 mL water
E. 2 oz egg whites, 2 slices white bread, 30 g strawberry jam, 120 mL water
F. 2 oz egg whites, 2 slices white bread, 30 g peanut butter, 120 mL water

2 A patient presents for the gastric emptying study. The technologist calls and informs you that only one of the camera head is working. In what projection should you instruct the technologist to perform the examination?

A. Anterior
B. Posterior
C. Right anterior oblique
D. Left anterior oblique
E. Right lateral
F. Left lateral

3 Which of the following corrections needs to be applied to the data acquired for the gastric emptying study?

A. CT-based attenuation correction
B. Uniformity correction
C. Linearity correction
D. Center of rotation correction
E. Decay correction

4 Which of the following curves most likely represents normal emptying of the liquids from the stomach?

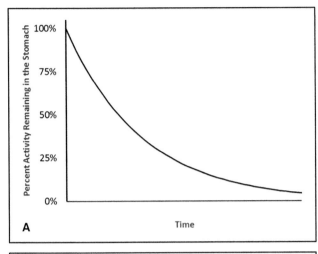

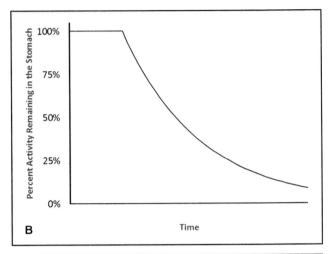

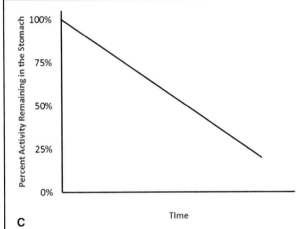

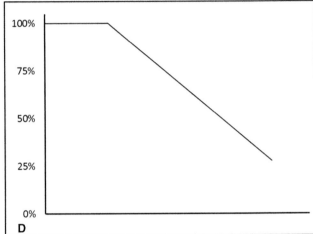

5 Based on the following image, what is the most likely diagnosis?

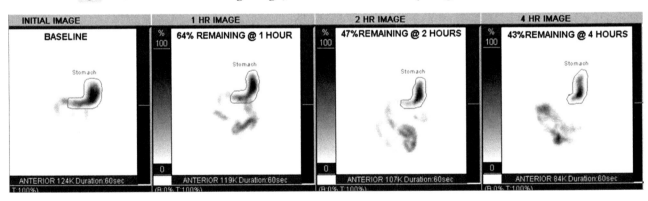

A. Normal gastric emptying
B. Gastroparesis
C. Gastric hypermotility
D. Gastroesophageal reflux

6 In the following patient with an acute gastrointestinal bleed, a branch supplied by which of the following major vessels is the most likely source of bleeding?

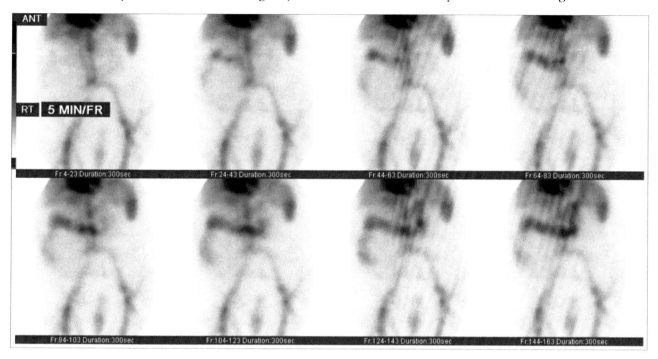

A. Celiac artery
B. Gastroduodenal artery
C. Superior mesenteric artery (SMA)
D. Inferior mesenteric artery (IMA)

7 The following image is from a 62-year-old lady who underwent splenectomy for idiopathic thrombocytopenic purpura (ITP) approximately 10 years ago. What is the most likely diagnosis?

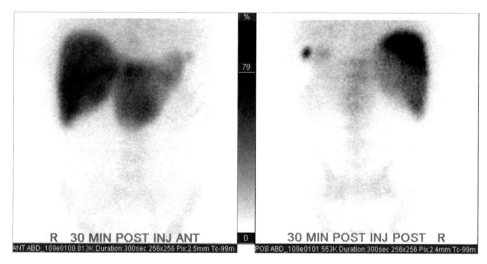

A. Focal nodular hyperplasia
B. Accessory spleen
C. Common bile duct obstruction
D. Acute cholecystitis
E. Intra-abdominal abscess
F. Lymphoma

8 The following image is from a patient who underwent Tc-99m RBC scintigraphy for the evaluation of gastrointestinal bleeding. What is the MOST likely diagnosis?

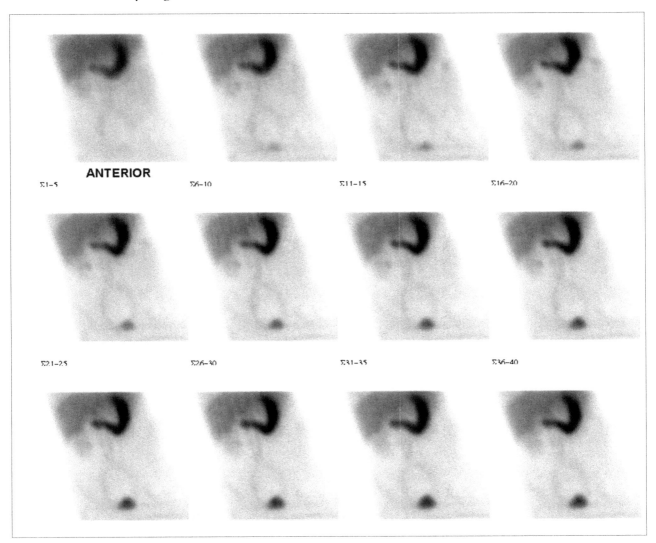

A. Bleeding gastric ulcer
B. Severe gastritis
C. Enterogastric reflux
D. Free pertechnetate
E. Aortogastric fistula

9 Tc-99m–tagged red blood cell (RBC) scintigraphy enables detection of gastrointestinal bleeding at the rate of as low as:

A. 0.01 to 0.04 mL/minute
B. 0.1 to 0.4 mL/minute
C. 1 to 4 mL/minute
D. 10 to 14 mL/minute

10 The following arterial phase CT as well as anterior and posterior planar images are from a patient with a mass within the lateral segment of the left hepatic lobe. What is the most likely diagnosis?

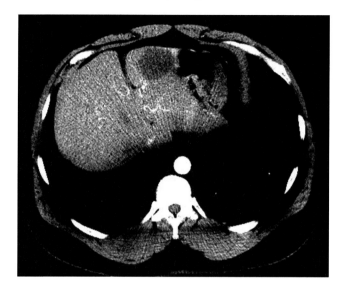

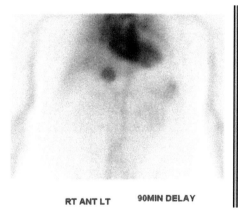 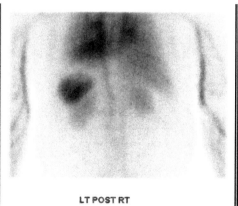

RT ANT LT   **90MIN DELAY**   **LT POST RT**

A. Focal nodular hyperplasia
B. Hepatocellular carcinoma
C. Cavernous hemangioma
D. Solitary metastasis
E. Hepatic adenoma
F. Hepatic abscess

11 The following axial, sagittal, and coronal SPECT images are from Tc-99m sulfurc colloid scan in a patient with a mass within the medial segment of the left hepatic lobe on the CT scan. What is the most likely diagnosis?

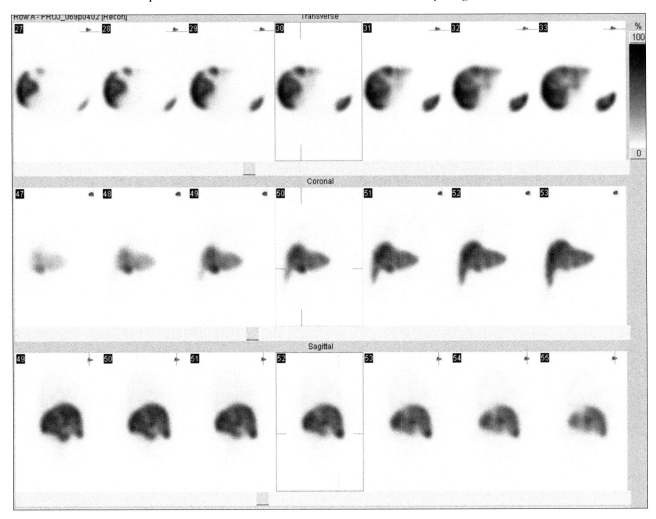

A. Hepatic adenoma
B. Solitary metastasis
C. Cavernous hemangioma
D. Hepatocellular carcinoma
E. Focal nodular hyperplasia

12 Which of the following is an indication for pretreatment with sincalide in a patient undergoing hepatobiliary scintigraphy?

A. Total parenteral nutrition
B. Fasting <24 hours
C. Fasting <2 hours
D. Biliary atresia
E. Biliary jaundice

13 The HIDA scan below is from a 26-year-old female with acute abdominal pain. Findings on the imaging are highly suggestive of what entity?

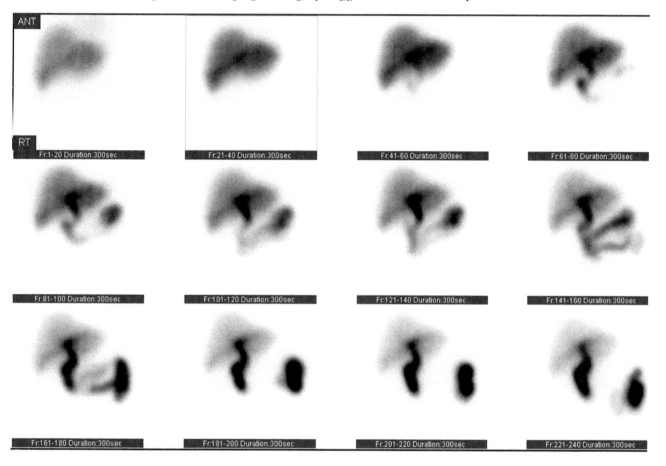

A. Partial common bile duct obstruction
B. Chronic cholecystitis
C. Acute cholecystitis
D. Pancreatitis
E. Bile leak

14 According to the most recent and best-validated prospective randomized study, what is the recommended infusion of sincalide that results in the least variability of the gallbladder ejection fraction in the healthy subjects?

A. 0.02 μg/kg infusion over 15 minutes
B. 0.02 μg/kg infusion over 30 minutes
C. 0.02 μg/kg infusion over 60 minutes
D. 0.02 μg/kg infusion over 90 minutes

15 Besides functional gallbladder disease, what can give delayed biliary to bowel transit?

A. Hypertension
B. Acute cholecystitis
C. Opiates
D. Hypothyroidism

16a A 52-year-old lady presents with elevated liver function tests. Ultrasound demonstrated gallbladder wall thickening and sludge. Based on the provided images, what is the most appropriate next step?

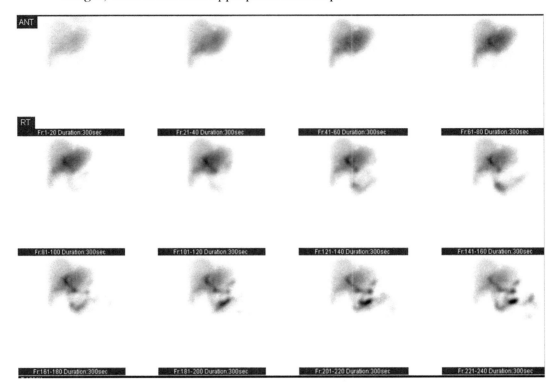

A. Acquire 24-hour delayed imaging
B. Recommend CT of the abdomen with IV contrast
C. Administer morphine
D. Administer booster dose
E. Administer phenobarbital

16b Postmorphine images of the same patient are shown below. What is the diagnosis?

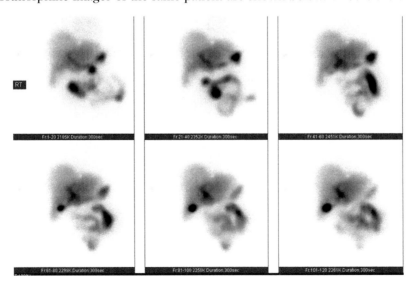

A. Bile leak
B. Focal nodular hyperplasia
C. Acute cholecystitis
D. Chronic cholecystitis

17 A 54-year-old female with a history of alcohol abuse presents for further evaluation with hepatobiliary scintigraphy (HIDA scan) due to right upper quadrant pain. What is the most likely diagnosis?

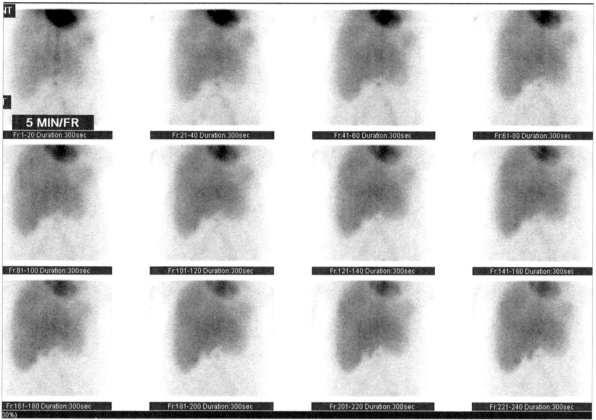

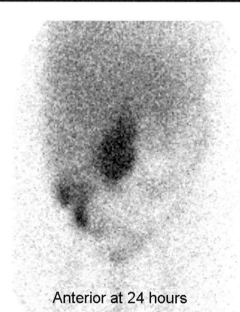

A. Common bile duct obstruction
B. Hepatocellular carcinoma
C. Cholecystitis
D. Pancreatitis
E. Hepatitis
F. Cirrhosis

18 What is the most likely diagnosis in this patient with the clinical history of a recent liver transplant?

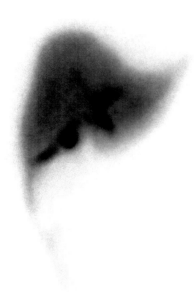

A. Biliary obstruction
B. Malignant ascites
C. Normal study
D. Biliary leak
E. Hepatic hydrothorax
F. Choledochoenteric fistula

19 The following images are from hepatobiliary scintigraphy performed on a 66-year-old gentleman with right upper quadrant pain. What is the most appropriate next step in management?

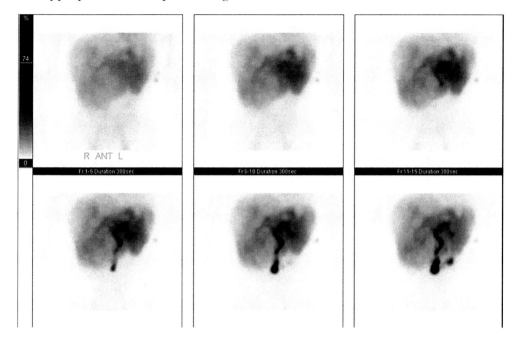

A. SPECT CT imaging

B. Surgical consultation for cholecystectomy

C. Contrast-enhanced CT of the abdomen and pelvis

D. Right upper quadrant ultrasound

20 A 47-year-old gentleman with cirrhosis and recurrent ascites presents for evaluation of his LeVeen/Denver shunt. Based on the supplied images below, what radiopharmaceutical was injected into the peritoneal cavity to evaluate the shunt function.

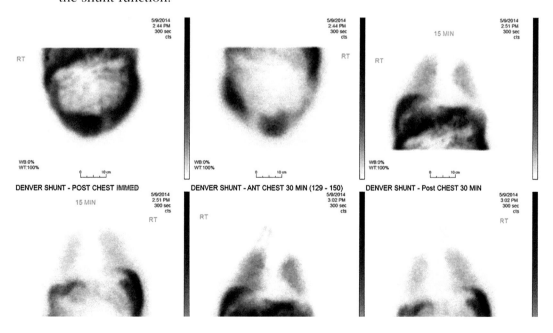

A. TC-99m sulfur colloid

B. Tc-99m DTPA

C. Tc-99m MAA

D. Tc-99m pertechnetate

21 A 26-year-old patient admitted after a motor vehicle accident undergoes a HIDA scan for right upper quadrant pain. Based on the following images, what is the most likely diagnosis?

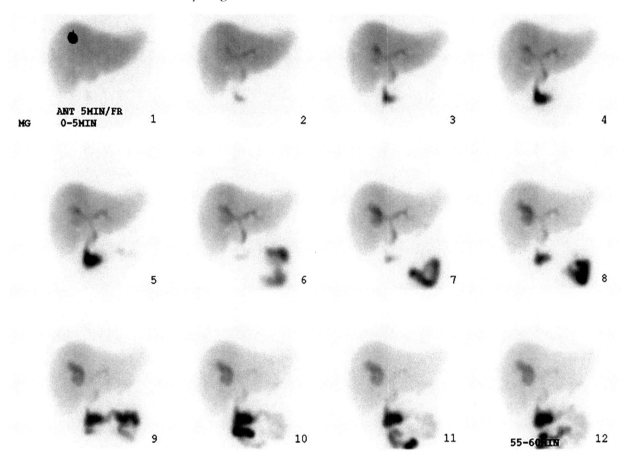

A. Cholangiocarcinoma
B. Metastasis
C. Hemangioma
D. Biloma
E. Hepatocellular carcinoma

ANSWERS AND EXPLANATIONS

1 **Answer A.** Gastric emptying study is commonly performed for the evaluation of gastroparesis. While it had been the standard for measuring gastric emptying, the gastric emptying study suffered from a lack of standardization regarding the meal composition, patient positioning, as well as the frequency and duration of imaging across the country. This prompted the American Neurogastroenterology and Motility Society and the Society of Nuclear Medicine and Molecular Imaging to publish consensus recommendations for standardizing these parameters in 2008. The meal's composition affects gastric emptying, with meals in high fat and protein content emptying slower than those composed of mainly simple carbohydrates. To reduce this variability, the composition of the meal was standardized. Approximately 1 mCi of Tc-99m sulfur colloid (SC) is cooked with 4 oz of egg whites only and served with 2 slices of bread, 30 g of strawberry jam, and 120 mL of water. Tc-99m SC remains bound to the ovalbumin in the egg white and does not dissociate into the liquid when in the stomach, thus allowing for accurate measurement of the solid emptying. Anterior and posterior planar images with the distal esophagus, stomach, and small bowel in the field of view are acquired for 1 minute immediately after the meal ingestion and at a minimum of 1 hour, 2 hours, and 4 hours after the meal ingestion with the patient standing upright. The images should be acquired with the same camera.

References: Abell TL, Camilleri M, Donohoe K, et al. Consensus recommendations for gastric emptying scintigraphy: a joint report of the American Neurogastroenterology and Motility Society and the Society of Nuclear Medicine. *Am J Gastroenterol* 2008;103(3):753–763.

O'Malley JP, Ziessman HA, Thrall JH. *Nuclear medicine: the requisites*, 5th ed. Philadelphia, PA: Saunders, 2020:220–229.

2 **Answer D.** While counts from the left anterior oblique (LAO) projection can be used as an alternative, geometric mean (GM) is the more accurate and preferred method of the two. If you only have one camera head, your best option is to take the anterior image immediately followed by the posterior image. The second-best option would be the LAO projection.

Anterior and posterior views allow for the calculation of the geometric mean (GM) using the following formula: geometric mean = square root (anterior counts × posterior counts). GM more accurately represents the amount of tracer in the stomach since it accounts for the posterior-to-anterior movement of the food as it travels from the fundus to the antrum, thus allowing for mathematical attenuation correction. With a dual-head gamma camera, anterior and posterior data are obtained simultaneously.

References: Abell TL, Camilleri M, Donohoe K, et al. Consensus recommendations for gastric emptying scintigraphy: a joint report of the American Neurogastroenterology and Motility Society and the Society of Nuclear Medicine. *Am J Gastroenterol* 2008;103(3):753–763.

O'Malley JP, Ziessman HA, Thrall JH. *Nuclear medicine: the requisites*, 5th ed. Philadelphia, PA: Saunders, 2020:220–229.

3 **Answer E.** The half-life of Tc-99m sulfur colloid is 6 hours. Given that the standard protocol for gastric emptying study requires imaging for 4 hours, one must correct for radioactive decay to ensure that accurate count statistics are used to determine the gastric retention/emptying. Uniformity and linearity are quality control measures that are done on a daily and weekly basis, respectively. The center of rotation calibration matches the axis of camera rotation to the center of the image matrix. This quality control is for SPECT imaging and is typically performed every month.

References: Abell TL, Camilleri M, Donohoe K, et al. Consensus recommendations for gastric emptying scintigraphy: a joint report of the American Neurogastroenterology and Motility Society and the Society of Nuclear Medicine. *Am J Gastroenterol* 2008;103(3):753–763.

O'Malley JP, Ziessman HA, Thrall JH. *Nuclear medicine: the requisites*, 5th ed. Philadelphia, PA: Saunders, 2020:220–229.

4 **Answer A.** Liquid normally empties from the stomach in a monoexponential pattern soon after it enters the stomach, as shown by the curve in choice A. On the other hand, ingested solid food gets converted into smaller particles (chyme) by mechanical grinding and by chemical digestion before it begins to empty from the stomach. The length of time required for this to occur is referred to as the lag phase, a period of time when there is no significant emptying of the solids from the stomach. It usually lasts for 5 to 20 minutes. Once initiated, the emptying of the solid food from the stomach normally occurs in a linear fashion. As such, a normal solid gastric emptying curve would look like that seen on choice D.

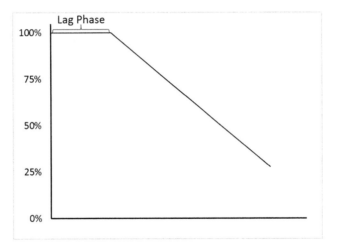

References: Mettler FA, Guiberteau MJ. *Essentials of nuclear medicine imaging*, 7th ed. Philadelphia, PA: Saunders, 2019:236–239.

O'Malley JP, Ziessman HA, Thrall JH. *Nuclear medicine: the requisites*, 5th ed. Philadelphia, PA: Saunders, 2020:220–229.

5 **Answer B.** Normal values for the standardized solid meal gastric emptying study are shown in the table below. Forty-three percent remaining activity in the stomach at 4 hours suggests gastroparesis. The 4-hour time point is more sensitive for the detection of delayed gastric emptying compared to the 2-hour time point. In this patient, 47% remaining at 2 hours would have been normal, and the diagnosis of gastroparesis would have been missed if 4-hour imaging was not acquired. Gastric hypermotility is suggested if there is <30% retention at 1 hour (>70% emptying).

It is important to know the causes of false-positive and false-negative gastric emptying study. Opiate analgesic medications (e.g., morphine, codeine, Demerol, and oxycodone), calcium channel blockers, antacids, and anticholinergic agents delay gastric emptying (GE); they can result in a false-positive study if not discontinued for the appropriate amount of time prior to the examination. Prokinetics such as domperidone and metoclopramide

(Reglan) may lead to a false-negative GE study in a patient with gastroparesis and should be stopped before the study as well. Serotonin receptor (5-HT-3) antagonists, such as ondansetron, have little effect on GE and may be given for severe symptoms of nausea and vomiting before the GE study. Insulin-dependent diabetics should be scheduled for an early morning study and should generally take 1/2 of their usual morning insulin dose, followed by the radiolabeled meal. Patients on oral hypoglycemic should be instructed to take their usual morning dose of hypoglycemic medication shortly before the radiolabeled meal. Since hyperglycemia may delay gastric emptying independently, the study should be rescheduled if the fasting blood glucose level is >200 mg/dL.

Normal Values for Standardized Solid Gastric Emptying Study		
Time	% Gastric Retention	% Gastric Emptying
1 h	<90 but >30	>10 but <70
2 h	<60	>40
4 h	<10	>90

References: Abell TL, Camilleri M, Donohoe K, et al. Consensus recommendations for gastric emptying scintigraphy: a joint report of the American Neurogastroenterology and Motility Society and The Society of Nuclear Medicine. *Am J Gastroenterol* 2008;103(3):753–763.

O'Malley JP, Ziessman HA, Thrall JH. *Nuclear medicine: the requisites*, 5th ed. Philadelphia, PA: Saunders, 2020:220–229.

6 **Answer C.** Since gastrointestinal (GI) bleeding can be an intermittent process, a tagged red blood cell (RBC) study helps identify patients who are bleeding at the time of examination (thus suitable for angiography) and helps localize the probable site of bleeding. Dynamic acquisition and review of images in the cine mode allows for better localization and increased sensitivity. GI bleeding is marked by (1) accumulation of radiolabeled RBCs outside the normal area of the vascular blood pool, (2) increasing intensity over time, and (3) movement within the bowel either in an antegrade or in a retrograde direction. At 10 minutes (frame 2), focal uptake in the hepatic flexure is seen, which increases in intensity over time, conforms to the large bowel, and moves in the antegrade and retrograde directions. This area is typically supplied by the superior mesenteric artery (SMA). The SMA supplies the bowel from the second portion of the duodenum as far distally as the splenic flexure of the transverse colon. The celiac artery supplies the distal esophagus, stomach, and the first portion of the duodenum. The inferior mesenteric artery (IMA) supplies from the distal third of the transverse colon to the proximal rectum. Accurate localization of GI bleeding on tagged RBC study helps direct the interventional radiologist to a specific vascular territory. This allows for prompt localization, reduced contrast load, reduced procedure time, and reduced patient radiation exposure. Quick localization should also minimize the chance that intermittent bleeding would have stopped by the time of contrast injection.

References: Mettler FA, Guiberteau MJ. *Essentials of nuclear medicine imaging*, 7th ed. Philadelphia, PA: Saunders, 2019:220–223.

O'Malley JP, Ziessman HA, Thrall JH. *Nuclear medicine: the requisites*, 5th ed. Philadelphia, PA: Saunders, 2020:242–246.

7 **Answer B.** A small focus of intense uptake is seen in the left upper quadrant on the posterior image of this heat-damaged Tc-99m–tagged red blood cell

(RBC) scan. This is consistent with an accessory spleen or residual splenic tissue. Removal of abnormal erythrocytes by the reticuloendothelial system is the basis for denatured RBC uptake by the functioning splenic tissue. In this study, the Tc-99m–labeled RBCs are heat damaged for 20 minutes in a water bath at 49°C to 50°C. This causes them to become rigid spherocytes that, upon reinjection, are phagocytosed by the reticuloendothelial system. Normal physiologic distribution of denatured RBCs is in the liver, spleen, and bone marrow. In cases of ITP, recurrence after splenectomy prompts an evaluation for residual splenic tissue. This examination can also be used in the diagnosis of splenosis after trauma (arrows in the image below).

Tc-99m sulfur colloid (SC) is taken up by the reticuloendothelial system and is commonly used for the evaluation of residual splenic tissue as well. Only 5% to 10% of the injected SC localizes in the normal spleen; 80% to 90% is sequestered by the liver, and <5% localizes in the bone marrow. This high liver uptake makes evaluation of the splenic tissue adjacent to the liver parenchyma difficult. Heat-damaged Tc-99m–labeled red blood cell (RBC) scan is more sensitive for the evaluation of residual splenic tissue as the denatured RBCs are sequestered by the splenic tissue in high concentration. This is due to their larger size compared to SC. Relatively higher uptake of denatured RBCs by the splenic tissue compared to the liver allows for better differentiation of a splenule from the adjacent liver parenchyma.

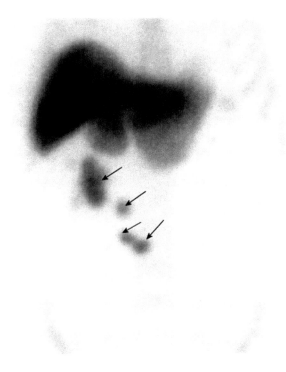

References: Mettler FA, Guiberteau MJ. *Essentials of nuclear medicine imaging*, 7th ed. Philadelphia, PA: Saunders, 2019:220.

O'Malley JP, Ziessman HA, Thrall JH. *Nuclear medicine: the requisites*, 5th ed. Philadelphia, PA: Saunders, 2020:218–219.

8 **Answer D.** The supplied images demonstrate persistent diffuse radiotracer uptake in the stomach, which does not move. The blood pool activity is markedly reduced. Activity is also seen in the renal collecting system and bladder (more so than usual). The findings are consistent with free pertechnetate. Gastric mucosal, salivary gland, thyroid gland, and renal activities are seen when free Tc-99m pertechnetate is present. When free Tc-99m pertechnetate is suspected, an image of the thyroid and salivary glands should be obtained to confirm that it is the source of this artifact (see below). Of the methods for labeling autologous RBCs, the in vivo technique has the worst labeling efficiency (~75%) and higher chance of free pertechnetate. This can be avoided by using the in vitro RBC-labeling method (labeling efficiency of 98%) and performing quality control to check for the free pertechnetate. In the event of gastric hemorrhage, a significant amount of activity would transit into the small bowel on the subsequent images.

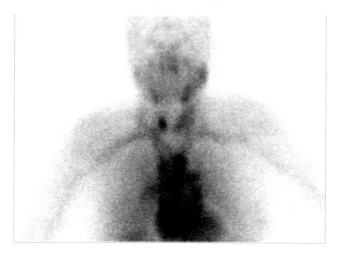

Reference: O'Malley JP, Ziessman HA, Thrall JH. *Nuclear medicine: the requisites*, 5th ed. Philadelphia, PA: Saunders, 2020:242–246.

9 **Answer B.** Tc-99m–tagged RBC scintigraphy has a high sensitivity in detecting bleeding rates as low as 0.04 to 0.2 mL/minute, although a total volume of 2 to 3 mL is necessary for scintigraphic detection. Comparatively, angiography will locate GI bleeding sites in up to 65% of cases when bleeding occurs at a rate >1 mL/minute. Also, the bleeding must be occurring during the 20 to 30 seconds of contrast injection for the angiography to localize the bleeding site. Compared to angiography, tagged RBC scintigraphy is easy to perform, requires no patient preparation, and is noninvasive. It also provides prognostic information as patients with negative scintigraphy will rarely require urgent surgery. CT angiography is less sensitive than tagged RBC but more sensitive than conventional angiography with an ability to detect bleeding at the rate of 0.3 to 0.5 mL/minute. CT angiography has the added ability to detect other causes of GI bleeding such as a tumor, diverticulosis, etc.

References: Mettler FA, Guiberteau MJ. *Essentials of nuclear medicine imaging*, 7th ed. Philadelphia, PA: Saunders, 2019:220–223.

O'Malley JP, Ziessman HA, Thrall JH. *Nuclear medicine: the requisites*, 5th ed. Philadelphia, PA: Saunders, 2020:237–250.

Wells ML, Hansel SL, Bruining DH, et al. CT for evaluation of acute gastrointestinal bleeding. *Radiographics* 2018;38(4):1089–1107.

10 **Answer C.** The anterior and posterior projection images from a 90-minute delayed Tc-99m RBC scan demonstrate intense physiologic activity in the blood pool and spleen with mild-to-moderate physiologic activity in the liver and kidneys. A moderate-sized focus of intense uptake in the lateral segment of the left hepatic lobe (arrow in the anterior image below) is consistent with a hemangioma.

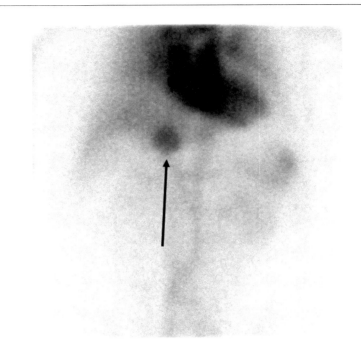

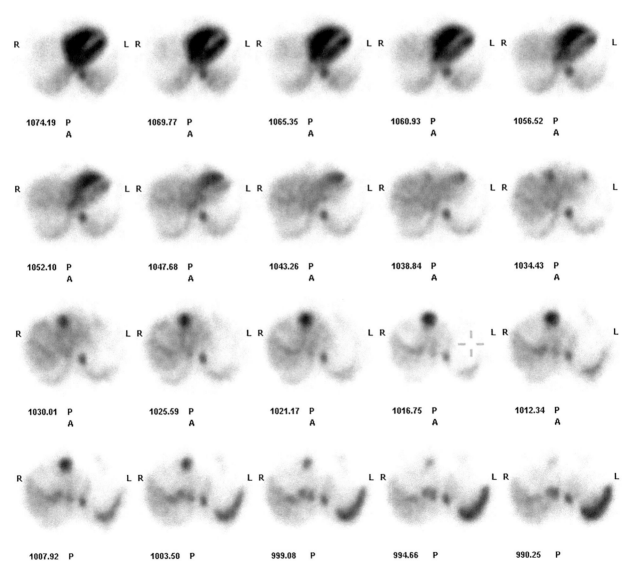

1074.19 P A	1069.77 P A	1065.35 P A	1060.93 P A	1056.52 P A
1052.10 P A	1047.68 P A	1043.26 P A	1038.84 P A	1034.43 P A
1030.01 P A	1025.59 P A	1021.17 P A	1016.75 P A	1012.34 P A
1007.92 P	1003.50 P	999.08 P	994.66 P	990.25 P

On the Tc-99m RBC scan, hemangioma generally has decreased intensity compared to the adjacent liver on the early flow images and increased intensity compared to the adjacent liver on the 90- to 120-minute delayed images. Radiotracer uptake of hemangioma is often equal to that of the blood pool, but heterogeneous uptake can be seen with giant cavernous hemangioma. Tc-99m RBC scintigraphy has a near 100% positive predictive value for diagnosing hemangioma. Other lesions present as areas of reduced tracer uptake ("cold") on the tagged RBC scans.

The most common cause of a false-negative Tc-99m RBC scintigraphy for hemangioma is its small size. Performing SPECT significantly improves the sensitivity of tagged RBC scan for hemangioma detection when compared to the planar imaging, especially if the lesions measure <2.5 to 3.0 cm in diameter. The SPECT imaging using Tc-99m RBCs has close to 100% sensitivity for lesions >1.5 cm in diameter, which decreases to <50% for lesions <1 cm. SPECT imaging also helps in confirming the anatomic localization of central lesions and allows for better differentiation from adjacent vascular structures. Other reported causes of false-negative study include the hemangioma being adjacent to a vascular structure (such as the heart, portal vein, or IVC), extensive fibrosis within the hemangioma, and perceived increased activity on the flow images.

Diagnostic features of hemangioma on multiphase liver CT or MRI include discontinuous peripheral nodular enhancement with progressive filling in on later phases with contrast enhancement following that of the vasculature. Tc-99m RBC scans are typically used when CT or MRI characteristics are not diagnostic or when contrast is contraindicated.

References: Mettler FA, Guiberteau MJ. *Essentials of nuclear medicine imaging*, 7th ed. Philadelphia, PA: Saunders, 2019:218–219.

O'Malley JP, Ziessman HA, Thrall JH. *Nuclear medicine: the requisites*, 5th ed. Philadelphia, PA: Saunders, 2020:211, 214.

11 **Answer E.** The SPECT images from a Tc-99m sulfur colloid (SC) scintigraphy demonstrate physiologic radiopharmaceutical distribution in the liver and spleen. Unlike Tc-99m RBC scintigraphy (used to diagnose cavernous hemangioma), there is no activity in the blood pool (aorta, IVC, or heart). The supplied images show a lesion with increased tracer uptake (more than that of the adjacent liver) in the medial segment of the left hepatic lobe (arrows in the image below). This is consistent with focal nodular hyperplasia (FNH). The liver spleen scan using Tc-99m SC is a specific but nonsensitive method for diagnosing FNH. Approximately 40% of the FNHs demonstrate increased radiotracer uptake, 30% demonstrate uptake similar to the remaining liver parenchyma, while the remaining 30% demonstrate decreased uptake. Other causes of focal "hot spots" on Tc-99m SC scintigraphy include regenerating nodules, hot quadrate lobe (seen with SVC/innominate vein obstruction), and hot caudate lobe (seen with the Budd-Chiari syndrome). A lesion without functioning Kupffer cells would demonstrate decreased SC uptake (i.e., cyst, hemangioma, hepatic adenoma, hepatoma, and metastasis). Contrast-enhanced MRI has a reported sensitivity of approximately 70% with a specificity of 98% for FNH.

For the Tc-99m SC scan, approximately 2 to 6 mCi of SC is injected intravenously. It undergoes rapid clearance from the intravascular space by the reticuloendothelial system with the intravascular half time of about 2 to 3 minutes. The majority (>98.4%) of the radiopharmaceutical would be removed from the intravascular blood pool in six half-lives (18 minutes). As such, imaging is usually commenced 20 minutes after the IV injection of

Tc-99m SC. The average particle size of the Tc-99m sulfur colloid (SC) is about 0.3 to 1.0 μm. Given its particulate nature, Tc-99m SC is phagocytosed by the reticuloendothelial system: Kupffer cells in the liver and macrophages in the spleen and bone marrow.

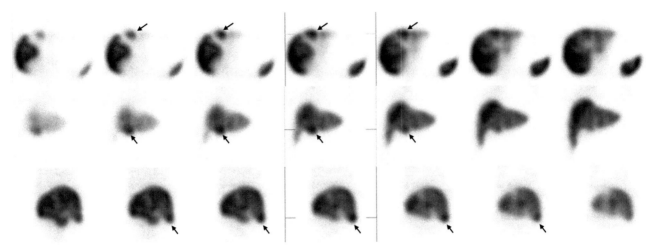

References: Mettler FA, Guiberteau MJ. *Essentials of nuclear medicine imaging*, 7th ed. Philadelphia, PA: Saunders, 2019:214–217.

O'Malley JP, Ziessman HA, Thrall JH. *Nuclear medicine: the requisites*, 5th ed. Philadelphia, PA: Saunders, 2020:213–218.

12 **Answer A.** Prolonged fasting and recent meal are some of the common causes of false-positive hepatobiliary scintigraphy. When the patient fasts for more than 24 hours, lack of endogenous CCK secretion/stimulation results in lack of gallbladder contraction. As such, gallbladder fills with viscous bile, resulting in increased intracholecystic pressure and lack of backflow of radiotracer into the gallbladder. In order to minimize the potential of a false-positive study, patients who have fasted for longer than 24 hours, are on parenteral hyperalimentation, or have a severe intercurrent illness should be pretreated with a 30- to 60-minute infusion of 0.02 μg/kg of sincalide 15 to 30 minutes before the injection of the hepatobiliary radiotracer. Sincalide is a polypeptide analog of CCK. It increases biliary secretion by contracting the gallbladder and relaxing the sphincter of Oddi.

Recent meal within 2 hours would result in gallbladder contraction; if the gallbladder is contracted at the time of examination, it will not fill in with radiotracer and result in a false-positive examination. As such, fasting for at least 2 hours, preferably 4 to 6 hours, should be required prior to the initiation of hepatobiliary scintigraphy.

Reference: Tulchinsky M, Ciak BW, Delbeke D, et al. SNM practice guideline for hepatobiliary scintigraphy 4.0. *J Nucl Med Technol* 2010;38(4):210–218.

13 **Answer C.** Sequential anterior images acquired for 60 minutes after the IV administration of Tc-99m mebrofenin demonstrate prompt clearance of blood pool activity within 5 minutes (normal <10 minutes), hepatic ducts are visualized at 15 minutes (normal <20 minutes), and common bile duct/ duodenum are visualized by 20 minutes (normal for CBD <30 minutes and for bowel <60 minutes). The gallbladder is not visualized. Increased radiopharmaceutical uptake is identified in a curvilinear fashion within the hepatic parenchyma adjacent to the gallbladder fossa (arrowheads in the image below). This is known as the rim sign. It is felt to be secondary to a combination of hyperemia from the inflammation (resulting in increased radiotracer delivery) and possible obstruction of biliary radicals owing to the inflammation. When present, it is a reliable indicator of acute cholecystitis, and no further imaging (delayed time point or postmorphine augmentation) is necessary. The rim sign indicates severe late-stage acute cholecystitis and has been associated with phlegmonous or gangrenous acute cholecystitis. The benefit of reporting this finding is that open cholecystectomy rather than routine laparoscopic cholecystectomy may be favored in these patients. Also seen is a cystic duct sign (arrow in the image below) where a small meniscus of activity is seen in the cystic duct distal to the obstruction.

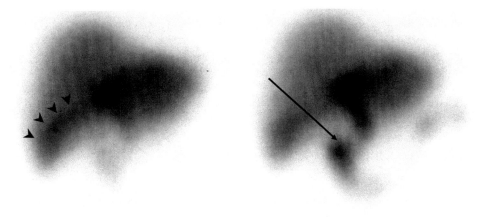

References: Mettler FA, Guiberteau MJ. *Essentials of nuclear medicine imaging*, 7th ed. Philadelphia, PA: Saunders, 2019:226–228.

O'Malley JP, Ziessman HA, Thrall JH. *Nuclear medicine: the requisites*, 5th ed. Philadelphia, PA: Saunders, 2020:190–192.

Tulchinsky M, Colletti PM, Allen TW. Hepatobiliary scintigraphy in acute cholecystitis. *Semin Nucl Med* 2012;42(2):84–100.

14 **Answer C.** In a study by Ziessman et al. published in 2010, a sincalide infusion of 0.02 µg/kg over 60 minutes resulted in the least variability and best-defined normal values of gallbladder ejection fraction (GBEF) in healthy volunteers. The calculated lower range of normal GBEF for 60-minute infusion was 38% (first percentile).

A prospective randomized investigation by Yap et al. utilized a 45-minute infusion of sincalide at a rate of 0.02 µg/kg/h with GBEF calculated at 1 hour. In this study, abnormal EF of <40% correlated well with the presence of chronic acalculous gallbladder disease and alleviation of the patient's symptoms after cholecystectomy. Reduced GBEF in response to sincalide, however, is a nonspecific finding, and correlation with the patient's presentation/clinical history is critical. Besides chronic gallbladder disease, it has been associated with acute medical illness from other causes, irritable bowel syndrome, obesity, achalasia, truncal vagotomy, as well as several medications (e.g., morphine, atropine, calcium channel blockers, octreotide, progesterone, indomethacin, theophylline, benzodiazepines, and histamine 2 receptor antagonists).

References: Yap L, Wycherley AG, Morphett AD, et al. Acalculous biliary pain: cholecystectomy alleviates symptoms in patients with abnormal cholescintigraphy. *Gastroenterology* 1991;101:786–793.

Ziessman HA, Tulchinsky M, Lavely WC, et al. Sincalide-stimulated cholescintigraphy: a multicenter investigation to determine optimal infusion methodology and gallbladder ejection fraction normal values. *J Nucl Med* 2010;51(2):277–281.

15 **Answer C.** Morphine and other opiates constrict the sphincter of Oddi and may delay the biliary to bowel transit. The practice guidelines recommend delaying hepatobiliary scintigraphy for the time equal to four half-lives of the opiate used. Delayed biliary to bowel transit is commonly associated with chronic cholecystitis/functional gallbladder disease. However, by itself, it is not diagnostic as it can be seen in up to 20% of the normal population as well as in patients with diabetes, pregnancy, truncal vagotomy, progesterone, and oral contraceptives. Partial common bile duct obstruction and severe hepatic dysfunction would also present with delayed biliary to bowel transit. As such, an attempt should be made to assess the patient's history, clinical presentation, and medications to help determine the specific cause.

References: Mettler FA, Guiberteau MJ. *Essentials of nuclear medicine imaging*, 7th ed. Philadelphia, PA: Saunders, 2019:224–225.

O'Malley JP, Ziessman HA, Thrall JH. *Nuclear medicine: the requisites*, 5th ed. Philadelphia, PA: Saunders, 2020:190–198.

Tulchinsky M, Ciak BW, Delbeke D, et al. SNM practice guideline for hepatobiliary scintigraphy 4.0. *J Nucl Med Technol* 2010;38(4):210–218.

16a **Answer C.** Images from hepatobiliary scintigraphy (HBS) demonstrate nonvisualization of the gallbladder at 60 minutes. This is a nonspecific finding and can be seen with acute cholecystitis, chronic cholecystitis, or physiologic failure of the gallbladder to fill with the radiotracer (e.g., GB contraction from a recent meal or CCK administration, fasting for >24 to 48 hours, severely ill or postoperative patients). In most of these cases, a specific diagnosis can be made based on the patient's clinical presentation. If not, and when the gallbladder is not visualized within 60 minutes, either 3- to 4-hour delayed images or images with morphine augmentation (0.04 mg/kg, maximum 3 mg) may be obtained. The radiotracer must be present in the intrahepatic biliary tree, common bile duct, and the small bowel prior to morphine injection. Morphine increases the tone of the sphincter of Oddi, in turn increasing the intraluminal bile duct pressure. This results in the backflow of the bile into the gallbladder if the cystic duct is patent. Contraindications to the use of morphine include increased intracranial pressure in children (absolute), respiratory depression in nonventilated patients (absolute), morphine allergy (absolute), and acute pancreatitis (relative). A second injection of the radiopharmaceutical, "booster dose," should be given at the end of the 60 minutes if there is an insufficient amount of radiotracer in the liver and biliary tree to permit the gallbladder visualization.

Phenobarbital, 5 mg/kg/day, may be given for 3 to 5 days before imaging infants in whom biliary atresia is suspected.

References: Mettler FA, Guiberteau MJ. *Essentials of nuclear medicine imaging*, 7th ed. Philadelphia, PA: Saunders, 2019:229.

O'Malley JP, Ziessman HA, Thrall JH. *Nuclear medicine: the requisites*, 5th ed. Philadelphia, PA: Saunders, 2020:190–198.

Tulchinsky M, Ciak BW, Delbeke D, et al. SNM practice guideline for hepatobiliary scintigraphy 4.0. *J Nucl Med Technol* 2010;38(4):210–218.

16b **Answer D.** Postmorphine images demonstrate radiotracer uptake in the gallbladder, excluding the diagnosis of acute cholecystitis. Delayed visualization of the gallbladder in the right clinical settings suggests chronic cholecystitis. Nonvisualization of the gallbladder within 30 minutes of morphine administration or on delayed 3- to 4-hour imaging would indicate acute cholecystitis. FNH will present as a lesion with increased radiopharmaceutical uptake on the HIDA scan as it contains functioning hepatocytes without connection into the biliary system. Activity in the left upper quadrant (adjacent to the left hepatic lobe) is from bile reflux into the stomach (double arrow in the image below) and not bile leak. Bile reflux that is marked and occurs in a symptomatic patient correlates strongly with bile gastritis. Of note, a relative regional decrease in activity along the superior lateral aspect of the right hepatic lobe (arrowheads in the image below) is secondary to breast attenuation artifact. A small area of photopenia at the junction of the left and right hepatic lobes in the hepatic dome (arrow in the image below) corresponded to a cyst on CT (not shown).

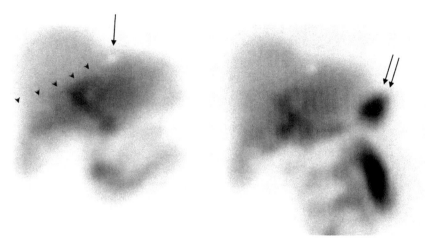

References: Mettler FA, Guiberteau MJ. *Essentials of nuclear medicine imaging*, 7th ed. Philadelphia, PA: Saunders, 2019:229.

O'Malley JP, Ziessman HA, Thrall JH. *Nuclear medicine: the requisites*, 5th ed. Philadelphia, PA: Saunders, 2020:190–198.

Tulchinsky M, Ciak BW, Delbeke D, et al. SNM practice guideline for hepatobiliary scintigraphy 4.0. *J Nucl Med Technol* 2010;38(4):210–218.

17 **Answer E.** The images demonstrate persistent blood pool activity (>60 minutes) consistent with severely impaired hepatic extraction. The liver is enlarged, and there is no excretion of the radiopharmaceutical into the bile ducts, the gallbladder, or the small bowel at 60 minutes. Differential considerations for poor hepatic extraction and biliary excretion include causes of hepatic dysfunction such as hepatitis or biliary obstruction. In this setting, delayed images should be obtained at 4 and/or 24 hours. The delayed 24-hour image demonstrates radiotracer in the gallbladder and small bowel, excluding acute cholecystitis and complete CBD obstruction, respectively. Delayed visualization of the gallbladder and small bowel, in this case, is most likely related to underlying poor liver function from acute alcoholic hepatitis. Delayed 24-hour imaging with hepatobiliary scintigraphy may be necessary in the setting of severe hepatocellular dysfunction, suspected common bile duct obstruction, or suspected biliary atresia because the hepatocellular dysfunction typically results in delayed extraction from the blood pool and excretion of the radiopharmaceutical into the biliary radicals, resulting in prolonged hepatic to biliary and hepatic to bowel transit times.

Reference: O'Malley JP, Ziessman HA, Thrall JH. *Nuclear medicine: the requisites*, 5th ed. Philadelphia, PA: Saunders, 2020:203.

18 **Answer D.** A single hepatobiliary scintigraphy (HBS) image demonstrates the pooling of the radiotracer in the gallbladder fossa, tracking along the inferior edge of the liver into the right paracolic gutter. This is consistent with a bile leak. Bile leak and biliary obstruction are two of the common complications after a liver transplant. A bile leak is present when the radiotracer is found in a location other than the liver, gallbladder, bile ducts, bowel, or urine. Using cinematic display or decubitus positioning may help with the diagnosis of a bile leak. Extravasation of a small quantity of bile occurs commonly after biliary surgery and is of little clinical significance. However, patients who develop profuse bilious drainage should be suspected of having a significant bile leak. Ultrasonography and CT detect the presence of fluid collections in these patients, but they cannot demonstrate if the collection communicates with the biliary tree. HBS can easily confirm bile leak as the etiology of the fluid collection (as opposed to infection, hemorrhage, or other postoperative fluid collections) and establish the primary route of bile flow. HBS is also useful in following these patients overtime to ensure the resolution of the leak.

References: Mettler FA, Guiberteau MJ. *Essentials of nuclear medicine imaging*, 7th ed. Philadelphia, PA: Saunders, 2019:231–235.

O'Malley JP, Ziessman HA, Thrall JH. *Nuclear medicine: the requisites*, 5th ed. Philadelphia, PA: Saunders, 2020:203.

19 **Answer C.** Sequential anterior images acquired after the IV administration of Tc-99m mebrofenin demonstrate markedly enlarged liver with heterogeneous radiotracer distribution. Focal areas of photopenia are noted throughout the liver and are more prominent along the superior aspect and in the right hepatic lobe (arrows in the image below). Normally there is homogeneous radiotracer uptake throughout the liver parenchyma. Any lesions that do not contain functioning hepatocytes (cysts, hemangioma, metastasis, and hepatocellular carcinoma, to name a few) will have decreased activity on the HIDA scan. Since hepatic adenoma and FNH contain functioning hepatocytes, these lesions will have increased activity on the HIDA scan. In this patient with markedly heterogeneous uptake and enlarged liver, the findings are highly suspicious for neoplasm. As such, contrast-enhanced CT to evaluate the liver lesions and potential primary would be the most appropriate next step. While right upper quadrant ultrasound may help confirm liver metastasis, CT scan has the added advantage of finding a potential primary malignancy. In this case, the medially displaced gallbladder due to right hepatic lobe enlargement fills with the radiotracer. Therefore, there is no need for cholecystectomy. Contrast-enhanced CT in this patient confirmed multiple liver metastases (shown below) with primary colon cancer (not shown).

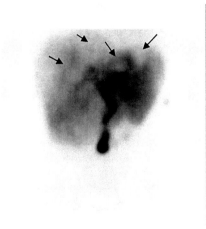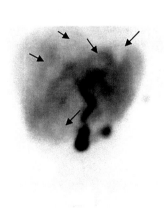

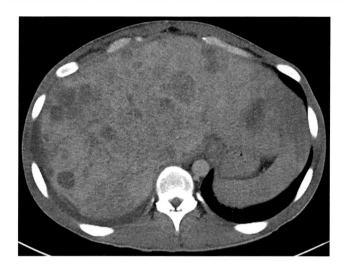

Reference: Mettler FA, Guiberteau MJ. *Essentials of nuclear medicine imaging*, 7th ed. Philadelphia, PA: Saunders, 2019:216.

20 **Answer C.** The acquired anterior images demonstrate the presence of radiopharmaceutical throughout the peritoneal cavity. Radiotracer is visualized in the lung on the chest images. Findings indicate a patent peritoneovenous shunt. Patients with recurrent ascites can be treated with a Denver or LeVeen peritoneovenous shunt, which transfer the fluid from the peritoneal cavity into the central vein through tubing with a one-way valve. This will take the fluid from the abdomen and transport it to the superior vena cava.

For evaluation of the shunt patency, the radiotracer is injected into the peritoneal cavity. The patient then rolls around on the table to distribute the radiopharmaceutical. Either Tc-99m sulfur colloid (SC) or macro aggregated albumin (MAA) can be utilized for this purpose. Physiologic distribution depends on which radiopharmaceutical is injected. If Tc-99m MAA is injected, it will get trapped in the pulmonary capillaries and will result in a visualization of the lungs (such as in this case). If Tc-99m SC is used and the shunt is functioning appropriately, the activity will be visualized in the liver. MAA is preferred over SC due to the potential of activity within the ascites making visualization of activity within the liver difficult. MAA and SC are used because they are large particles and will not diffuse into the blood pool through the peritoneal surfaces.

Reference: O'Malley JP, Ziessman HA, Thrall JH. *Nuclear medicine: the requisites*, 5th ed. Philadelphia, PA: Saunders, 2020:253–254.

21 **Answer D.** Sequential anterior images from the hepatobiliary scintigraphy demonstrate a moderate-sized area of progressive radiotracer accumulation within the right hepatic lobe, which increases in size and uptake throughout the examination. It appears to be in communication with the right bile duct. In a patient with a recent history of trauma, the imaging characteristics are most compatible with a biloma (see CT image below). Differential diagnosis of liver lesions with increased radiotracer uptake on hepatobiliary scintigraphy includes focal nodular hyperplasia and hepatic adenoma. Both of which contain functioning hepatocytes. Other liver lesions such as cyst, hemangioma, hepatocellular carcinoma, cholangiocarcinoma, and metastasis do not contain functioning hepatocytes. As such, they present as areas of photopenia on hepatobiliary scintigraphy.

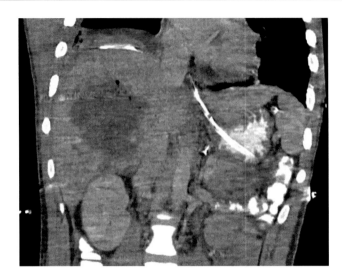

Reference: Habibian MR, Delbeke D, Martin WH, et al. *Nuclear medicine imaging: a teaching file*. Philadelphia, PA: LWW, 1999:276.

QUESTIONS

1 A 35-year-old potential renal transplant donor presents for the evaluation of glomerular filtration rate (GFR) as a part of the preoperative workup. Which of the following radiopharmaceuticals would be most appropriate to use in this situation?

A. MAG3
B. DTPA
C. DMSA
D. Glucoheptonate

2 In the following diagram of the renal nephron, where does DMSA localize on the 2- to 4-hour images acquired for the renal cortical imaging?

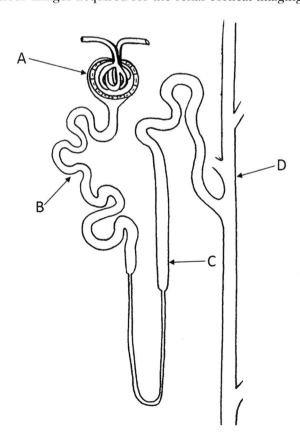

3 Based on the following renal function images and accompanying time–activity curve (renogram) from a MAG3 dynamic renography, what is the most likely diagnosis?

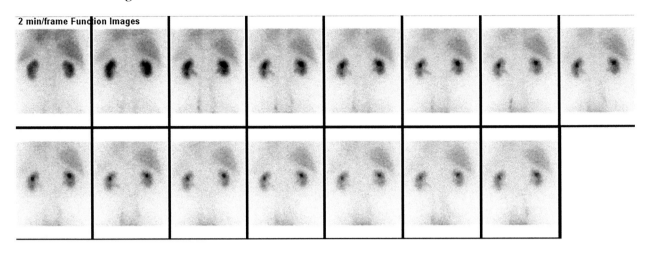

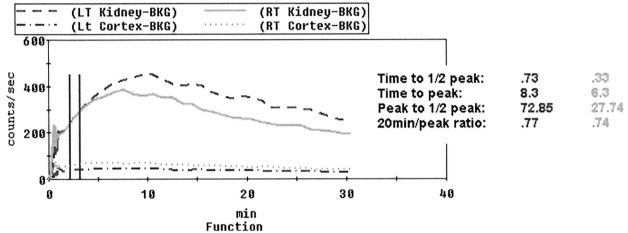

A. Normal renal function
B. Mildly impaired renal function
C. Moderately impaired renal function
D. Severely impaired renal function
E. Bilateral renal artery stenosis
F. Bilateral obstructive hydronephrosis

4 The following Tc-99m MAG3 functional renal scintigraphy images, as well as time–activity curves, are from a 60-year-old who was admitted with dehydration and elevated creatine kinase levels. What is the most likely diagnosis?

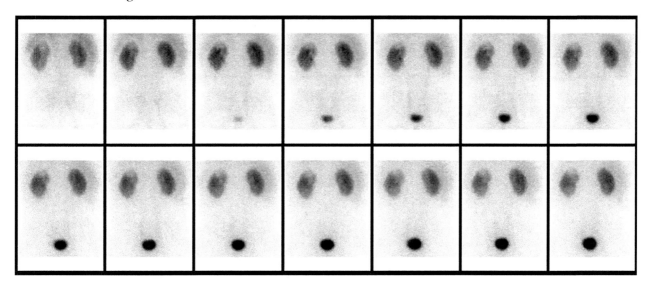

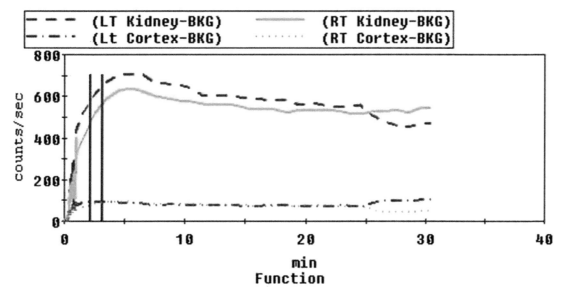

A. Acute tubular necrosis
B. Severe chronic renal disease
C. Bilateral hydronephrosis
D. Bilateral renal artery stenosis

5 In the setting of renal artery stenosis, how does the renin–angiotensin axis maintain the glomerular filtration rate (GFR)?

A. Afferent arteriolar vasoconstriction
B. Afferent arteriolar vasodilatation
C. Efferent arteriolar vasoconstriction
D. Efferent arteriolar vasodilatation
E. Diffuse dilation throughout the capillary bed
F. Diffuse constriction throughout the capillary bed

6   What is the most appropriate management in this patient with the following renal scintigraphy findings?

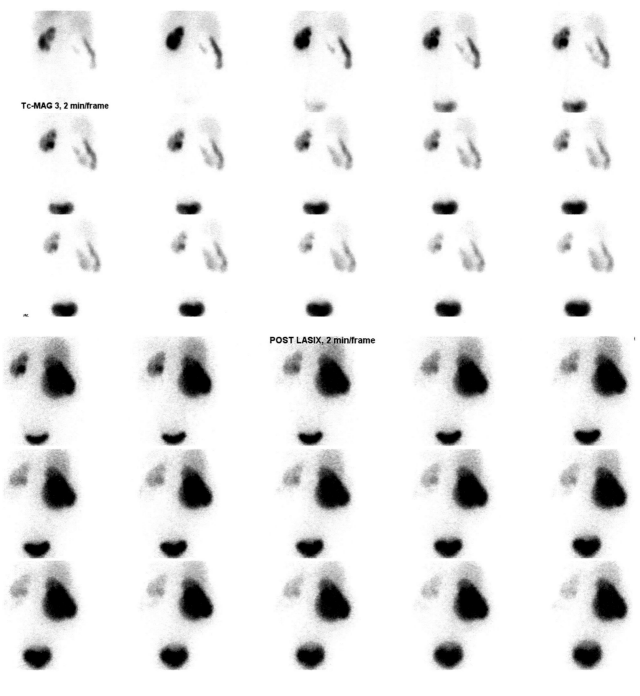

Tc-MAG 3, 2 min/frame

POST LASIX, 2 min/frame

A. Nephrectomy
B. Pyeloplasty
C. Ureteral reimplantation
D. Cystectomy
E. Ileal conduit

7 A 45-year-old lady with hypertension and back pain was found to have an abnormality on a recent contrast-enhanced CT scan. Based on the supplied images, which of the following is the most likely diagnosis?

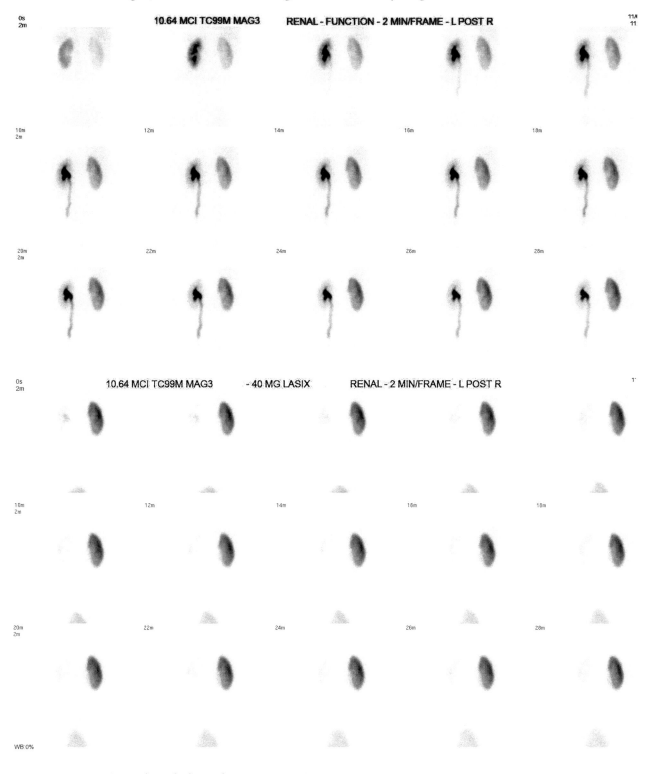

A. Right-sided renal artery stenosis
B. Right-sided hydronephrosis without obstruction
C. Right-sided high-grade obstruction
D. Left-sided renal artery stenosis
E. Left-sided hydronephrosis with obstruction
F. Left-sided high-grade obstruction

8   A 3-year-old male presents for further workup of left-sided hydronephrosis. Based on the following post-Lasix images and time–activity curve, what is the most appropriate next step?

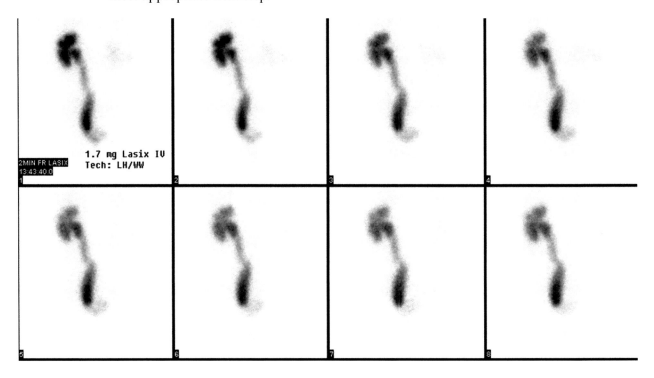

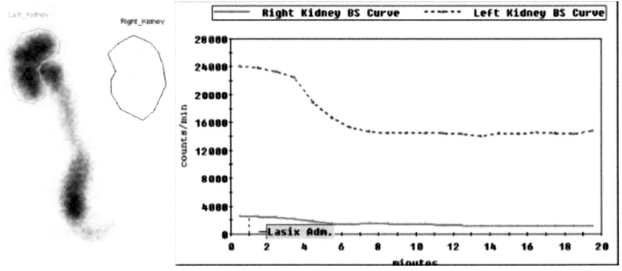

A. Do nothing; the study is diagnostic for hydronephrosis with obstruction.
B. Do nothing; the study is diagnostic for hydronephrosis without obstruction.
C. Do nothing; the study is indeterminate for obstruction.
D. Ask the technologist to reprocess the images.
E. Recommend correlation with a VCUG.
F. Recommend correlation with a contrast-enhanced CT.

9 Which of the following sets of renogram curves represent a positive study for renovascular hypertension using MAG3 or DTPA? The dotted line (– – –) represents the baseline, while the solid line represents the captopril study.

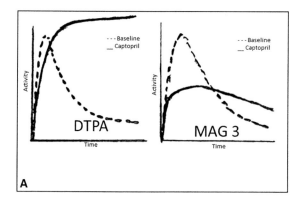

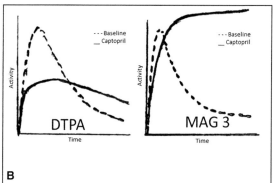

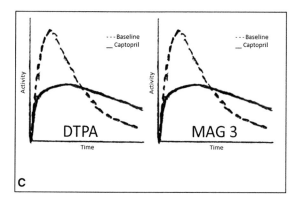

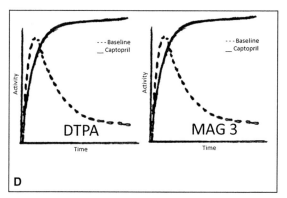

10 What is the most likely diagnosis in this patient with the following Tc-99m MAG3 captopril (top) and baseline (bottom) renography?

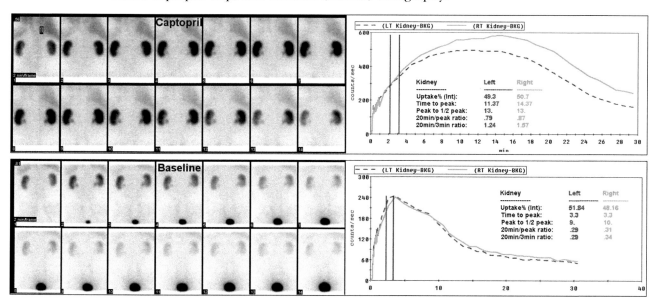

A. Severe hydronephrosis

B. Ca channel blocker intake

C. Beta-blocker intake

D. Alpha-blocker intake

11 The following images are from a 53-year-old who underwent renal scintigraphy to rule out obstruction. What is the most appropriate next step?

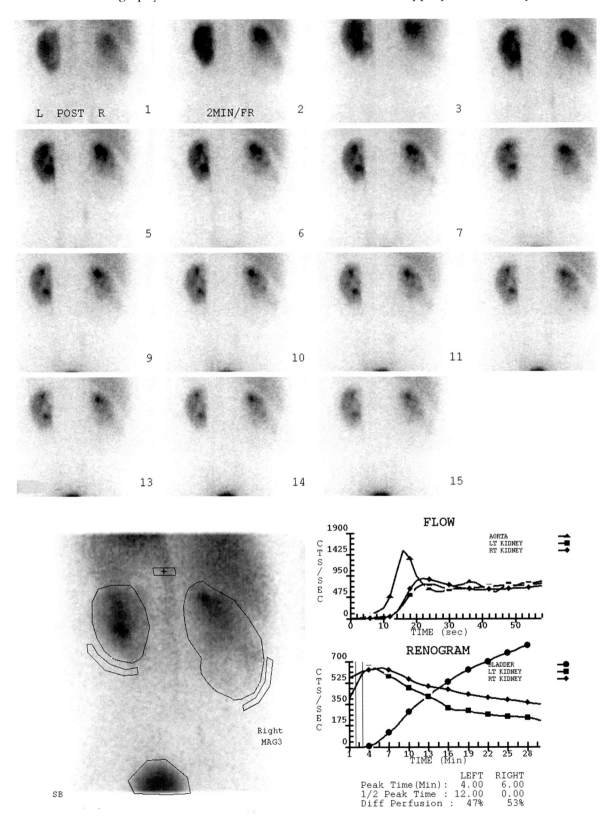

A. Administer Lasix.
B. Ask the technologist to reprocess the images.
C. Ask the technologist to provide anterior images.
D. Recommend ultrasound.

12 The following examination was performed on a 57-year-old who underwent renal transplantation a few days ago. What is your interpretation?

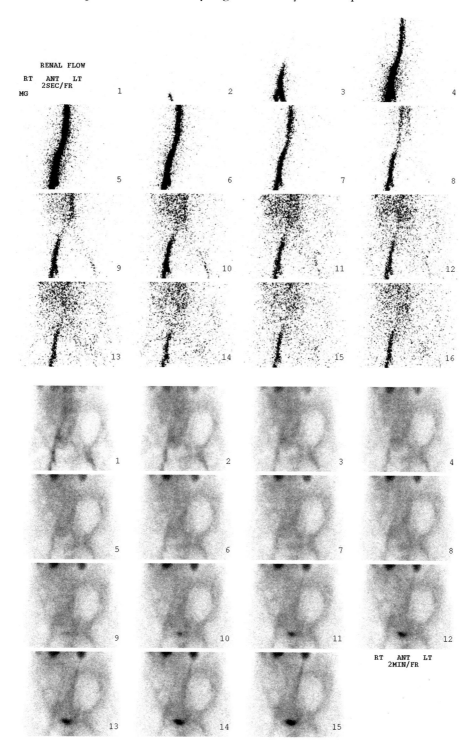

A. Left lower extremity deep venous thrombosis
B. Vasomotor nephropathy
C. Acute transplant rejection
D. Vascular occlusion
E. Hydronephrosis
F. Lymphocele
G. Hematoma

13 Two days after renal transplantation, a 45-year-old female presents with decreased urine output. What is the most likely diagnosis based on the following images?

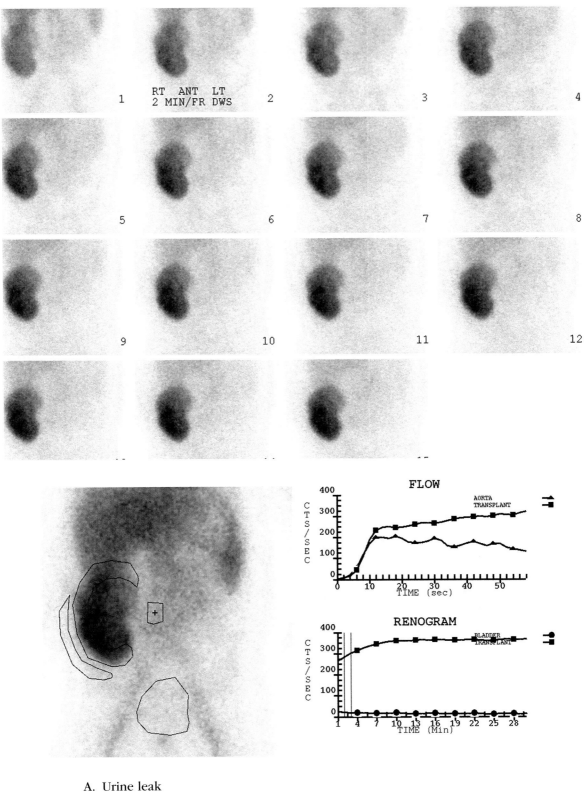

A. Urine leak

B. Lymphocele

C. Hydronephrosis

D. Vascular occlusion

E. Vasomotor nephropathy

F. Acute transplant rejection

14 The following renal scintigraphy images are from a 37-year-old woman with abdominal pain and decreased urine output. What is the most likely diagnosis?

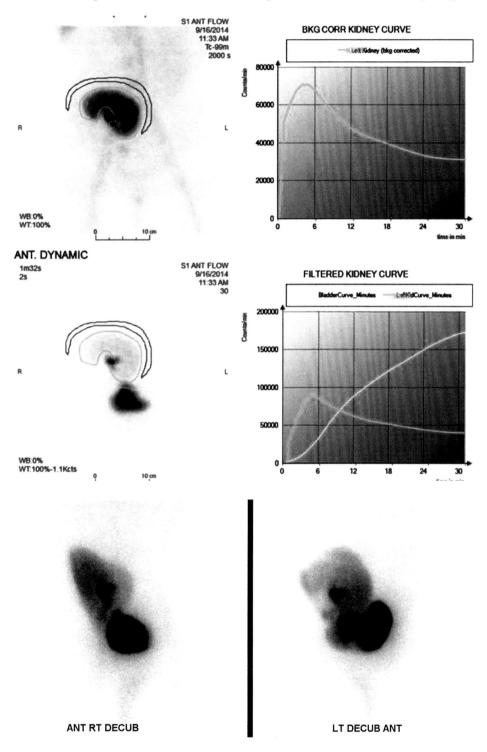

A. Normal
B. Urine leak
C. Lymphocele
D. Bowel uptake
E. Hydronephrosis
F. Vasomotor nephropathy
G. Acute transplant rejection

15 The following patient with a recently diagnosed enhancing soft tissue renal lesion on a recent CT undergoes evaluation with a Tc-99m sestamibi scan. What is the most likely diagnosis based on the provided SPECT/CT images?

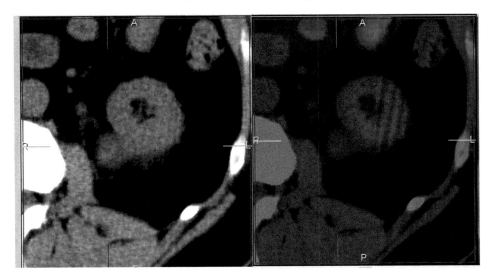

A. Renal cell carcinoma
B. Renal cyst
C. Lymphoma
D. Oncocytoma

ANSWERS AND EXPLANATIONS

1 **Answer B.** Diethylenetriamine pentaacetic acid (DTPA) is filtered through the glomeruli and can, therefore, be used to estimate GFR. Approximately 5% to 10% of DTPA is bound to plasma protein, resulting in a slight underestimation of GFR. Twenty percent of renal plasma flow is cleared by glomerular filtration, and 80% is cleared by the tubular secretion.

Mercaptoacetyltriglycine (MAG3) is cleared predominantly via proximal tubular secretion with minimal filtration. Higher extraction efficiency and plasma protein binding of MAG3 make it a better agent for evaluation of renal flow and function, but it cannot measure GFR (although complicated camera based techniques can be used to estimate GFR). In the setting of obstruction, GFR typically declines before tubular secretion. Additionally, the extraction fraction of MAG3 is 40% to 50%, more than twice that of DTPA. As such, MAG3 is preferred over DTPA in patients with suspected obstruction and impaired renal function. MAG3 is also the preferred radiopharmaceutical for renal function evaluation in the pediatric population because glomerular filtration is incompletely developed in the neonates. The alternative path of MAG3 excretion is by the hepatobiliary system. So, bowel activity may be visualized on the delayed images in patients with severely diminished renal function.

Dimercaptosuccinic acid (DMSA) is a renal cortical imaging agent, which is primarily used in the pediatric population for evaluation of pyelonephritis, renal cortical scarring, and differential renal function. DMSA is cortically bound and demonstrates very little renal excretion compared to the other renal agents. For this reason, it is the best agent to determine differential renal function. This lack of significant renal excretion is particularly useful for differential function evaluation in the setting of hydronephrosis.

Glucoheptonate is cleared via both glomerular filtration and renal tubule secretion and cannot be used to calculate GFR. The measured GFR is used as a confirmatory test for the estimated GFR in certain clinical situations such as severe malnutrition or obesity or diseases of skeletal muscle, or in the evaluation of donor renal function prior to transplantation.

References: Mettler FA, Guiberteau MJ. *Essentials of nuclear medicine imaging*, 7th ed. Philadelphia, PA: Saunders, 2019:28.

O'Malley JP, Ziessman HA, Thrall JH. *Nuclear medicine: the requisites*, 5th ed. Philadelphia, PA: Saunders, 2020:18, 258.

2 **Answer B.** DMSA is a renal cortical imaging agent that localizes in the renal cortex by binding to the sulfhydryl groups in the proximal renal tubules. Glomerular filtration followed by tubular reabsorption is the predominant route of DMSA uptake by the kidney. MAG3 is primarily removed from the plasma by active transport in the proximal renal tubules (choice B). DTPA is filtered through the glomerulus (choice A). Tc-99m glucoheptonate (GH) is both filtered by the glomerulus and secreted by the renal tubules, allowing for evaluation of renal function and collecting system. Approximately 10% to 15% of the injected GH dose remains bound to the renal tubules at 1 to 2 hours after the injection, and thus, it can also be used for renal cortical imaging. Loop diuretics (i.e., furosemide and bumetanide) block the $Na^+/K^+/2Cl^-$

cotransporter that is present in the loop of Henle. The following diagram shows the location of the localization of different radiopharmaceuticals in the renal nephron.

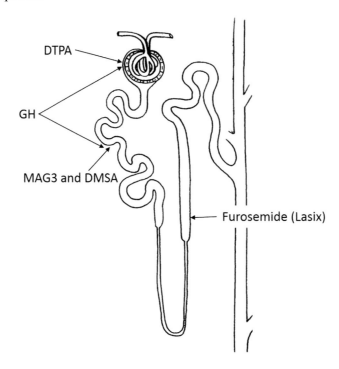

References: Mettler FA, Guiberteau MJ. *Essentials of nuclear medicine imaging*, 7th ed. Philadelphia, PA: Saunders, 2019:288.

Taylor AT. Radionuclides in nephrology, part 1: radiopharmaceuticals, quality control, and quantitative indices. *J Nucl Med* 2014;55(4):608–615.

3 **Answer C.** A normal MAG3 time–activity curve (renogram) demonstrates prompt tubular extraction (time to peak 3 to 5 minutes) with good renal clearance/excretion (time to half peak 6 to 10 minutes or 20 minutes to peak ratio of <0.3) as shown in the image below. Mild renal function impairment demonstrates normal tubular extraction with normal time to peak and slightly prolonged renal clearance (slightly prolonged 20 minutes to peak ratio), which would manifest as mild retention of radiotracer in the renal parenchyma at the end of 30 minutes. With moderate renal function impairment, there is tubular dysfunction (prolonged time to peak) and moderate cortical retention (prolonged 20 minutes to peak ratio). With severe renal function impairment, there is poor uptake with progressive accumulation and no significant clearance of the radiopharmaceutical (markedly prolonged time to peak). While renal scintigraphy and renogram are good in determining the degree of renal dysfunction, the exact cause of dysfunction (i.e., ATN, pyelonephritis, drug toxicity, or chronic medical renal disease) depends on the patient's medical history. Of note, the patient should be well hydrated for dynamic renography. While blood flow and radiopharmaceutical uptake are not altered by dehydration, excretion and washout may be delayed, simulating poor function or obstruction. Renogram curves must be interpreted in conjunction with the images as they can be affected by numerous factors, including hydronephrosis.

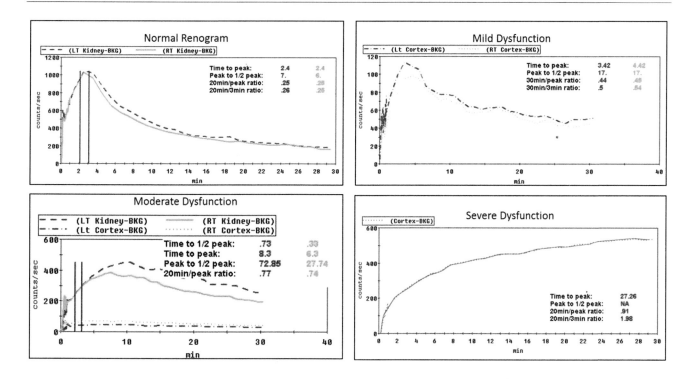

References: Mettler FA, Guiberteau MJ. *Essentials of nuclear medicine imaging,* 7th ed. Philadelphia, PA: Saunders, 2019:293–299.

O'Malley JP, Ziessman HA, Thrall JH. *Nuclear medicine: the requisites,* 5th ed. Philadelphia, PA: Saunders, 2020:258–270.

4 **Answer A.** Dynamic posterior images acquired after the IV administration of MAG3 demonstrate brisk uptake of the radiopharmaceutical within both kidneys. However, there is minimal excretion. Findings are most compatible with acute tubular necrosis in this patient with dehydration and rhabdomyolysis. In severe chronic renal disease, due to chronic tubular dysfunction, the rate of radiopharmaceutical concentration would be lower with gradual upslope instead of brisk upstroke (see renograms below). There is no evidence of a dilated renal collecting system on the supplied images to suggest hydronephrosis. Since captopril was not given for the examination, renal artery stenosis is not a possibility. Of note, a small area of photopenia within the upper pole of the left kidney (arrow on images below) corresponded to a renal cyst. Since the peak uptake in normal kidney occurs between 2 and 5 minutes, nonfunctioning renal tissue or photopenic defects (i.e., cyst, renal cell carcinoma, or metastasis) are best appreciated during this time period.

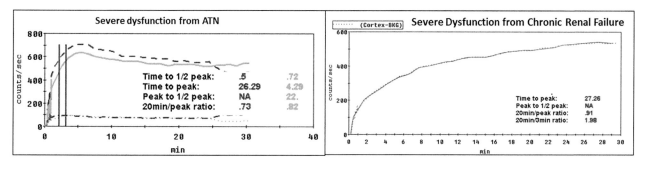

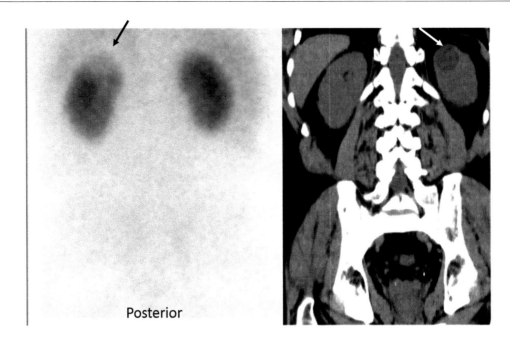

Posterior

References: Mettler FA, Guiberteau MJ. *Essentials of nuclear medicine imaging*, 7th ed. Philadelphia, PA: Saunders, 2019:293–310.

O'Malley JP, Ziessman HA, Thrall JH. *Nuclear medicine: the requisites*, 5th ed. Philadelphia, PA: Saunders, 2020:274–277.

5 **Answer C.** In the setting of renal artery stenosis, the juxtaglomerular apparatus of the kidneys produce renin, which converts angiotensinogen to angiotensin in the liver. Angiotensin I gets converted to angiotensin II by the angiotensin-converting enzyme (ACE) in the lung parenchyma. One of the actions of angiotensin II is efferent arteriolar constriction. This increases the net gradient pressure across the glomerulus and helps maintain the GFR. ACE inhibitors block the conversion of angiotensin I to angiotensin II in the lung parenchyma. The resultant inhibition of efferent arterial constriction causes a decrease in the GFR with resultant renal function impairment.

References: Mettler FA, Guiberteau MJ. *Essentials of nuclear medicine imaging*, 7th ed. Philadelphia, PA: Saunders, 2019:301–306.

O'Malley JP, Ziessman HA, Thrall JH. *Nuclear medicine: the requisites*, 5th ed. Philadelphia, PA: Saunders, 2020:268–271.

Saha GB. *Fundamentals of nuclear pharmacy*, 6th ed. New York, NY: Springer, 2010:296.

6 **Answer B.** Posterior dynamic MAG3 renal scintigraphy images demonstrate an enlarged right kidney with a large central area of photopenia, which fills in with the radiotracer on the delayed images. There is no significant emptying of radiotracer after administration of Lasix. Findings represent hydronephrosis with right ureteropelvic junction (UPJ) obstruction. The left kidney appears normal.

Pyeloplasty is typically the initial management in patients with UPJ obstruction. If corrected promptly, renal function can recover fully. Nephrectomy is reserved for cases with minimal residual renal function; in this case, the function may be mildly impaired. Ureteral reimplantation, cystectomy, and ileal conduit would not help in the management of a UPJ obstruction.

Diuretic renography can help distinguish obstructive from nonobstructive hydronephrosis. An increase in the urine flow caused by Lasix administration in a dilated but nonobstructed system would lead to washout of the accumulated radiopharmaceutical. In obstructive hydronephrosis, there would be progressive filling of the dilated collecting system, which does not empty after Lasix administration. This can be quantified using the time–activity curve by measuring the amount of time it takes to reach half the level of the activity, known as the diuretic T1/2 time. Diuretic T1/2 time of <10 minutes suggests nonobstructive hydronephrosis, while that >20 minutes suggests obstructive hydronephrosis. Diuretic T1/2 time of 10 to 20 minutes is indeterminate for obstruction.

References: Mettler FA, Guiberteau MJ. *Essentials of nuclear medicine imaging*, 7th ed. Philadelphia, PA: Saunders, 2019:295–301.

O'Malley JP, Ziessman HA, Thrall JH. *Nuclear medicine: the requisites*, 5th ed. Philadelphia, PA: Saunders, 2020:265–268.

7 **Answer C.** Thirty-minute posterior dynamic images demonstrate a central area of photopenia within the right kidney (arrowheads), which is secondary to a dilated pelvicalyceal system filled with nonradiolabeled urine. The right kidney is slightly enlarged compared to the left kidney. There is progressive tubular extraction by the right kidney without excretion into the renal collecting system, representing severely impaired right renal function. Findings are likely secondary to a high-grade obstruction with resultant renal dysfunction. Normally functioning left kidney is seen with the accumulation of the radiopharmaceutical in the dilated left pelvicalyceal system and ureter. This empties promptly after the administration of Lasix, indicating left hydroureteronephrosis without obstruction. Prolonged high-grade obstruction, if left untreated, can result in progressive loss of nephrons, causing diminished renal function and eventual atrophy. If corrected, a significant portion of the function can recover. As such, renal scintigraphy is helpful not only in the diagnosis of obstruction but also in the assessment of the functional significance of the obstruction and in the evaluation of recovered residual function after proper treatment of the obstruction. Serial examinations may also be performed to monitor patients with partial obstruction or patients at risk for worsening obstruction.

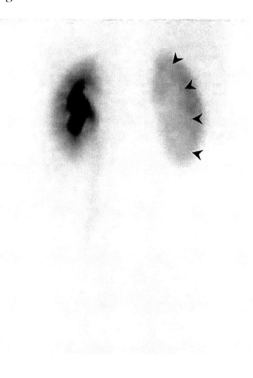

References: Mettler FA, Guiberteau MJ. *Essentials of nuclear medicine imaging*, 7th ed. Philadelphia, PA: Saunders, 2019:293–299.

O'Malley JP, Ziessman HA, Thrall JH. *Nuclear medicine: the requisites*, 5th ed. Philadelphia, PA: Saunders, 2020:263–270.

8 **Answer D.** Post-Lasix posterior dynamic images demonstrate marked left hydroureteronephrosis. The Lasix renogram suggests partial emptying of the renal collecting system. However, the left kidney region of interest (ROI) only includes the renal pelvicalyceal system, which is inaccurate. The data were reprocessed including the dilated ureter and the pelvicalyceal system in the region of interest. The generated time–activity curve demonstrated no emptying with Lasix (image below). Findings represent hydroureteronephrosis in the setting of left ureterovesical junction obstruction. Quantitative values and time–activity curves should always be interpreted in conjunction with the images of the renal function. Attention should be paid to the regions of interest drawn around the kidney and the collecting system, especially if there is evidence of dilatation. In the case of UVJ obstruction, ureter should be included in the collecting system ROI.

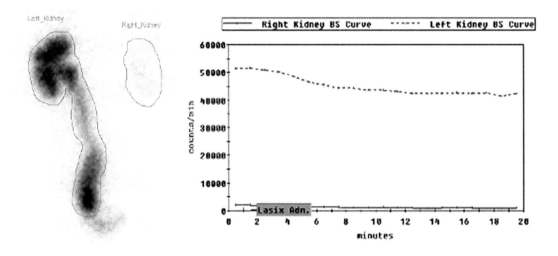

References: Mettler FA, Guiberteau MJ. *Essentials of nuclear medicine imaging*, 7th ed. Philadelphia, PA: Saunders, 2019:293–299.

O'Malley JP, Ziessman HA, Thrall JH. *Nuclear medicine: the requisites*, 5th ed. Philadelphia, PA: Saunders, 2020:258–270.

Taylor AT, Brandon DC, de Palma D, et al. SNMMI Procedure Standard/EANM Practice Guideline for Diuretic Renal Scintigraphy in Adults With Suspected Upper Urinary Tract Obstruction 1.0. *Semin Nucl Med* 2018;48(4):377–390.

9 **Answer B.** If a patient has renovascular hypertension, then the administration of captopril will cause a decrease in the GFR. This will manifest as an overall decrease in the renal accumulation and excretion of the agent that is filtered by the glomerulus, that is, DTPA. On the other hand, the rate of tubular extraction is not significantly affected. As such, the rate of accumulation of the tubular agent, that is, MAG3 will be slightly delayed but not decreased. However, due to the decrease in GFR, this tubular accumulated agent will not demonstrate washout. As such, the correct pair of renogram curves for DTPA and MAG3 is identified by the choice B.

References: Mettler FA, Guiberteau MJ. *Essentials of nuclear medicine imaging*, 7th ed. Philadelphia, PA: Saunders, 2019:301–306.

O'Malley JP, Ziessman HA, Thrall JH. *Nuclear medicine: the requisites*, 5th ed. Philadelphia, PA: Saunders, 2020:268–271.

10 **Answer B.** The supplied images demonstrate severe captopril-induced renal dysfunction bilaterally. Captopril renogram is a noninvasive screening test of choice for the diagnosis of renovascular hypertension. It is highly sensitive (93%) and specific (95%). However, when bilateral captopril-induced renal dysfunction is seen, artifactual causes of false-positive captopril renography should be considered as they are more common than bilateral renal artery stenosis. These artifactual causes of bilateral false-positive study include dehydration, captopril-induced hypotension, and calcium channel blockers. If possible, the patient should stop Ca channel blockers prior to captopril renogram. If artifactual causes for false-positive captopril renography are excluded, then bilateral renal artery stenosis should be presumed as a bilateral involvement may be present in approximately 30% of patients greater than 55 years of age. Alpha- and beta-blockers do not interfere with ACE inhibitor renography.

References: Claveau-Tremblay R, Turpin S, De Braekeleer M, et al. False-positive captopril renography in patients taking calcium antagonists. *J Nucl Med* 1998;39(9):1621–1626.

Ludwig V, Martin WH, Delbeke D. Calcium channel blockers: a potential cause of false-positive captopril renography. *Clin Nucl Med* 2003;28(2):108–112.

11 **Answer D.** The sequential dynamic posterior images demonstrate an enlarged right kidney with a large area of relative photopenia occupying its lower pole. Nonfunctioning renal tissue will not concentrate the radiopharmaceutical and appear as a photopenic, space-occupying lesion. Since the peak uptake in a normal kidney occurs between 2 and 5 minutes, photopenic lesions are usually best visualized during this time. While the most common photopenic lesions are renal cysts, renal cell carcinoma and other malignancies may appear similarly. As such, correlation with anatomic imaging such as ultrasound, CT, or MRI should be considered for further evaluation. Since there is no evidence of obstruction, the administration of Lasix is not necessary. There are no processing errors, and providing anterior images would not change the management in this patient. This patient had a large renal cell carcinoma involving the lower pole of the right kidney.

References: Mettler FA, Guiberteau MJ. *Essentials of nuclear medicine imaging,* 7th ed. Philadelphia, PA: Saunders, 2019:292–293.

O'Malley JP, Ziessman HA, Thrall JH. *Nuclear medicine: the requisites,* 5th ed. Philadelphia, PA: Saunders, 2020:260–263.

12 **Answer D.** Anterior flow images acquired after the IV administration of Tc-99m MAG3 for the evaluation of transplant renal function demonstrate no significant flow through the left common iliac artery (arrow). The functional images show absent perfusion to the transplanted kidney in the left hemipelvis with a round area of photopenia (arrowheads). Findings are most compatible with a nonviable transplant from acute arterial occlusion. Since there is no collateral venous drainage in the transplanted kidney, renal vein thrombosis will also demonstrate a similar appearance with a lack of perfusion and function owing to the absence of venous collaterals in the transplanted kidney; however, flow through the left common iliac artery would be visualized.

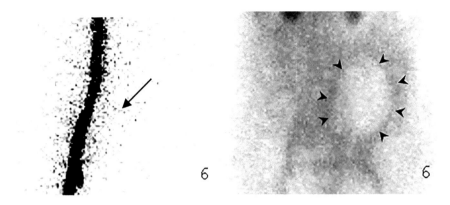

References: Mettler FA, Guiberteau MJ. Essentials of nuclear medicine imaging, 7th ed. Philadelphia, PA: Saunders, 2019:308–309.

O'Malley JP, Ziessman HA, Thrall JH. *Nuclear medicine: the requisites*, 5th ed. Philadelphia, PA: Saunders, 2020:271–277, 280.

13 **Answer E.** Anterior dynamic images acquired after the IV administration of Tc-99m MAG3 demonstrates brisk but progressive uptake of the radiopharmaceutical without significant excretion into the renal collecting system. Time–activity curve from the renal flow (perfusion) images demonstrates good flow to the transplanted kidney with the slope of the renal flow similar to that of the aorta/iliac artery at that level (arrow). The functional time–activity curve (renogram) demonstrates a progressive increase in activity without significant excretion. Findings are compatible with vasomotor nephropathy, also known as ischemic nephropathy, delayed graft function, or acute tubular necrosis.

Transplant renogram must be interpreted in the context of clinical history. Renal dysfunction in the early posttransplant period is due to either vasomotor nephropathy or acute rejection. Vasomotor nephropathy occurs immediately after surgery and should recover during the first 2 weeks. On the other hand, acute rejection does not typically occur until after a few weeks and is most common in the first three months. While severe renal dysfunction from obstruction could have a similar appearance, there would typically be photopenia related to the dilated collecting system and some excretion into the collecting system. Renal artery or renal vein occlusion would present with absent renal flow and function of the allograft. Urine leak would demonstrate activity outside the kidney or bladder that layers on decubitus images.

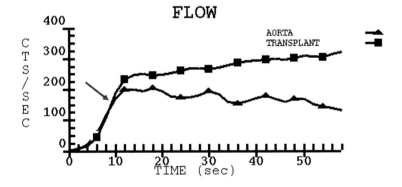

References: Mettler FA, Guiberteau MJ. *Essentials of nuclear medicine imaging*, 7th ed. Philadelphia, PA: Saunders, 2019:308–309.

O'Malley JP, Ziessman HA, Thrall JH. *Nuclear medicine: the requisites*, 5th ed. Philadelphia, PA: Saunders, 2020:274–276.

14 **Answer B.** The anterior Tc-99m MAG3 renogram images of renal transplant in the right iliac fossa show good uptake and excretion by the transplanted kidney. However, the decubitus images demonstrate activity external to the kidney and renal collecting system (arrowheads). This is most compatible with a urine leak. If there is a clinical suspicion of a possible urine leak, decubitus imaging as well as delayed 1- to 2-hour imaging should be considered. At some institutions, decubitus images are routinely done to demonstrate the shifting of the activity and to increase the sensitivity of the examination for urine leak. If needed, SPECT/CT images would also help with the confirmation. A postoperative urine leak may occur at the anastomotic site or result from the rupture of an obstructed allograft. The pattern of the shown uptake does not conform to the bowel and, as such, is not of GI origin. Renal scintigraphy is a simple, sensitive, and reliable way of diagnosing and following patients with a urinary leak. Other fluid collections associated with renal transplant include hematoma and lymphocele. Both of these would demonstrate photopenia on renal scintigraphy. Hematoma is typically seen in the early postoperative period, and lymphocele is typically seen 2 to 3 months after the transplant due to a lack of lymphatic drainage from the transplanted kidney.

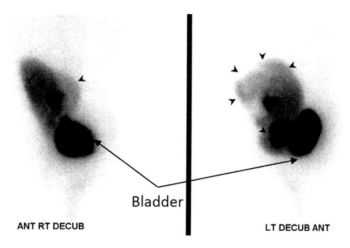

Bladder

ANT RT DECUB   LT DECUB ANT

References: Mettler FA, Guiberteau MJ. *Essentials of nuclear medicine imaging,* 7th ed. Philadelphia, PA: Saunders, 2019:300, 308–309.

O'Malley JP, Ziessman HA, Thrall JH. *Nuclear medicine: the requisites,* 5th ed. Philadelphia, PA: Saunders, 2020:271–277.

Schillaci O, Danieli R, Manni C, et al. Technetium-99m-labelled red blood cell imaging in the diagnosis of hepatic haemangiomas: the role of SPECT/CT with a hybrid camera. *Eur J Nucl Med Mol Imaging* 2004;31(7):1011–1015. PubMed PMID: 15057491.

15 **Answer A.** Fused SPECT/CT and CT images demonstrate a soft tissue lesion emanating from the posteromedial aspect of the left kidney (arrows below), which demonstrates no significant Tc-99m sestamibi uptake (arrow on the fused image below). Tc-99m sestamibi is used for the differentiation of oncocytoma from renal cell carcinoma. Tc-99m sestamibi is a lipophilic cation that localizes in the cells based on their mitochondrial content. Renal oncocytomas have large numbers of mitochondria, especially in comparison to renal cell carcinoma (RCC), which has a relative paucity of mitochondria. RCCs also often possess multidrug-resistant (MDR) pumps. These pumps eliminate Tc-99m sestamibi out of the cells. Renal parenchyma has high physiologic uptake of Tc-99m sestamibi. RCCs generally show a distinct decrease in uptake relative to adjacent normal parenchyma. In contrast, oncocytomas display uptake that is similar to or above that of the adjacent renal parenchyma. Masses displaying variable uptake (uptake similar to or higher than the adjacent renal parenchyma) are likely to be of benign etiology, such as oncocytoma. This patient had a partial nephrectomy, which showed clear cell renal carcinoma.

Increased utilization of cross-sectional imaging has led to an increase in the diagnosis of incidental renal masses on conventional imaging. While most of the incidental soft tissue renal masses represent RCC, of the benign solid masses, oncocytoma is the most common (up to 15% of all renal masses). Tc-99m sestamibi scan is used to allow for differentiation of RCC from oncocytoma when conventional imaging is not conclusive.

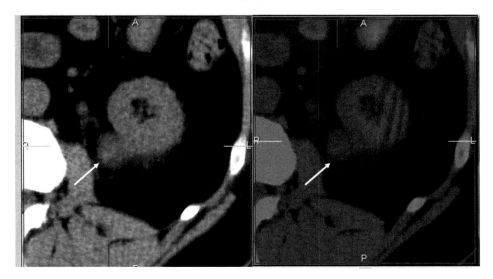

Reference: Rowe SP, Gorin MA, Gordetsky J, et al. Initial experience using 99mTc-MIBI SPECT/CT for the differentiation of oncocytoma from renal cell carcinoma. *Clin Nucl Med* 2015;40(4):309–313.

QUESTIONS

1a The following renal scintigraphy was performed on a 7-year-old patient with fever. What radiopharmaceutical was used for this examination?

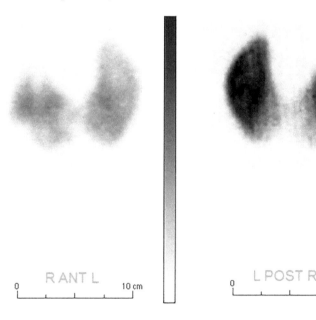

R ANT L   0   10 cm

L POST R   0   10 cm

    A. Tc-99m DMSA
    B. Tc-99m DTPA
    C. Tc-99m MAG3
    D. I-123 hippuran

1b What is the most likely diagnosis?

    A. Severe renal dysfunction
    B. Bilateral hydronephrosis
    C. Pyelonephritis
    D. Wilms tumor
    E. Lymphoma

2   What is an advantage of the contrast voiding cystourethrogram (VCUG) compared to the direct radionuclide cystogram (RNC)?

A. Lower radiation
B. Better anatomic detail
C. Greater sensitivity
D. Bladder volume calculation

3   Grade the vesicoureteral reflux based on the following images.

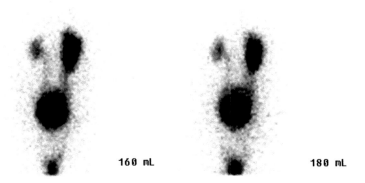

160 mL   180 mL

A. Mild left, moderate right
B. Moderate left, mild right
C. Severe left, moderate right
D. Moderate left, severe right
E. Mild bilateral
F. Moderate bilateral
G. Severe bilateral

4   A 7-year-old male presents with left knee pain and fever for 2 days with negative radiographs. The patient was unable to undergo MR due to cochlear implants. Instead, three-phase bone scintigraphy was performed. What is the most likely diagnosis?

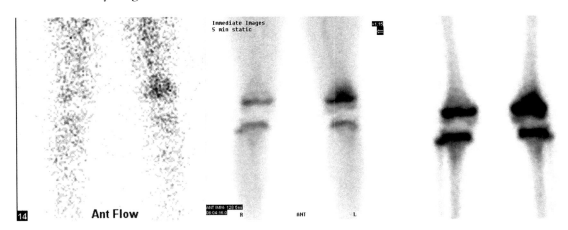

A. Septic arthritis
B. Osteosarcoma
C. Fracture
D. Osteomyelitis

5 A 2-year-old girl has a known renal anomaly on ultrasound. Renal scintigraphy was performed to evaluate the renal function. What is the most likely diagnosis?

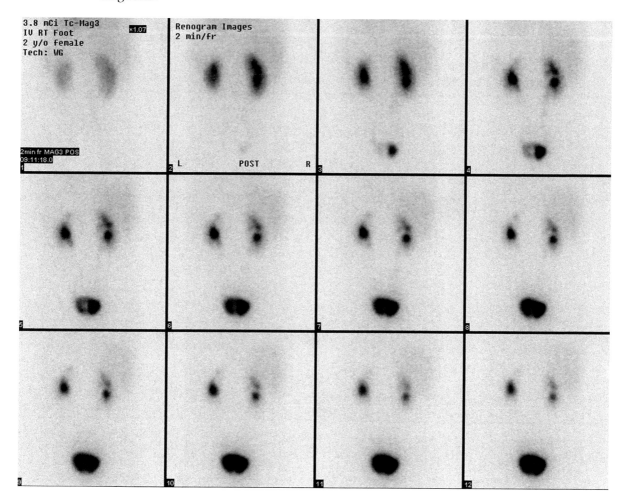

A. Calculus

B. Diverticulum

C. Ureterocele

D. Rhabdomyosarcoma

6 An 18-month-old patient presents with a high clinical suspicion for child abuse and equivocal findings on the skeletal survey. What site of fracture has the highest specificity for the nonaccidental trauma on bone scintigraphy?

A. Skull

B. Scapula

C. Clavicle

D. Long bone diaphysis

7 The following anterior and posterior bone scintigraphy images were acquired on a 19-year-old with low back pain. The nuclear medicine technologist asks you to review the images prior to the patient leaving the department. What is the most appropriate next step?

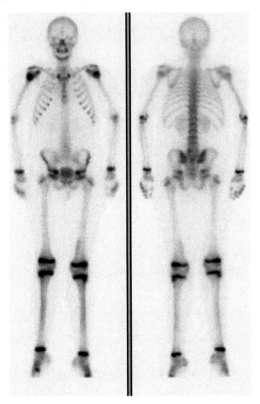

A. MRI of the lumbar spine
B. CT of the lumbar spine
C. Radiographs of the lumbar spine
D. SPECT images of the lumbar spine
E. No further imaging necessary

8 The shown examination was performed on a child with neurologic impairment. Which of the following is the most likely indication?

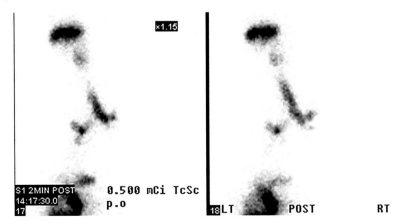

A. Gastroesophageal reflux
B. Esophageal dysmotility
C. Gastric emptying
D. Aspiration

9a Which of the following statements is most accurate regarding the findings in this 6-month-old infant?

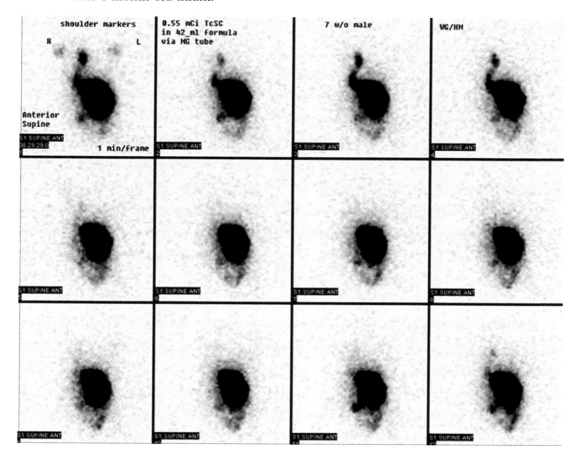

A. This is the gold standard test.
B. Provocative maneuvers were performed.
C. Barium esophagogram is more sensitive.
D. Findings may be physiologic in young infants.

9b Semiquantitative parameters can be used to assess gastroesophageal reflux in a milk scan. The above patient should be categorized as:

A. Low level, <10 seconds
B. Low level, 10 seconds or longer
C. High level, <10 seconds
D. High level, 10 seconds or longer

10 The following nuclear scintigraphy was performed on a 2-year-old with painless rectal bleeding. What is the most common cause of a false-positive examination?

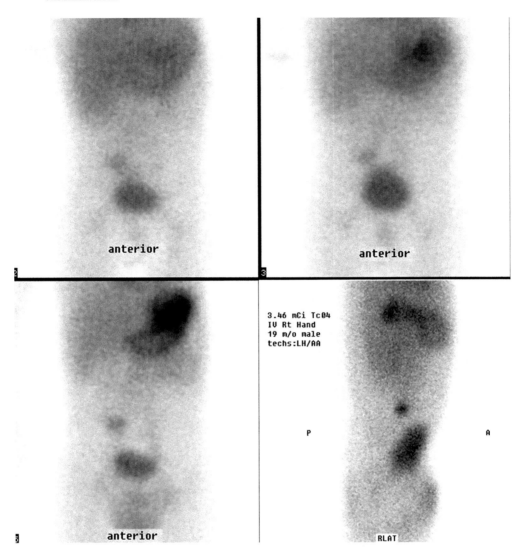

A. Appendicitis
B. Duplication cyst
C. Genitourinary uptake
D. Inflammatory bowel disease

11 What is the most appropriate conclusion for this child with cholestatic jaundice and the following 60-minute Tc-99m IDA analog scan?

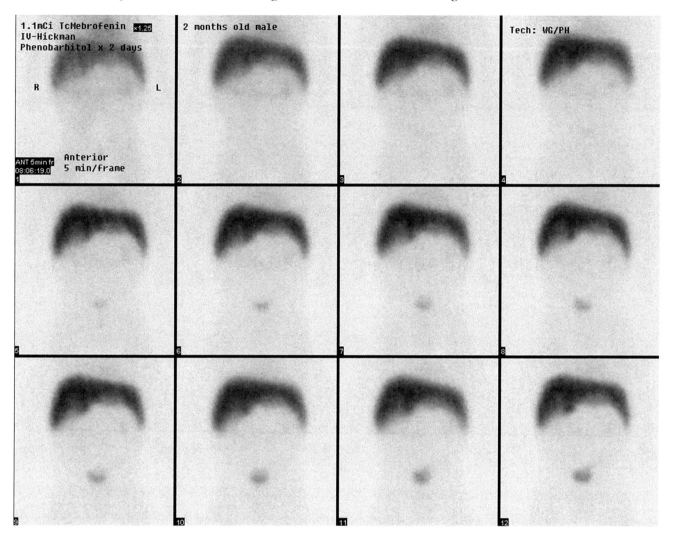

A. Biliary atresia
B. Neonatal hepatitis
C. Nondiagnostic examination
D. Alpha-1 antitrypsin deficiency

12 Anterior and lateral images from Tc-99m scintigraphy are shown below. Which of the following is associated with this entity?

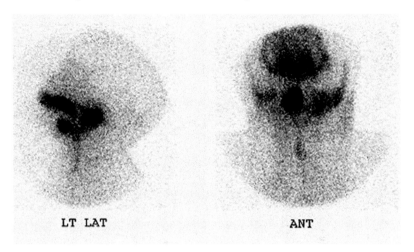

A. Normal eutopic tissue
B. Permanent hypothyroidism
C. Elevated T4 levels
D. Peroxidase deficiency
E. Abnormal perchlorate washout test

ANSWERS AND EXPLANATIONS

1a **Answer A.** Tc-99m DMSA (dimercaptosuccinic acid) is commonly used to detect acute pyelonephritis and renal scarring due to vesicoureteral reflux or pyelonephritis in the pediatric population. Approximately 40% of the injected radiopharmaceutical binds to the sulfhydryl groups of the proximal renal tubules and remains there, thus allowing for high-count renal cortical imaging. MAG3 (mercaptoacetyltriglycine) is a tubular-secreting agent; it is the most commonly used radiopharmaceutical for the evaluation of renal flow and function. DTPA (diethylenetriaminepentaacetic acid) is a glomerular filtration agent, which can be used to calculate the glomerular filtration rate (GFR); while DTPA can also be used to examine the renal flow and function, it has poor image quality compared to MAG3 due to significantly higher background activity and slower renal clearance. I-123 hippuran undergoes tubular secretion and glomerular filtration allowing for assessment of renal function. It has been replaced by MAG3.

References: Mettler FA, Guiberteau MJ. *Essentials of nuclear medicine imaging*, 7th ed. Philadelphia, PA: Saunders, 2019:306.

O'Malley JP, Ziessman HA, Thrall JH. *Nuclear medicine: the requisites*, 5th ed. Philadelphia, PA: Saunders, 2020:278, 279, 282, 283.

1b **Answer C.** Anterior and posterior Tc-99m DMSA planar images demonstrate abnormal renal axis with tissue joining the lower poles of each kidney (arrow) consistent with a horseshoe kidney. Additionally, multiple areas of decreased radiotracer uptake (arrowheads) are identified within the upper and lower pole of the right kidney. In the setting of acute febrile illness, the findings are most compatible with pyelonephritis. In the absence of an acute illness, the cortical findings would be consistent with renal parenchymal scarring. While other lesions would present similarly, they are less likely.

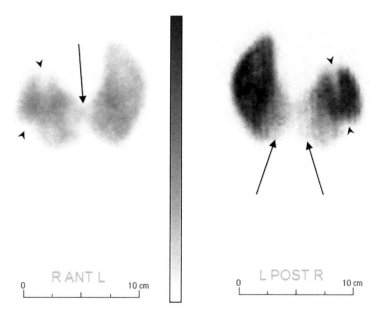

References: Mettler FA, Guiberteau MJ. *Essentials of nuclear medicine imaging*, 7th ed. Philadelphia, PA: Saunders, 2019:306.

O'Malley JP, Ziessman HA, Thrall JH. *Nuclear medicine: the requisites*, 5th ed. Philadelphia, PA: Saunders, 2020:278, 279, 282, 283.

2 **Answer B.** The main advantages of contrast voiding cystourethrogram (VCUG) are superior anatomic detail and more accurate grading of the vesicoureteral reflux (VUR). VCUG is recommended for the initial workup of boys with vesicoureteral reflux to exclude an anatomic cause of the reflux (i.e., posterior urethral valve). The advantages of direct radionuclide cystography (RNC) include greater sensitivity for the detection of reflux, lower radiation, and the ability to calculate the residual bladder volume. RNC allows for continuous imaging of the urinary tract throughout the examination and thus may be more sensitive in the diagnosis of significant VUR. However, due to low anatomic resolution, it is more likely to miss low-grade reflux. While the use of modern grid-controlled variable-rate pulsed fluoroscopy reduces the effective radiation dose by about eightfold compared to the older continuous fluoroscopy units, an effective dose of VCUG performed with this technique is still about ninefold higher than that received during RNC.

References: Mettler FA, Guiberteau MJ. *Essentials of nuclear medicine imaging*, 7th ed. Philadelphia, PA: Saunders, 2019:306, 308.

O'Malley JP, Ziessman HA, Thrall JH. *Nuclear medicine: the requisites*, 5th ed. Philadelphia, PA: Saunders, 2020:282, 284–285.

Ward VL, Strauss K, Barnewolt C, et al. Pediatric radiation exposure and effective dose reduction during voiding cystourethrography. *Radiology* 2008;249(3):1002–1009.

3 **Answer D.** Posterior images acquired during the direct radionuclide cystography (RNC) demonstrate reflux of radiopharmaceutical into bilateral renal pelvicalyceal systems. There is dilatation of the right collecting system. Findings represent moderate left-sided and severe right-sided vesicoureteral reflux (VUR). Direct RNC with bladder catheterization is the most commonly used technique for diagnosing reflux. Dynamic posterior imaging is acquired during the bladder filling, during voiding, and after voiding. Grading of VUR is as follows: mild—visualization of the ureters (* in the image below); moderate—visualization of the pelvicalyceal system (# in the image below); and severe—visualization of the pelvicalyceal system with dilated collecting system (## in the image below). Grading is important as renal damage is more likely in severe VUR compared to mild or moderate grades. RNC is the technique of choice for the evaluation and follow-up of the children with UTIs and suspected vesicoureteral reflux. It is also used in screening the siblings of the patients with VUR. Tc-99m sulfur colloid and Tc-99m DTPA are the radiopharmaceuticals most commonly used as they do not get absorbed by the epithelial lining of the bladder or ureters.

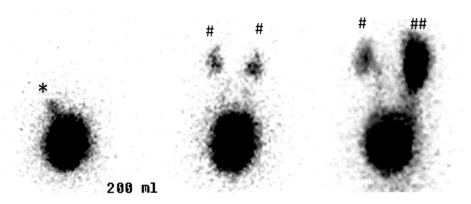

References: Mettler FA, Guiberteau MJ. *Essentials of nuclear medicine imaging*, 7th ed. Philadelphia, PA: Saunders, 2019:306, 308.

O'Malley JP, Ziessman HA, Thrall JH. *Nuclear medicine: the requisites*, 5th ed. Philadelphia, PA: Saunders, 2020:282, 284–285.

Sandler M. *Diagnostic nuclear medicine*, 4th ed. Philadelphia, PA: Lippincott Williams & Wilkins, 2003:1100–1102.

4 **Answer D.** The supplied three-phase images acquired after the IV injection of diphosphonate demonstrate a regional area of increased blood flow to the distal left femur, which further localizes to the distal femoral metaphysis on the blood pool and the delayed images. Findings represent osteomyelitis. While this is the most common appearance of osteomyelitis on bone scintigraphy, it is important to remember that early osteomyelitis in children may present as a cold or photopenic defect of the metaphysis with increased activity in the adjacent diaphysis; this is thought to result from increased intramedullary pressure or thrombosed vessels.

Osteomyelitis is a common pediatric problem and frequently involves the highly vascularized metaphysis of fast-growing bones. The distal femur and proximal tibia are the most common locations. Initial radiographs for osteomyelitis are often negative, especially in the first few weeks. MRI is regarded as the optimum imaging modality in the evaluation of infection. However, if there is a concern for multifocal infection, bone scintigraphy can offer an advantage over MRI because whole-body images are routinely included with scintigraphy. If there are contraindications to MR imaging or if sedation may be required for the MRI, then bone scintigraphy should be considered since it offers greater sensitivity than radiograph and can detect changes as early as 24 hours.

References: Coley B. *Caffey's pediatric diagnostic imaging*, 12th ed. Philadelphia, PA: Elsevier Saunders, 2013:1471–1474.

O'Malley JP, Ziessman HA, Thrall JH. *Nuclear medicine: the requisites*, 5th ed. Philadelphia, PA: Saunders, 2020:111–113.

Sandler M. *Diagnostic nuclear medicine*, 4th ed. Philadelphia, PA: Lippincott Williams & Wilkins, 2003:1108.

5 **Answer C.** The early images demonstrate a rounded area of photopenia within the left side of the bladder (long arrow), which is most compatible with a ureterocele. On more delayed images, a left upper pole moiety (short arrows) with a central area of photopenia (arrowhead) is identified. This is most compatible with a hydronephrotic left upper pole moiety with a moderately impaired renal function. Normal functioning left lower pole moiety is seen without hydronephrosis. Duplex collecting system is also identified on the right side with normal functioning, nondilated upper and lower pole moieties.

An ectopic ureterocele is commonly found in the setting of a duplicated system and is almost always associated with the upper pole moiety. Lower pole moiety is typically associated with reflux. As the Weigert-Meyer rule states, the ureter from the upper pole moiety of a completely duplicated collecting system inserts inferior and medial to the normal insertion site of the lower pole moiety in the trigone. In patients with duplication, the MAG3 renogram is typically done to assess the function of the obstructed upper pole moiety. Bladder calculus and rhabdomyosarcoma may also cause a photopenic defect in the bladder but are not associated with renal duplication. A diverticulum would appear as an intense outpouching from the bladder.

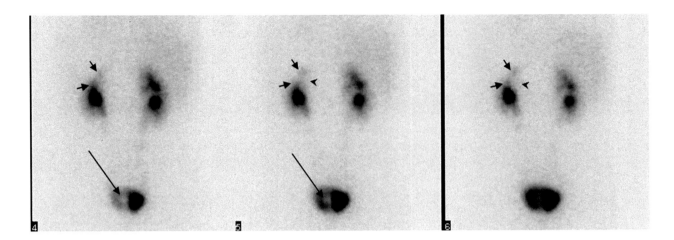

References: Coley B. *Caffey's pediatric diagnostic imaging*, 12th ed. Philadelphia, PA: Elsevier Saunders, 2013:1091.

Sandler M. *Diagnostic nuclear medicine*, 4th ed. Philadelphia, PA: Lippincott Williams & Wilkins, 2003:1200–1202.

6 **Answer B.** Shaking injury may result in scapular fractures, which have high specificity for child abuse. Skull, diaphyseal long bone, and clavicle fractures have lower specificity. While skull fractures are seen on the radiographs, they may be difficult to see on the bone scan. Also, subtle fractures along the growth plates are best seen on radiographs owing to the intense physiologic physeal uptake on the bone scan. As such, the skeletal survey using radiographs is more sensitive than bone scintigraphy. Bone scintigraphy is best utilized when the clinical suspicion for nonaccidental trauma is high, but the skeletal survey is inconclusive.

References: Coley B. *Caffey's pediatric diagnostic imaging*, 12th ed. Philadelphia, PA: Elsevier Saunders, 2013:1588.

Habibian MR. *Nuclear medicine imaging: a teaching file*, 2nd ed. Philadelphia, PA: Lippincott Williams & Wilkins, 2009:377–378.

7 **Answer D.** Spondylolysis is a common cause of lower back pain in young adults, especially athletes. Repetitive trauma is thought to be the precipitating factor leading to a stress reaction and eventual disruption of the par interarticularis. This may occur unilaterally or bilaterally, and occurs most commonly at the L5 level. Bone scintigraphy is more sensitive than radiographs for localizing the site of bone stress, and in this patient, the initial radiographs were negative. At the initial workup, both plain films of the lumbar spine and planar bone scintigraphy may be unrevealing. In these instances, SPECT or SPECT/CT imaging may show increased uptake at the par interarticularis. Additionally, SPECT can provide further anatomic localization allowing for the distinction of uptake at the pars abnormality or that at the facet joints. Furthermore, SPECT/CT will demonstrate the presence or absence of a pars defect and its associated changes, such as sclerosis. As seen with this case, a subtle abnormality on planar bone imaging is readily visible on the SPECT images (arrows in image below), which revealed a focus of intense uptake at the left L5 level consistent with spondylolysis.

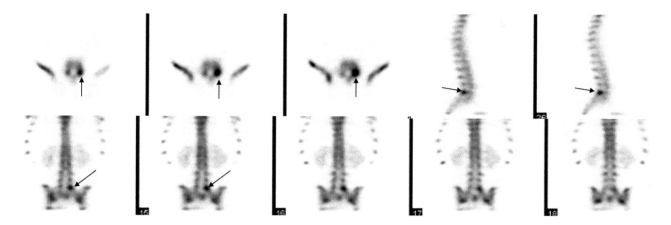

References: O'Malley JP, Ziessman HA, Thrall JH. *Nuclear medicine: the requisites*, 5th ed. Philadelphia, PA: Saunders, 2020:107, 111.

Sandler M. *Diagnostic nuclear medicine*, 4th ed. Philadelphia, PA: Lippincott Williams & Wilkins, 2003:1112.

Zukotynski K, Curtis C, Grant FD, et al. The value of SPECT in the detection of stress injury to the pars interarticularis in patients with low back pain. *J Orthop Surg Res* 2010;5:13.

8 **Answer D.** The salivagram is a simple yet sensitive nuclear medicine study to evaluate for aspiration. At our institution, Tc-99m sulfur colloid (0.3 to 0.4 mCi) is mixed in water and placed on the back of the tongue with the patient in the supine position. Dynamic acquisition for 1 hour is performed, followed by static images at 1 and 3 hours. This case is grossly positive with an abrupt aspiration of the radiotracer into the tracheobronchial tree (arrows below). Gastroesophageal reflux, gastric emptying, and esophageal motility are not evaluated on the salivagram scintigraphy. This examination is more sensitive than reflux scintigraphy in detecting aspiration.

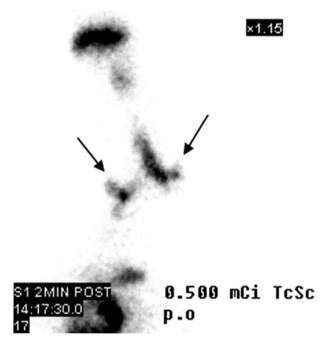

Reference: O'Malley JP, Ziessman HA, Thrall JH. *Nuclear medicine: the requisites*, 5th ed. Philadelphia, PA: Saunders, 2020:235–237.

9a **Answer D.** This study represents a typical "milk" scan where the infant is administered Tc-99m sulfur colloid mixed in formula or milk and imaged in the supine position for up to 60 minutes using dynamic acquisition. Gastroesophageal reflux (GER) is a normal physiologic finding in neonates, which resolves by late infancy. Reflux scintigraphy does not evaluate complications of gastroesophageal reflux disease (GERD), and the presence of GER on scintigraphy does not correlate with the symptoms of GERD. However, given that persistent GER can lead to serious complications such as strictures, recurrent pneumonia, and failure to thrive, it is important to diagnose this condition. Reflux scintigraphy represents a physiologic, sensitive, and noninvasive modality to detect GER. While intraesophageal pH monitoring is considered the gold standard in the evaluation of GERD, it is an invasive and technically demanding procedure. Barium esophagogram has a low sensitivity for detecting reflux and is mainly used to evaluate an anatomic cause of obstruction (i.e., stricture, malignancy, vascular anomalies). Furthermore, gastric emptying scintigraphy can be performed simultaneously with reflux scintigraphy providing additional information. Provocative maneuvers, such as the utilization of an abdominal binder to increase intra-abdominal pressure during imaging, are no longer recommended.

References: Coley B. *Caffey's pediatric diagnostic imaging*, 12th ed. Philadelphia, PA: Elsevier Saunders, 2013:1019–1020.

O'Malley JP, Ziessman HA, Thrall JH. *Nuclear medicine: the requisites*, 5th ed. Philadelphia, PA: Saunders, 2020:232–236.

9b **Answer D.** This patient had multiple episodes of high reflux (> mid esophagus), which lasted longer than 10 seconds. The frames on this study are 1 minute each, illustrating just how long each episode of reflux persisted. Semiquantitative parameters used to evaluate reflux on a milk scan include duration, height, and temporal relationship to the meal. Episodes with higher transit (> mid esophagus), longer duration (>10 seconds), and at lower stomach volumes are thought to reflect a higher severity of the GER. While pulmonary aspiration may be detected on delayed reflux scintigraphy images, a salivagram is more sensitive for its evaluation.

Reference: O'Malley JP, Ziessman HA, Thrall JH. *Nuclear medicine: the requisites*, 5th ed. Philadelphia, PA: Saunders, 2020:232–236.

10 **Answer C.** Anterior and lateral images acquired after the IV administration of Tc-99m pertechnetate demonstrate a moderate-sized focus of moderate-to-intense activity in the right lower quadrant, which appears at the same time as the gastric mucosa. Also, it is anteriorly located on the lateral image, excluding activity in the distal ureter (arrows in the image below). This finding represents heterotopic gastric mucosa in the Meckel diverticulum, the most common congenital anomaly of the GI tract. While heterotopic gastric mucosa has been reported to be present in only 10% to 30% of the Meckel diverticula, it is present in 95% to 98% of the bleeding Meckel diverticula. Genitourinary uptake is the most common cause of a false-positive result on the Meckel scan. Duplication cyst, inflammatory bowel disease, and appendicitis also represent potential causes of a false-positive examination but are less common.

Several strategies can be implemented to increase the sensitivity of the Meckel's scan. H-2 receptor antagonists (cimetidine, famotidine, or ranitidine) block the release of Tc-99m pertechnetate from the mucin-producing cells of the ectopic gastric mucosa in the Meckel diverticulum, increasing the sensitivity of the study. Other medications used for this purpose include pentagastrin and glucagon. Pentagastrin increases the mucosal uptake of pertechnetate while glucagon decreases the bowel motility (preventing radiotracer migration).

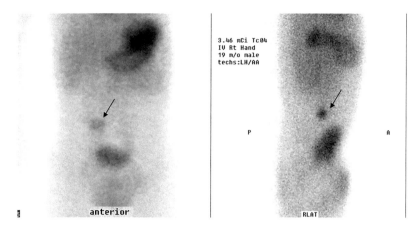

References: Mettler FA, Guiberteau MJ. *Essentials of nuclear medicine imaging*, 7th ed. Philadelphia, PA: Saunders, 2019:223–224.

O'Malley JP, Ziessman HA, Thrall JH. *Nuclear medicine: the requisites*, 5th ed. Philadelphia, PA: Saunders, 2020:250–252.

11 **Answer C.** On the anterior images acquired for 60 minutes after IV administration of Tc-99m mebrofenin, there is no evidence of radiopharmaceutical in the biliary tree or bowel. However, this 1-hour study cannot distinguish between biliary atresia and other etiologies causing poor hepatocellular function. As such, these patients should undergo additional imaging for up to 24 hours after the radiopharmaceutical injection. Patients with biliary atresia will have good blood pool clearance with retention of activity in the liver without biliary excretion. On the other hand, patients with neonatal hepatitis will typically have delayed blood pool clearance (decreased hepatic uptake) with visualization of bowel on 24-hour images. Once extrahepatic biliary or bowel activity is visualized, the diagnosis of biliary atresia is excluded. The sensitivity of this examination for detecting biliary atresia is approximately 100%, with a specificity of 75% to 80%. This infant with midline liver and visceral heterotaxy was found to have biliary atresia on 24-hour images, which was confirmed intraoperatively.

Phenobarbital-enhanced hepatobiliary scintigraphy is highly accurate in differentiating biliary atresia from other causes of neonatal jaundice. Prior to the radiopharmaceutical injection, the infant typically receives 5 mg/kg/day of phenobarbital for 5 days to achieve a serum level of ≥15 µg/mL. Phenobarbital is believed to stimulate the hepatic secretion of the IDA analog by activating liver enzymes and increasing the bile flow. This increases the likelihood of hepatobiliary excretion of the radiopharmaceutical and visualization of the biliary tree, thus reducing false negatives and improving the specificity. The sensitivity of hepatobiliary scintigraphy in detecting biliary atresia is 100%, with specificity approaching 93% when phenobarbital is utilized.

References: Mettler FA, Guiberteau MJ. *Essentials of nuclear medicine imaging*, 7th ed. Philadelphia, PA: Saunders, 2019:235–236.

O'Malley JP, Ziessman HA, Thrall JH. *Nuclear medicine: the requisites*, 5th ed. Philadelphia, PA: Saunders, 2020:198–200, 202–203.

12 **Answer B.** Anterior and lateral images acquired after IV administration of Tc-99m pertechnetate demonstrate a focus of intense activity in the floor of the mouth (large arrow), which is most compatible with a lingual thyroid. Another focus of intense activity more inferiorly and anteriorly (small arrow) likely represents ectopic thyroid tissue at the level of the hyoid bone. Physiologic uptake is present within the oral cavity as well as lingual and submandibular salivary glands (arrowheads). Ectopic thyroid is nearly always associated with lifelong hypothyroidism and typically requires higher doses of ʟ-thyroxine. T4 levels are low in congenital hypothyroidism. Eutopic thyroid is almost never seen in addition to a lingual thyroid. Thyroid peroxidase deficiency represents thyroid dyshormonogenesis and is associated with normally positioned glands.

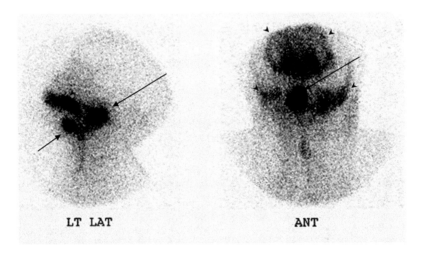

References: Coley B. *Caffey's pediatric diagnostic imaging*, 12th ed. Philadelphia, PA: Elsevier Saunders, 2013:151–155.

Habibian MR. *Nuclear medicine imaging: a teaching file*, 2nd ed. Philadelphia, PA: Lippincott Williams & Wilkins, 2009:24–25.

QUESTIONS

1 Which of the following interventions would **LEAST** likely help in reducing the abnormal F-18 FDG uptake seen in the following patient?

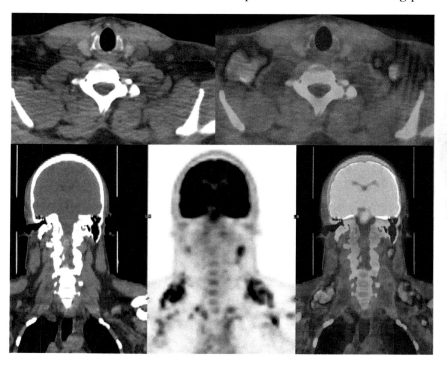

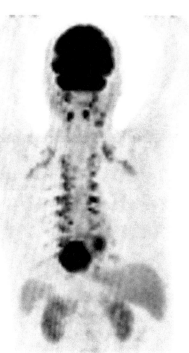

A. Beta-blockers such as propranolol
B. Raising the ambient temperature
C. Phenylephrine
D. Diazepam

2 With regard to breast cancer, F-18 FDG is **LEAST** likely to be helpful in which of the following clinical scenarios?

A. Initial staging in patients with advanced breast cancer
B. Evaluation of lymph node status in a patient with newly diagnosed breast cancer
C. Evaluating the response to treatment in locally advanced and metastatic breast cancer
D. Staging recurrent or metastatic breast cancer

3 Which of the following statements is MOST correct regarding the preparation instructions for a patient undergoing F-18 FDG-PET/CT for tumor imaging?

A. The patient should fast for at least 12 to 24 hours prior to the examination.
B. Hydration with dextrose-containing solutions does not need to be discontinued.
C. Diabetic medications should be discontinued for 12 hours prior to the examination.
D. Strenuous exercise should be avoided for 24 hours prior to the FDG-PET/CT examination.
E. The fasting blood glucose levels should be <250 mg/dL prior to the injection of FDG.

4 The following FDG-PET/CT images were acquired from a patient with a clinical history of head and neck squamous cell carcinoma. What is the most likely etiology for the abnormal intracardiac uptake?

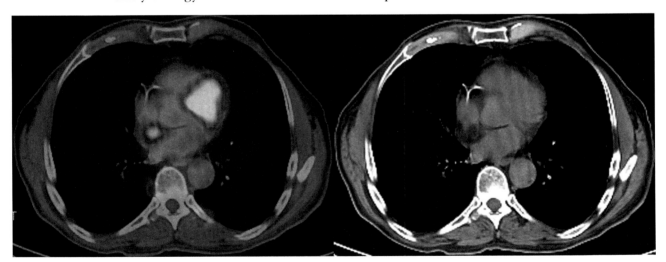

A. Atrial thrombus
B. Ventricular thrombus
C. Primary cardiac malignancy
D. Infectious endocarditis
E. Physiologic variant
F. Metastasis
G. Sarcoidosis

5 F-18 FDG-PET can be false negative in the evaluation of which of the following malignancies?

A. Squamous cell carcinoma of the head and neck
B. Squamous cell carcinoma of the lung
C. Esophageal adenocarcinoma
D. Adenocarcinoma of the lung
E. Small cell lung carcinoma
F. Lung carcinoid

6 Which of the following is the most likely cause of abnormal findings on the following examination?

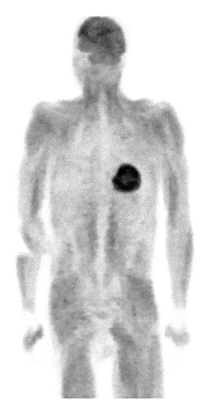

A. Infection
B. Inflammation
C. Wrong radiopharmaceutical
D. Endogenous or exogenous insulin
E. Exercise

7 What degree of FDG uptake is typically observed in low-grade gliomas?

A. Higher than normal cortical gray matter
B. Same as normal cortical gray matter
C. Lower than normal cortical gray matter but greater than white matter
D. Similar to the white matter

8 What is the most appropriate next step in this patient with an enlarging pulmonary nodule?

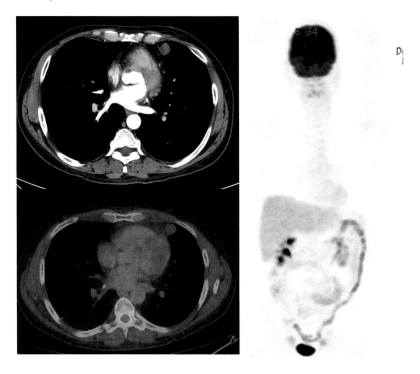

A. Follow-up FDG-PET/CT in 1 year
B. No further follow-up necessary
C. Follow-up CT scan in 1 year
D. Image-guided biopsy

9 The following patient with HIV/AIDS presents with a headache. Based on the supplied images, what is the most likely diagnosis?

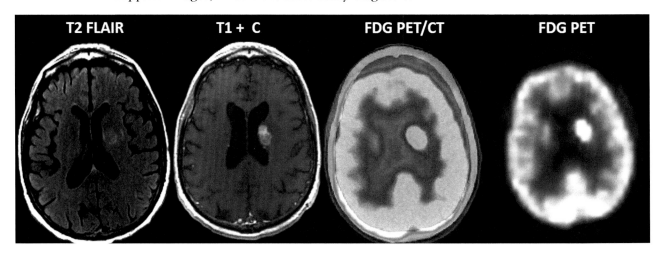

A. Progressive multifocal leukoencephalopathy
B. Intracerebral abscess
C. Toxoplasmosis
D. Metastasis
E. Lymphoma

10 The following images are from a 30-year-old male with a clinical history of retroperitoneal lymphoma (arrows) before and after initiation of chemotherapy. Which of the following is the most likely etiology of the abnormal finding on the follow-up FDG-PET scan?

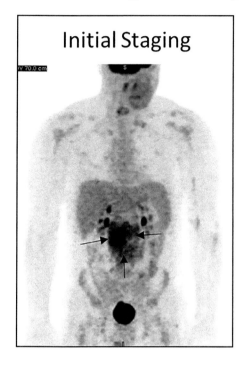
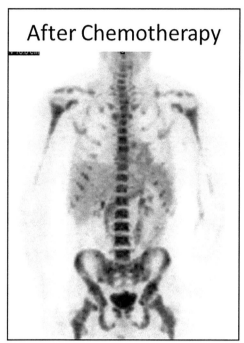

A. Malignant
B. Infectious
C. Physiologic
D. Inflammatory

11 The following F-18 FDG-PET/CT images are from a 55-year-old gentleman with newly diagnosed lung cancer. What is the most likely cause of abnormal uptake in the neck marked by the arrow on the MIP image?

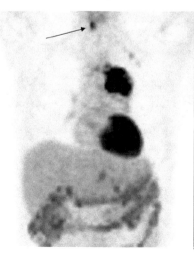
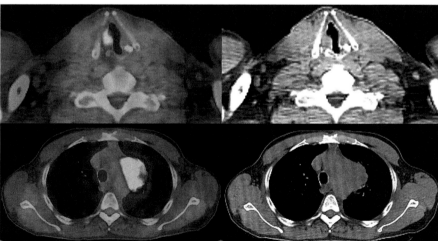

A. Metastasis
B. Second primary malignancy
C. Physiologic
D. Infection
E. Inflammation

12 The following FDG-PET/CT is from a 67-year-old gentleman with extensive history of smoking and newly diagnosed right upper lobe lung mass. Which of the following is the most likely cause of abnormal FDG uptake within the right parotid gland?

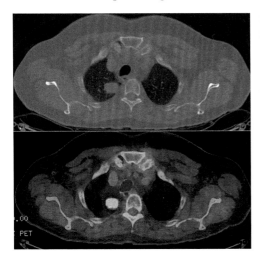 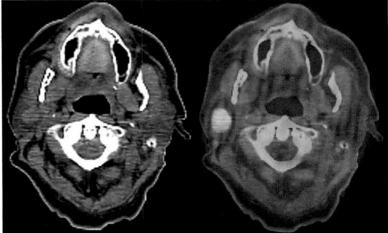

A. Infection
B. Metastasis
C. Warthin tumor
D. Adenoid cystic carcinoma

13 A 25-year-old gentleman with Hodgkin lymphoma presents for evaluation of response to treatment with F-18 FDG-PET/CT. Based on the pretreatment and posttreatment images provided, what is the most appropriate Deauville score on the posttreatment scan?

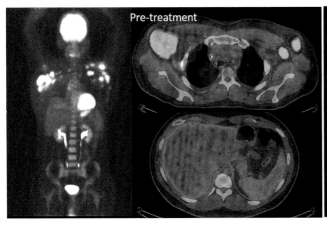 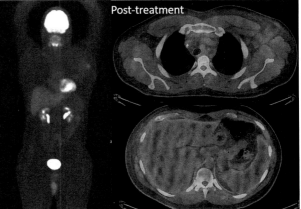

A. 0
B. 1
C. 2
D. 3
E. 4
F. 5

14 A 36-year-old gentleman presents with a history of frequent nontraumatic fractures. Based on the following OctreoScan images, what is the most likely diagnosis?

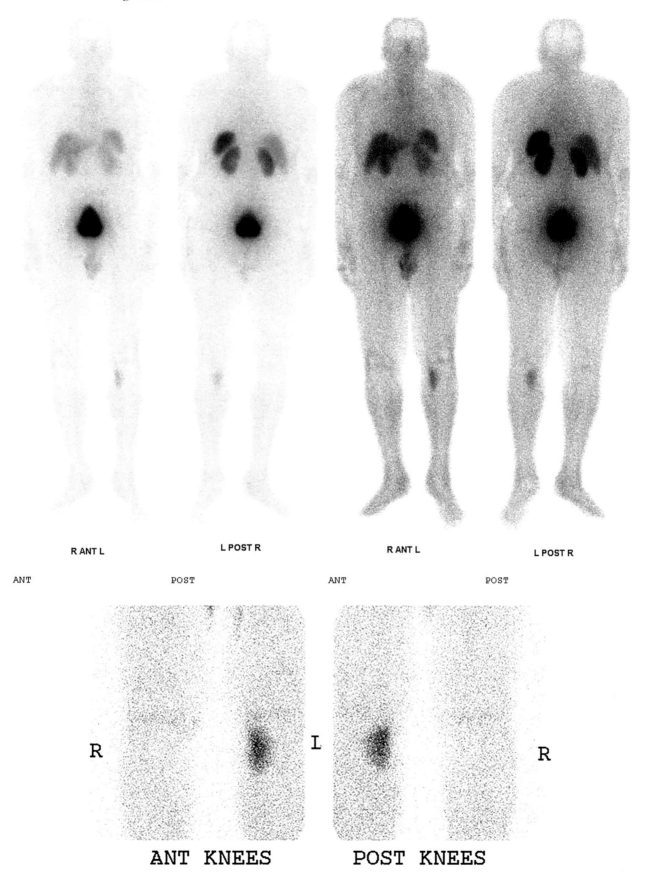

R ANT L   L POST R   R ANT L   L POST R

ANT   POST   ANT   POST

R   L   R

ANT KNEES   **POST KNEES**

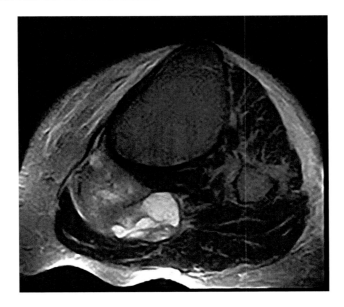

A. Carcinoid
B. Neuroblastoma
C. Infection
D. Oncogenic osteomalacia
E. Metastatic small cell carcinoma

15 Lutathera (lutetium-177 DOTATATE) is indicated for the treatment of what type of malignancy?

A. Estrogen receptor–positive tumor
B. Somatostatin receptor–positive tumor
C. Prostate-specific membrane antigen receptor–positive tumors
D. Dopamine receptor–positive tumors

16 What is the most likely cause for the findings shown below in this patient who is undergoing evaluation of metastatic carcinoid with Ga-68 DOTATATE PET/CT?

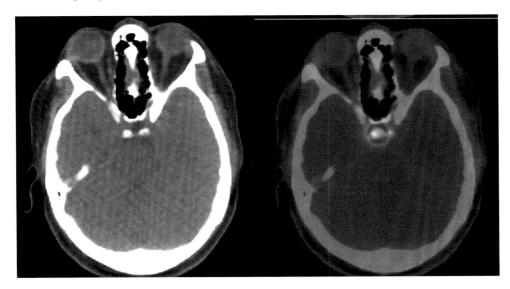

A. Macroadenoma
B. Hypophysitis
C. Meningioma
D. Physiologic
E. Metastatic

17 Based on the following supplied MIP image from a Ga-68 DOTATATE PET/CT scan, what is the most likely diagnosis?

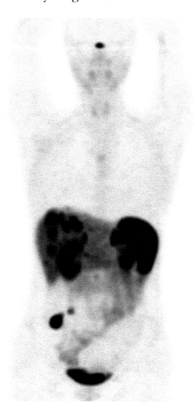

A. Metastatic colon cancer
B. Metastatic carcinoid
C. Metastatic ovarian carcinoma
D. Metastatic pancreatic neuroendocrine tumor
E. Splenosis

18 The following CT, fused F-18 FDG-PET/CT, and PET axial images are from a 68-year-old gentleman with a history of colon cancer. What is the most likely diagnosis?

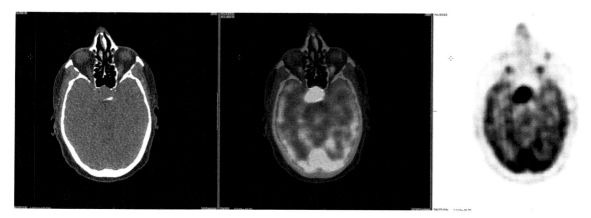

A. Physiologic uptake
B. Pituitary adenoma
C. Metastasis
D. Contamination
E. Pituitary melanoma

19 What is the most likely cause for the following findings?

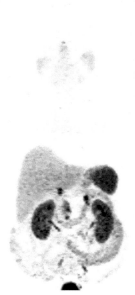
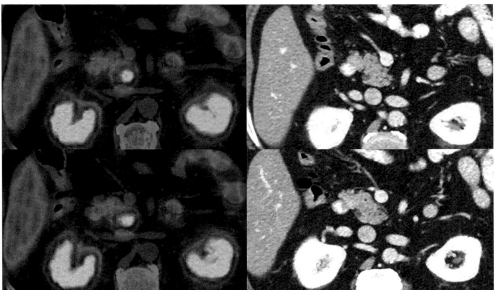

A. Primary pancreatic neuroendocrine tumor
B. Metastatic carcinoid to the pancreas
C. Metastatic renal cell carcinoma to the pancreas
D. Primary pancreatic adenocarcinoma
E. Physiologic pancreatic activity
F. Bilateral renal involvement by lymphoma with a retroperitoneal lymph node metastasis

20 Which of the following radiopharmaceuticals is a hypoxia imaging agent?

A. Cu-144 ATSM
B. F-18 FES
C. C-11 choline
D. F-18 FDG

21 Several adverse reactions are associated with immune checkpoint inhibitors. Most of them are readily reversed by stopping the agent. Which type of immune-related adverse event (irAE) is irreversible?

A. Pneumonitis
B. Hypophysitis
C. Colitis
D. Rash

22 The following images are from a 48-year-old gentleman with a past medical history of small bowel carcinoid status postresection. Which of the following is the most likely diagnosis based on the images provided?

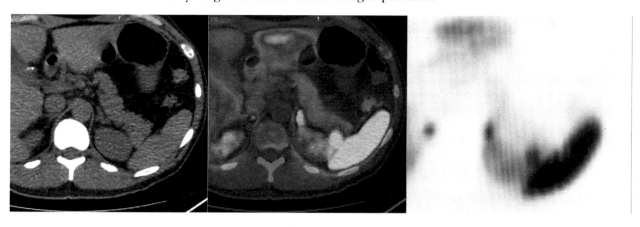

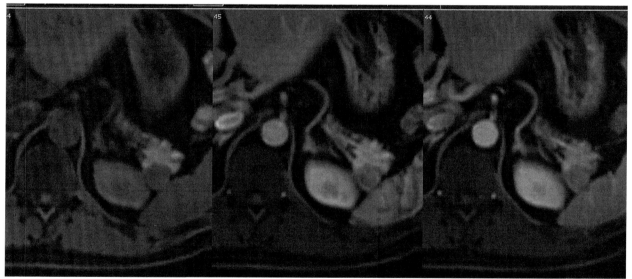

    A. Primary pancreatic neuroendocrine tumor
    B. Pancreatic metastasis from carcinoid
    C. Pancreatic adenocarcinoma
    D. Ectopic splenic tissue in the pancreas
    E. Left adrenal metastasis

23 Which of the following radiotracers should be considered in the workup of a patient with poorly differentiated neuroendocrine tumors?

    A. I-123 MIBG
    B. Ga-68 PSMA
    C. F-18 FDG
    D. In-111 pentetreotide

24 The mechanism of action for Axumin (fluciclovine F-18) PET scans for the detection of prostate cancer involves which of the following?

    A. Prostate-specific membrane antigen binding
    B. Amino acid transporters
    C. Fluorodeoxyglucose metabolism
    D. Somatostatin receptor binding

25 Which of the following is an indication for Ga-68 PSMA PET imaging?

A. Sarcoid
B. Prostate cancer
C. Lymphoma
D. Neuroendocrine tumor

26 What radiotracer was utilized for generating the following scintimammography image?

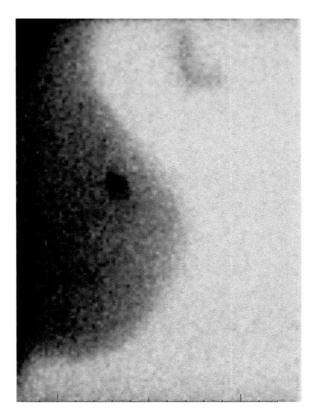

A. Tc-99m sestamibi
B. Tl-201
C. Tc-99m MDP
D. F-18 FDG

27 Which of the following immune checkpoint inhibitor agents is an anti-CTLA-4 monoclonal antibody?

A. Nivolumab
B. Pembrolizumab
C. Ipilimumab
D. Durvalumab

28 Which of the following disease processes can result in a false-positive finding on a Ga-68 DOTATATE scan?

A. Meningioma
B. Primitive neuroectodermal tumors (PNET)
C. Ependymoma
D. Astrocytoma

29 The following F-18 FDG-PET/CT images are from an 18-year-old female with a history of ulcerative colitis and resulting colon cancer who is status post colectomy as well as chemotherapy. The patient now presents for restaging in the setting of rising CEA levels. The intensely FDG avid presacral mass shown below was subsequently proven to be recurrent colon cancer. What is the most likely explanation for the abnormal findings in the chest?

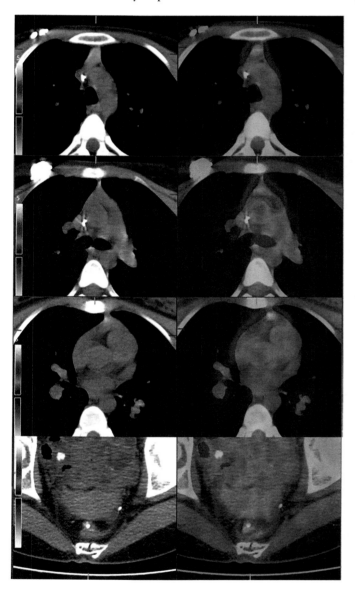 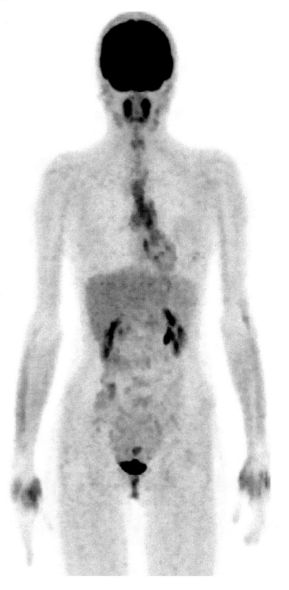

A. Metastatic colon cancer
B. Lymphoma
C. Thymic hyperplasia
D. Teratoma

30   What is the most likely etiology responsible for the following F-18 FDG PET/CT findings in a 90-year-old patient with a history of pelvic radiation for treatment of malignancy?

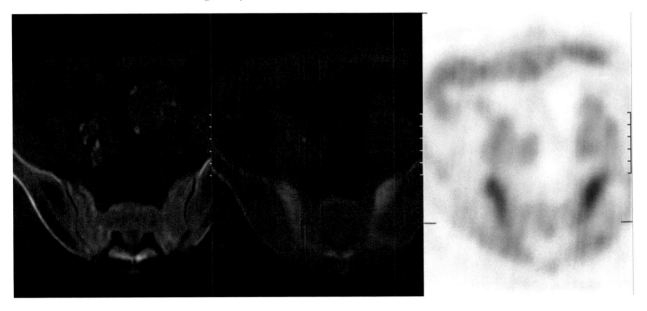

    A. Sacral insufficiency fracture
    B. Radiation-induced sarcoma
    C. Osseous metastases
    D. Paget disease

31   A 59-year-old gentleman undergoes F-18 FDG-PET/CT for initial staging of non–small cell lung carcinoma. Based on the following images, what is the most likely stage of this patient's malignancy?

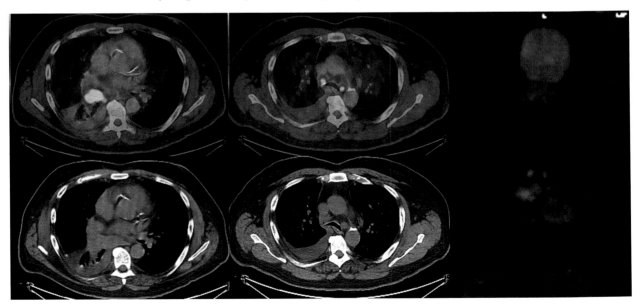

    A. II
    B. IIIA
    C. IIIB
    D. IV

32 What is the most likely reason for intense F-18 fluciclovine uptake in the pancreas for the following patient?

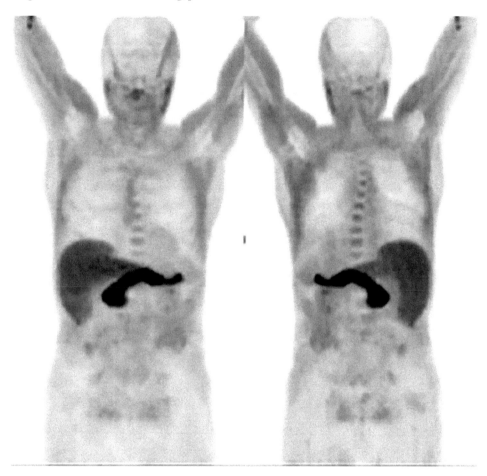

A. Physiologic receptor binding
B. Physiologic amino acid metabolism
C. Physiologic fatty acid metabolism
D. Pancreatitis

33 What is the most likely diagnosis in the following 67-year-old patient with a history of prostatectomy and a rising PSA of 2.7?

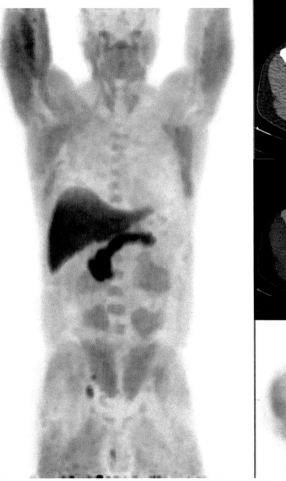

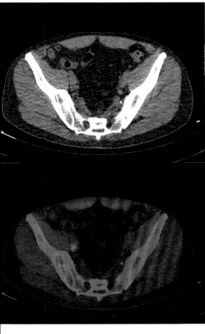

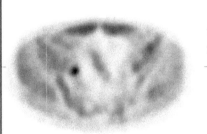

A. Postprandial state
B. Exercise within 24 hours of scan
C. Recurrent prostate cancer
D. Liver metastasis

ANSWERS AND EXPLANATIONS

1 **Answer C.** The supplied images demonstrate intense FDG uptake in bilateral cervical, supraclavicular, subpectoral, and paravertebral regions corresponding to fat attenuation on CT scan. Findings are consistent with physiologic brown adipose tissue (BAT) uptake. BAT is a sympathetically innervated tissue that plays an important role in cold-induced and diet-induced thermogenesis. Physiologic BAT uptake is typically identified in bilateral cervical, supraclavicular, axillary, subpectoral, costovertebral, and retroperitoneal/retrocrural regions. It occurs more commonly in cold weather, young females, and children. Successful strategies to reduce brown fat uptake include preventing exposure to cold temperature, controlling environment temperature prior to and after FDG injection (warm clothing, warm blankets, temperature-controlled rooms at 75°F, etc.), avoiding sympathetic stimulants (nicotine, phenylephrine, ephedrine, etc.), pharmacologically by reducing sympathetic activity (beta-blockers such as propranolol), or pharmacologically by using sedatives such as oral or intravenous diazepam. In a study done by Agrawal et al., 40 mg propranolol PO administered 60 minutes prior to F-18 FDG injection resulted in complete resolution of BAT uptake in 90% of patients. Although mixed results have been reported with the success of diazepam in reducing BAT uptake, Rakheja et al. observed a significant reduction in brown fat activity following premedication with 5 mg of diazepam intravenously 10 minutes prior to F-18 FDG administration. Sympathetic stimulants such as phenylephrine are known to cause brown fat activation and increase its FDG uptake.

References: Agrawal A, Nair N, Baghel NS. A novel approach for reduction of brown fat uptake on FDG PET. *Br J Radiol* 2009;82(980):626–631.

Garcia C, Bandaru V, Van Nostrand D, et al. Effective reduction of brown fat FDG uptake by controlling environmental temperature prior to PET scan: an expanded case series. *Mol Imaging Biol* 2010;12(6):652–656.

Rakheja R, Ciarallo A, Alabed YZ, et al. Intravenous administration of diazepam significantly reduces brown fat activity on 18F-FDG PET/CT. *Am J Nucl Med Mol Imaging* 2011;1(1): 29–35.

2 **Answer B.** Sentinel node localization with Tc-99m sulfur colloid, with or without blue dye, is the preferred method for evaluating nonpalpable lymph nodes in a patient with newly diagnosed breast cancer. Since a negative F-18 FDG-PET scan does not exclude the need for further workup, it has no role in this scenario. Mammography, MRI, and ultrasound are the primary modalities used in screening and diagnosing breast cancer. F-18 FDG-PET is most useful in the initial staging of patients with advanced breast cancer, in monitoring response to therapy, and in the evaluation of patients with suspected recurrence or residual active disease.

References: O'Malley JP, Ziessman HA, Thrall JH. *Nuclear medicine: the requisites*, 5th ed. Philadelphia, PA: Saunders, 2020:320–327.

Rosen EL, Eubank WB, Mankoff DA. FDG PET, PET/CT, and breast cancer imaging. *RadioGraphics* 2007;27(suppl 1):S215–S229.

3 **Answer D.** Patient preparation is critical for individuals undergoing evaluation of malignancy by FDG-PET/CT. The goal of patient preparation is to maximize the F-18 FDG uptake by tumor and minimize the normal physiologic uptake in other tissues. The patient should be instructed to fast and not consume beverages, except for water, for at least 4 to 6 hours before the administration of F-18 FDG to decrease physiologic glucose levels and to reduce serum insulin levels. Similarly, IV fluids containing dextrose or parenteral feedings should be withheld for 4 to 6 hours. Since tumor uptake of F-18 FDG is reduced in hyperglycemic states, most institutes reschedule patients if the blood glucose level is >200 mg/dL. Both NCI and ACR recommend avoiding strenuous activities such as jogging, cycling, weight lifting, strenuous housework, and sexual activity for a minimum of 24 hours in order to reduce physiologic muscular uptake. All oral medications, including those for diabetes, can be taken as prescribed. While there are no current guidelines, at our institution patients taking long-acting insulin at night before the study are instructed to take half the dose to avoid an episode of hypoglycemia from a full dose.

Reference: Surasi DS, Bhambhvani P, Baldwin JA, et al. (1)(8)F-FDG PET and PET/CT patient preparation: a review of the literature. *J Nucl Med Technol* 2014;42(1):5–13.

4   **Answer E.** Axial fused F-18 FDG-PET/CT and CT images demonstrate a moderate-sized focus of intense FDG uptake corresponding to fat attenuation between left and right atrium (arrow). This is physiologic FDG uptake within lipomatous hypertrophy of the interatrial septum. Lipomatous hypertrophy of the interatrial septum may demonstrate variable degree of FDG uptake. This patient also had significant brown adipose tissue (BAT) uptake elsewhere in the body, and intense uptake within this lipomatous hypertrophy of interatrial septum is likely secondary to BAT within it. A large focus of intense activity in the location of the left ventricle (arrowhead) is physiologic glucose uptake in the anterior wall of the myocardium. Depending on the patient's nutritional status, myocardium can utilize either fatty acids or glucose for metabolism and demonstrate a variable degree of F-18 FDG uptake.

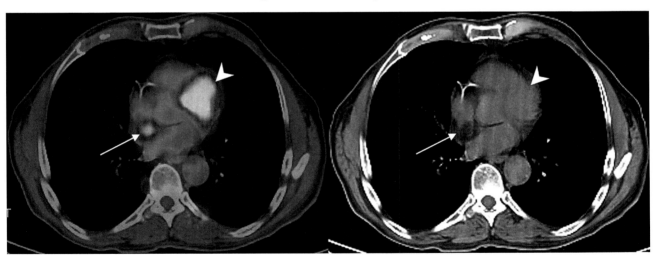

Reference: Rao PM, Woodard PK, Patterson GA, et al. Myocardial metastasis or benign brown fat? *Circ Cardiovasc Imaging* 2009;2(4):e25–e27.

5   **Answer F.** Tumors with low metabolic activity such as bronchioloalveolar carcinoma (adenocarcinoma in situ) and carcinoid tumors can give rise to false-negative FDG-PET results. A well-differentiated lepidic predominant adenocarcinoma and mucinous adenocarcinoma can also be falsely negative on FDG-PET. FDG-PET has been reported to have false-negative results with mucosa-associated lymphoid tissue (MALT), extranodal marginal zone lymphoma, and chronic lymphocytic leukemia (CLL). However, FDG-PET has been found to be useful in the detection of Richter transformation of CLL

to large cell lymphoma with a high sensitivity and specificity and negative predictive value. Lesions <1 cm in diameter may be below PET resolution and can be falsely negative on FDG-PET.

References: Bruzzi JF, Macapinlac H, Tsimberidou AM, et al. Detection of Richter's transformation of chronic lymphocytic leukemia by PET/CT. *J Nucl Med* 2006;47(8): 1267–1273.

Kostakoglu L, Agress H, Goldsmith SJ. Clinical role of FDG PET in evaluation of cancer patients. *RadioGraphics* 2003;23(2):315–340.

Weiler-Sagie M, Bushelev O, Epelbaum R, et al. (18)F-FDG avidity in lymphoma readdressed: a study of 766 patients. *J Nucl Med* 2010;51(1):25–30.

6   **Answer D.** A single anterior MIP image demonstrates the presence of increased FDG uptake diffusely throughout the musculature with intense FDG uptake within the myocardium. Relatively decreased FDG uptake is noted within the brain's gray matter as well as within the liver. This distribution pattern is typically seen with exposure to endogenous or exogenous insulin with resultant uptake of the FDG into the musculature. Causes of endogenous insulin release include recent ingestion of food or beverage containing carbohydrates, IV fluids containing dextrose, and tube feeds. Increased F-18 FDG uptake in the musculature results in decreased availability for tumor uptake, resulting in decreased sensitivity and standard uptake values (SUVs). As such the patients are asked to fast for at least 4 hours, preferably 6 hours prior to F-18 FDG administration. Differential considerations for diffuse muscular uptake include strenuous exercise within 24 hours. However, the FDG uptake would be less diffuse and only involve the muscle groups that were used during the exercise. Also, myocardial uptake would not be as prominent with exercise as with postprandial state. Strenuous exercise causes depletion of muscular glycogen storage, which may result in glucose uptake by the muscle over the next 24 hours. As such, the patients are asked to avoid strenuous exercise for 24 hours prior to the F-18 FDG PET scan.

References: Cohade C. Altered biodistribution on FDG-PET with emphasis on brown fat and insulin effect. *Semin Nucl Med* 2010;40(4):283–293. doi:10.1053/j.semnuclmed.2010.02.001. Review. PubMed PMID: 20513450.

Surasi DS, Bhambhvani P, Baldwin JA, et al. (1)(8)F-FDG PET and PET/CT patient preparation: a review of the literature. *J Nucl Med Technol* 2014;42(1):5–13.

7   **Answer D.** Low-grade gliomas typically demonstrate low FDG uptake, similar to or less than that of the white matter. On the other hand, high-grade gliomas such as glioblastoma multiforme demonstrate intense FDG uptake, similar to or slightly less than that of the cortical gray matter. Primary CNS lymphoma typically demonstrates the highest degree of FDG uptake, more than that of the cortical gray matter. A higher degree of FDG uptake is typically associated with a higher grade of malignancy and poorer prognosis. While FDG-PET has been reported to be able to differentiate between radiation necrosis and recurrence, several reports suggest that the ability of FDG-PET to differentiate between radiation necrosis and recurrence is limited.

References: Padma MV, Said S, Jacobs M, et al. Prediction of pathology and survival by FDG PET in gliomas. *J Neurooncol* 2003;64(3):227–237.

Ricci PE, Karis JP, Heiserman JE, et al. Differentiating recurrent tumor from radiation necrosis: time for re-evaluation of positron emission tomography? *Am J Neuroradiol* 1998;19(3):407–413.

8   **Answer D.** Axial CT, fused FDG-PET/CT, and MIP images demonstrate the presence of a large noncalcified, non-FDG avid pulmonary nodule within the anteromedial aspect of the left upper lung. Even though benign entities such as pulmonary hamartoma may present similarly, malignancies such as well-differentiated adenocarcinoma, adenocarcinoma in situ, carcinoid, and low-grade lymphoma can be falsely negative on FDG-PET/CT; as such, lack of FDG uptake does not confirm benignancy. In this patient with an enlarging pulmonary nodule, further evaluation with image-guided biopsy would be the most appropriate next step. If this was the initial imaging and prior comparisons were not available, a short-term follow-up CT may be a valid option. Lesions <1 cm may be below the FDG-PET resolution and also be false negative on FDG-PET in which case follow-up chest CT should be considered.

References: Chang JM, Lee HJ, Goo JM, et al. False-positive and false-negative FDG-PET scans in various thoracic diseases. *Korean J Radiol* 2006;7(1):57–69.

O'Malley JP, Ziessman HA, Thrall JH. *Nuclear medicine: the requisites*, 5th ed. Philadelphia, PA: Saunders, 2020:315–320.

Ziessman HA, O'Malley JP, Thrall JH. *Nuclear medicine: the requisites*, 4th ed. Philadelphia, PA: Saunders, 2014:248.

9 **Answer E.** Axial MRI (FLAIR and T1 postcontrast), PET/CT, and PET images demonstrate markedly hypermetabolic (greater than that of the gray matter), slightly heterogeneously enhancing mass within the subependymal region of the left periventricular white matter (arrows on image below). There is no significant surrounding T2 hyperintensity on FLAIR images. The appearance, location, and marked intense FDG uptake are characteristics of primary CNS lymphoma (PCNSL). PCNSL demonstrates the most pronounced metabolic activity, more than that seen with high-grade gliomas (GBM) or metastasis. Less likely differential for this appearance would include glioblastoma multiforme (GBM). Enhancement with GBM would be typically more heterogeneous, and it would usually demonstrate significant surrounding T2 hyperintensity on FLAIR from tumor infiltration/vasogenic edema. Also, FDG uptake in GBM would be more heterogeneous with the degree of FDG uptake, while intense (equal or slightly less than gray matter), not as intense as PCNSL. An abscess would demonstrate ring enhancement with T2-hypointense rim and surrounding edema on FLAIR. Although toxoplasmosis can produce enhancing brain lesions in a patient with HIV/AIDS, it would not demonstrate significant FDG uptake. Progressive multifocal leukoencephalopathy manifests as T2 hyperintensity without enhancement and typically involves subcortical U fibers and corpus callosum. Metastasis is more common at the gray–white matter junction, and the degree of FDG uptake is usually significantly lower than that of primary CNS lymphoma seen in this case.

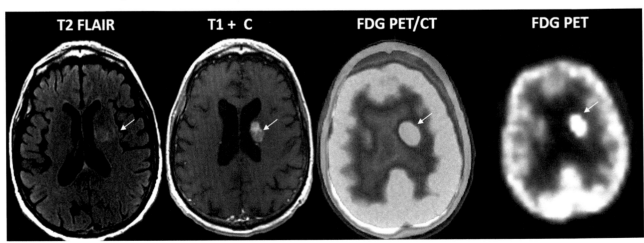

Reference: Haldorsen IS, Espeland A, Larsson E-M. Central nervous system lymphoma: characteristic findings on traditional and advanced imaging. *Am J Neuroradiol* 2011;32(6):984–992.

10 **Answer C.** The follow-up positron emission tomography images after chemotherapy demonstrate resolution of intense FDG uptake within the retroperitoneal lymphadenopathy. However, there is now diffuse slightly heterogeneous intense FDG uptake within the axial and proximal appendicular skeleton. These findings are most compatible with physiologic bone marrow hyperplasia (BMH) secondary to granulocyte colony-stimulating factor (G-CSF). Increased splenic activity may also be seen in BMH secondary to extramedullary hematopoiesis. Increased FDG uptake by bone marrow with G-CSF therapy is felt to be secondary to increase in bone marrow metabolism and cellularity in response to the treatment. It is important to recognize this as a physiologic finding and not to misinterpret it as progression of disease. Findings of BMH commonly persist for 2 to 4 weeks after cessation of therapy. BMH has also been reported in G-CSF–producing lung tumors. Similar findings can also be seen in patients with severe anemia.

References: Morooka M, Kubota K, Murata Y, et al. (18)F-FDG-PET/CT findings of granulocyte colony stimulating factor (G-CSF)-producing lung tumors. *Ann Nucl Med* 2008;22(7):635–639.

Sugawara Y, Fisher SJ, Zasadny KR, Kison PV, et al. Preclinical and clinical studies of bone marrow uptake of fluorine-1-fluorodeoxyglucose with or without granulocyte colony-stimulating factor during chemotherapy. *J Clin Oncol* 1998;16(1):173–180.

11 **Answer C.** A large intensely FDG-avid mass is present within the medial aspect of the left upper lobe, which invades into the mediastinum at the level of the aortic arch. Abnormal uptake in the neck corresponds to asymmetric intense FDG uptake within the right vocal cord (arrows in image below). No FDG uptake is present within the left vocal cord. Findings are due to physiologic FDG uptake in the right vocal cord with none in the left vocal cord secondary to the left vocal cord paralysis. The left recurrent laryngeal nerve (RLN) branches from the left vagus nerve in the thorax and travels inferior and posterior to the aortic arch before ascending into the neck. As such, any mass in the region of the aortic arch can result in its paralysis. The right RLN branches from the right vagus nerve in the neck anterior to the right subclavian artery at the level of T1–T2 and travels inferior and posterior to the right subclavian artery to ascend in the neck. There is no mass corresponding to the vocal cord on the CT, making second primary malignancy unlikely; slight asymmetry on CT is secondary to paralysis. Metastasis involving vocal cord would be highly unusual. Since there is no significant asymmetry or stranding, infection/inflammation is unlikely likewise.

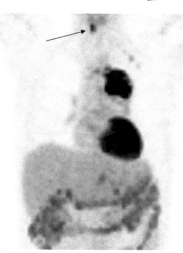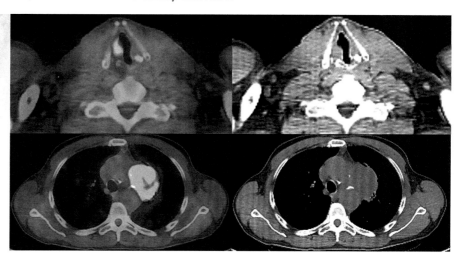

Reference: Komissarova M, Wong KK, et al. Spectrum of 18F-FDG PET/CT findings in oncology-related recurrent laryngeal nerve palsy. *Am J Roentgenol* 2009;192(1):288–294.

12 **Answer C.** About 80% of parotid tumors are benign, with benign mixed-cell tumors (pleomorphic adenomas) being the most common and Warthin tumor the second most common. Warthin tumor and pleomorphic adenoma are the most common causes of incidental FDG-avid parotid mass. An isolated parotid metastasis from a lung primary is unlikely. While adenoid cystic carcinoma is almost always FDG avid, it is rare. Given the focal nature of the abnormality and lack of surrounding stranding, infection is less likely. According to a recently published study in patients who underwent FDG-PET/CT for an oncologic indication by Makis et al., only 4% of the incidental FDG-positive parotid lesions were malignant. The degree of FDG uptake in the Warthin tumor (SUVmax 10.3) was considerably greater than that of the malignancy (SUVmax 7.4), and degree of FDG uptake did not differentiate benign from malignant lesions.

References: Dua SG, Purandare NC, Shah S, et al. Bilateral synchronous and multifocal Warthin's tumor mimicking metastases from lung cancer: a rare cause of false positive flourodeoxy glucose positron emission tomography/computed tomography. *Indian J Nucl Med* 2012;27(2):139–140.

Makis W, Ciarallo A, Gotra A. Clinical significance of parotid gland incidentalomas on F-FDG PET/CT. *Clin Imaging* 2015;39(4):667–671.

13 **Answer D.** F-18 FDG-PET/CT plays a crucial role in staging and restaging/treatment response evaluation of patients with Hodgkin and many non-Hodgkin lymphomas. In these patients, change in disease status is more accurately depicted by the changes in F-18 FDG metabolic activity when compared to anatomic measurements on CT or MRI. Deauville Criteria were established to standardize the grading of F-18 FDG metabolic activity, comparing maximal tumor uptake to that of the background structures (i.e., mediastinal blood pool and liver). The scoring is as follows:

Deauville Score	Maximal Lesion Metabolic Activity
1	No uptake above background
2	Uptake ≤ mediastinal blood pool
3	Uptake > mediastinum but ≤ liver
4	Uptake moderately increased compared to liver
5	Uptake markedly increased compared to liver
X	New areas of uptake unlikely to be related to lymphoma

Pretreatment scan in this patient shows markedly hypermetabolic (Deauville Score 5) lymphadenopathy in bilateral axillae. Posttreatment scan reveals marked interval reduction in the FDG uptake along with marked reduction in the size of the axillary lymph nodes. Residual left axillary lymph nodes show FDG uptake greater than that of the mediastinum but less than or equal to that of the liver (Deauville Score 3). No new FDG-avid lesions are seen on the MIP image. Findings represent complete response to treatment by Lugano criteria for lymphoma response assessment.

References: Mettler FA, Guiberteau MJ. *Essentials of nuclear medicine imaging*, 7th ed. Philadelphia, PA: Saunders, 2019:347–349.

O'Malley JP, Ziessman HA, Thrall JH. *Nuclear medicine: the requisites*, 5th ed. Philadelphia, PA: Saunders, 2020:306.

14 **Answer D.** The 24-hour anterior and posterior whole-body as well as spot images of bilateral lower extremities demonstrate a moderate-sized focus of intense activity in the medial aspect of the left proximal leg. This corresponds to a T2-hyperintense lesion in the calf muscle on the MRI. Physiologic activity is seen corresponding to the liver, spleen, kidneys, and bladder. In this patient with a clinical history of fragility fractures, the findings are most consistent with oncogenic osteomalacia secondary to mesenchymal tumor in the left calf muscle.

Oncogenic osteomalacia is a rare disease, but its awareness is important as it can result in significant morbidity secondary to repeated fractures. Decreased bone strength is secondary to the tumor secreting fibroblast growth factor 23, which inhibits the kidney's ability to absorb phosphate, resulting in tumor-induced hypophosphatemic osteomalacia. This is typically caused by mesenchymal tumors expressing high levels of somatostatin receptors (SSTR), allowing for their detection using In-111 OctreoScan or Ga-68 DOTATATE. Given better imaging characteristics, anatomic resolution, and anatomic localization offered by PET/CT, Ga-68 DOTATATE is now preferred over In-111 OctreoScan. Since osteoblasts express SSTR and increased osteoblastic activity is seen with fragility fractures, healing fractures may appear as areas of increased DOTATATE uptake. These should not be confused as areas of osseous metastasis. Correlation with CT scan characteristics would help differentiate fragility fractures from tumor involvement. While activated lymphocytes express SSTR (i.e., tuberculosis, sarcoidosis), pyogenic infection does not typically show increased activity on OctreoScan. Even though malignancies such as carcinoid, neuroblastoma, and small cell carcinoma express SSTR, they are unlikely given the patient's clinical presentation.

References: El-Maouche D, Sadowski SM, Papadakis GZ, et al. 68Ga-DOTATATE for tumor localization in tumor-induced osteomalacia. *J Clin Endocrinol Metab* 2016;101(10):3575–3581. doi:10.1210/jc.2016-2052

Wuying C, Jiang Y, et al. Performance of 68Ga-DOTA-SST PET/CT, octreoscan SPECT/CT and 18F-FDG PET/CT in the detection of culprit tumors causing osteomalacia: a meta-analysis. *Nucl Med Commun* 2020;41(4):370–376.

15 **Answer B.** Lu-177 DOTATATE (Lutathera) is a somatostatin analog approved for the treatment of somatostatin receptor–positive neuroendocrine tumors by the FDA in early 2018. Patients receive at least four doses of Lutathera, each dose about two months apart. In patients with normal renal function, approximately 200 mCi of Lu-177 DOTATATE is infused intravenously over 30 minutes. Amino acids are administered intravenously to reduce renal toxicity by decreasing the radiation dose to the kidney. Amino acid infusion begins 30 minutes before Lutathera infusion, continues during the 30-minute Lutathera infusion, and continues for 3 hours after. Severe nausea and vomiting are common side effects of amino acid solution infusion. These are more prominent with solutions containing all or most of the amino acids when compared to solutions containing only lysine and arginine. Pretreatment with an antiemetic is started 30 minutes prior to amino acid infusion to reduce nausea.

References: O'Malley JP, Ziessman HA, Thrall JH. *Nuclear medicine: the requisites*, 5th ed. Philadelphia, PA: Saunders, 2020:344.

Strosberg J, El-Haddad G, Wolin E, et al. Phase 3 trial of 177 Lu-dotatate for midgut neuroendocrine tumors. *NEJM* 2017;376(2):125–135.

16 **Answer D.** As shown on the image below, a normal Ga-68 DOTATATE scan shows highest physiologic activity in the spleen followed by the adrenal glands, kidneys, and pituitary gland. Moderate physiologic activity is seen in the liver, salivary glands, and bowel. Mild to moderate physiologic activity may also be present in the thyroid gland. This biodistribution is due to either specific receptor binding or nonspecific tissue handling of the peptide. While meningioma has high SSTR 2 receptor density and is readily visualized on DOTATATE scan, the location suggests physiologic pituitary uptake. Knowledge of the normal biodistribution of radiotracer distribution is important in its identification in cases of misadministration or altered biodistribution due to quality control, etc.

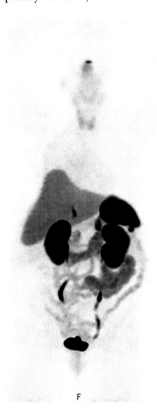

Reference: Deppen SA, Walker RC, et al. Safety and efficacy of 68Ga-DOTATATE PET/CT for diagnosis, staging, and treatment management of neuroendocrine tumors. *J Nucl Med* 2016;57(5):708–714.

17 **Answer B.** The supplied anterior projection MIP image from Ga-68 DOTATATE PET/CT demonstrates a large focus of intense activity within the right lower quadrant (arrow) with a smaller focus of intense activity more superomedial to it (arrowhead). Numerous foci of intense activity are seen within the liver parenchyma. This distribution pattern is most compatible with primary small bowel carcinoid in the right lower quadrant with associated right lower quadrant mesenteric lymph node metastases and numerous DOTATATE avid liver metastases. While a pancreatic neuroendocrine tumor (NET) would demonstrate DOTATATE avidity, the distribution pattern is that of carcinoid as no abnormal activity is seen in the pancreatic bed. While intense physiologic DOTATATE activity is seen in splenic tissue, again the pattern is not that of splenosis. The other mentioned malignancies are not typically DOTATATE avid and do not show a similar distribution pattern.

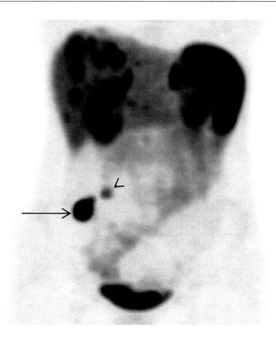

Ga-68 DOTATATE (DOTA-0-Tyr3-Octreotate) and Ga-68 DOTANOC and DOTATOC are PET tracers that bind to somatostatin receptors (SSTR) with high affinity. As such, like In-111 OctreoScan, they are useful in the evaluation of NETs. Compared to In-111 OctreoScan, PET agents have improved pharmacokinetics (faster tumor uptake and rapid clearance), higher sensitivity/resolution, less radiation, and less time (approximately 2 hours compared to 24 to 48 hours). In a study done by Deppen et al., Ga-68 DOTATATE was found to have greater sensitivity, specificity, and accuracy when compared to In-111 OctreoScan. Ga-68 DOTATATE is currently FDA approved for the localization of SSTR-positive NETs in adult and pediatric populations. It has also been proven superior to In-111 OctreoScan in the evaluation of tumor-induced osteomalacia and paraganglioma.

Reference: Deppen SA, Walker RC, et al. Safety and efficacy of 68Ga-DOTATATE PET/CT for diagnosis, staging, and treatment management of neuroendocrine tumors. *J Nucl Med* 2016;57(5):708–714.

18 **Answer B.** Axial CT, fused PET/CT, and PET images acquired after the intravenous administration of F-18 FDG reveal intense, focal uptake corresponding to an enlarged pituitary gland. On the CT scan image, widening of the sella is seen. The findings likely represent a pituitary macroadenoma for which further evaluation with contrast-enhanced MRI of the brain should be considered. Incidentally detected increased pituitary 18F-FDG PET uptake is usually associated with benign pituitary tumors such as adenoma. The most common cause of an abnormal pituitary uptake is generally a primary pituitary tumor including micro- and macroadenomas, followed by metastatic malignancy, Langerhans cell histiocytosis (LCH), and inflammatory hypophysitis. C and E are incorrect as metastasis from the colon cancer and a primary pituitary melanoma are both less likely than an adenoma. Under physiologic conditions, the pituitary gland shows FDG uptake less than that of the gray matter and is smaller in size than seen in this patient. Intense physiologic pituitary uptake is generally seen with Ga-68 DOTATATE scan and not F-18 FDG.

Reference: Ju H, Zhou J, Pan Y, et al. Evaluation of pituitary uptake incidentally identified on 18F-FDG PET/CT scan. *Oncotarget* 2017;8(33):55544–55549.

19 Answer E. Radiotracer distribution on the MIP image suggests that this is an image from Ga-68 DOTATATE scan. Fused PET/CT images show intense activity in the pancreatic uncinate process. However, no abnormal enhancement is seen in this region on an early-phase contrast-enhanced CT of the abdomen. No space-occupying lesions are seen in this region on the CT with preservation of fat planes surrounding the pancreatic lobules. As such, this finding is most consistent with physiologic pancreatic uncinate process activity. This is a normal variant and should not be confused with malignancy. Similar but less intense activity can also be seen in the pancreatic tail and has been associated with nonneoplastic islet cell hyperplasia. Careful correlation with patient's clinical history and contrast-enhanced multiphase CT or MRI must be performed to ascertain if the abnormal DOTATATE activity corresponds to any lesion. Image below shows focal intense radiotracer activity corresponding to an enhancing subcentimeter nodule on contrast enhanced CT scan in the anterior inferior aspect of the uncinate process (arrows below); finding is consistent with a primary pancreatic neuroendocrine tumor in the patient below.

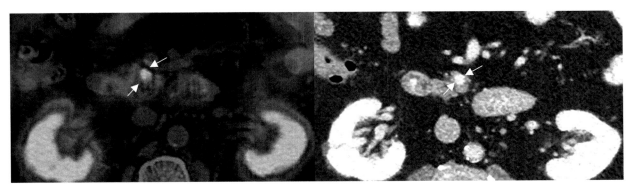

Reference: Hofman MS, Lau WF, Hicks RJ. Somatostatin receptor imaging with 68Ga DOTATATE PET/CT: clinical utility, normal patterns, pearls, and pitfalls in interpretation. *RadioGraphics* 2015;35(2):500–516.

20 Answer A. Tumor hypoxia is associated with malignant progression, radiotherapy resistance, and poor prognosis. As such, agents have been developed to image tumor hypoxia to assess tumor radiosensitivity and patient prognosis. Cu-144 ATSM and F-18 FMISO are two of the most commonly used agents for hypoxia imaging. The half-life of Cu-144 ATSM (12.7 hours) is well suited for hypoxia imaging. F-18 FES PET/CT influences the staging and management of patients with newly diagnosed estrogen receptor–positive breast cancer. C-11 and F-18 choline have been used in the workup for recurrent prostate cancer.

Reference: O'Malley JP, Ziessman HA, Thrall JH. *Nuclear medicine: the requisites*, 5th ed. Philadelphia, PA: Saunders, 2020:68–70, 67.

21 Answer B. Immune checkpoint inhibitors are monoclonal antibodies that block immune checkpoints to augment T–cell-mediated tumor destruction. In current clinical practice, they target the following cell surface proteins: programmed cell death protein 1 (PD-1), cytotoxic T- lymphocyte antigen-4 (CTLA-4), or the PD-1 ligand programmed cell death 1 ligand 1 (PD-L1). CTLA-4 and PD-1 are expressed by T cells. Ipilimumab is a monoclonal antibody that attaches to CTLA-4 and inhibits it. This drug was approved by FDA in 2011 for melanoma treatment. Nivolumab and pembrolizumab target PD-1, whereas durvalumab targets PD-L1. Adverse events associated with these agents are due to autoimmunity caused by hyperactivated T cells.

These are different from traditional chemotherapy and, in most of the cases, they are mild or moderate. Most common of them are dermatologic manifestations such as rash, erythema, or vitiligo. However, autoimmune pancreatitis, thyroiditis, colitis, and hypophysitis can also be seen. Most of these are readily reversed by stopping the agent and starting corticosteroids. However, endocrinopathies such as hypophysitis, adrenal insufficiency, and thyroid dysfunction are generally irreversible. Colitis and hypophysitis are more commonly seen with ipilimumab, and pneumonitis is seen with PD-1 inhibitors. Nivolumab-induced pneumonitis can have predominantly four CT patterns: Cryptogenic organizing pneumonia (COP), nonspecific interstitial pneumonia, hypersensitivity pneumonitis, and acute interstitial pneumonia (AIP)/acute respiratory distress syndrome (ARDS).

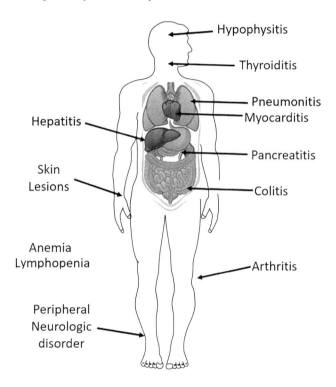

References: Nishino M, Ramaiya NH, et al. PD-1 inhibitor-related pneumonitis in advanced cancer patients: radiographic patterns and clinical course. *Clin Cancer Res* 2016;22(24):6051–6060.

Weber JS, Yang JC, Atkins MB, et al. Toxicities of Immunotherapy for the Practitioner. *J Clin Oncol* 2015;33(18):2092–2099.

22 **Answer D.** Axial CT and fused PET/CT images show a small focus of intense activity in the pancreatic tail. Early and delayed contrast-enhanced images from MRI demonstrate that the lesion within the pancreatic tail follows the contrast enhancement pattern of the spleen with signal intensity similar to that of the splenic tissue. As such, given the patient's clinical history and the lesion's imaging characteristics, the findings likely represent ectopic splenic tissue in the pancreatic tail. If needed, this can be confirmed with either denatured RBC SPECT-CT or sulfur colloid SPECT-CT. Physiologic pancreatic tail uptake tends to be less intense and less focal with no focal lesion on a dedicated multiphase CT or MRI. Primary pancreatic neuroendocrine tumor and metastatic carcinoid may appear similar on PET/CT, but the characteristic "tigroid" enhancement of splenic tissue on early contrast-enhanced phase would not be present. Physiologic DOTATATE activity in the adrenal glands should not be confused with malignant involvement.

References: Hofman MS, Lau WF, Hicks RJ. Somatostatin receptor imaging with 68Ga DOTATATE PET/CT: clinical utility, normal patterns, pearls, and pitfalls in interpretation. *RadioGraphics* 2015;35(2):500–516.

Mettler FA, Guiberteau MJ. *Essentials of nuclear medicine imaging*, 7th ed. Philadelphia, PA: Saunders, 2019:359–360.

O'Malley JP, Ziessman HA, Thrall JH. *Nuclear medicine: the requisites*, 5th ed. Philadelphia, PA: Saunders, 2020:342.

23 **Answer C.** Majority of neuroendocrine tumors are well differentiated (G1 and G2 with Ki-67 <5%) and are best visualized by Ga-68 DOTATATE PET/CT as they express somatostatin receptors (SSTR). These tumors are usually not FDG avid, and F-18 FDG-PET/CT is not a preferred modality for their evaluation. However, tumors or lesions that have undergone dedifferentiation are high-grade lesions that lack SSTR. For higher grade lesions with dedifferentiation, F-18 FDG PET/CT demonstrates increased sensitivity and plays a significant clinical role in combination with Ga-68 DOTATATE. Ga-68 PSMA is a prostate-specific antigen–binding agent that is used in the imaging of prostate cancer. In-111 pentetreotide (OctreoScan) is an SSTR-binding agent used for the imaging of well-differentiated neuroendocrine tumor, which has been superseded by DOTATATE due to increased sensitivity. While useful for imaging tumors of neural crest origin such as pheochromocytoma, paraganglioma, or neuroblastoma, I-123 MIBG has no role in the evaluation of the poorly differentiated neuroendocrine tumors.

The World Health Organization and the European Neuroendocrine Tumor Society (ENETS) have established grading systems for neuroendocrine tumors that are based on immunohistochemical staining of Ki-67 protein, a marker of cellular proliferation. These grading systems stratify tumors into one of three grades:

	G1	G2	G3
Ki-67	≤2	2–20	>20
Mitoses	<2	2-20	>20

Reference: O'Malley JP, Ziessman HA, Thrall JH. *Nuclear medicine: the requisites*, 5th ed. Philadelphia, PA: Saunders, 2020:342–343.

24 **Answer B.** F-18 fluciclovine (FACBC, Axumin) was approved by the FDA in 2016 for the diagnosis of suspected recurrent prostate cancer in patients with elevated PSA after initial therapy. It is a radiolabeled amino acid analog that takes advantage of the amino acid transport up-regulation that can be seen in many cancers including prostate cancer. Axumin is a radiolabeled analog of levorotatory leucine, which is an essential amino acid. Like L-leucine, FACBC is taken up via the human L-type amino acid transporter (LAT) and alanine–serine–cysteine (ASC2) transporter systems. Prostate-specific membrane antigen is the binding site for Ga-68 PSMA. PSMA is overexpressed in primary and metastatic adenocarcinomas of the prostate. FDG accumulation is nonspecific and seen in many different tumors. Most prostate cancers demonstrate no or very little FDG metabolism. Ga-68 DOTATATE and In-111 OctreoScan work by binding to the somatostatin receptors.

The interpretation of F-18 fluciclovine imaging is based on visual assessment rather than SUV values. A 1-cm or larger lesion/lymph node with avidity greater than or equal to that of bone marrow is suspicious for cancer. Lesion/lymph nodes smaller than 1 cm with avidity greater than that of the blood pool is suspicious for cancer. Pathologic activity in prostate cancer and nodal metastatic disease peaks rapidly, between 4 and 10 minutes, after the radiotracer injection. Because of the rapid influx and efflux of F-18 fluciclovine, imaging is generally obtained within 3 to 5 minutes after the injection rather than 60 minutes typical for the F-18 FDG PET. With Axumin, intense physiologic uptake is seen in the liver and pancreas. Mild diffuse uptake is seen in skeletal muscles.

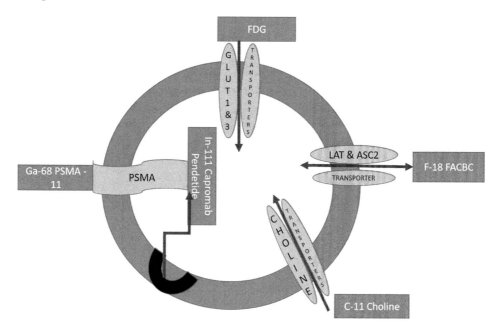

The image above demonstrates interaction of five commonly used radiotracers with prostate cancer cells. F-18 FDG enters through GLUT1 and 3 transporters. C-11 choline enters through choline transporters, while FACBC is transported by LAT and ASCT2 transporters. Out of these three, FACBC is the only one that is free to enter and exit the cells.

References: Gusman M, Aminsharifi JA, Peacock JG, et al. Review of 18F-fluciclovine PET for detection of recurrent prostate cancer. *RadioGraphics* 2019;39(3):822–841.

Mettler FA, Guiberteau MJ. *Essentials of nuclear medicine imaging*, 7th ed. Philadelphia, PA: Saunders, 2019:360.

O'Malley JP, Ziessman HA, Thrall JH. *Nuclear medicine: the requisites*, 5th ed. Philadelphia, PA: Saunders, 2020:352–353.

25 **Answer B.** Prostate-specific membrane antigen (PSMA) is a cell surface protein (glutamate carboxypeptidases, GCP, Type II) that is highly up-regulated in prostate carcinoma cells. Its active enzyme site within the extracellular domain is the target of small molecule radiopharmaceuticals such as Ga-68 PSMA 11 (Glu-NH-CO-NH-Lys-(Ahx)-[Ga-68 HBED-CC]), F-18 DCFPyL, etc. After antigen binding to PSMA on the cell membrane, these agents are internalized by endocytosis, leading to concentration and retention in the cells. This allows for a very high-contrast resolution image and the detection of even small-volume disease. Prostate-specific membrane antigen (PSMA) is overexpressed in the primary and metastatic adenocarcinomas of the prostate. The level of PSMA expression rises with increasing tumor dedifferentiation and in hormone refractory cancers.

References: Afshar-Oromieh A, et al. PET imaging with a [68Ga]gallium-labelled PSMA ligand for the diagnosis of prostate cancer: biodistribution in humans and first evaluation of tumour lesions. *Eur J Nucl Med Mol Imaging* 2013;40(4):486–495.

Bois F, Noirot C, Dietemann S, et al. [68Ga]Ga-PSMA-11 in prostate cancer: a comprehensive review. *Am J Nucl Med Mol Imaging* 2020;10(6):349–374.

Mettler FA, Guiberteau MJ. *Essentials of nuclear medicine imaging*, 7th ed. Philadelphia, PA: Saunders, 2019:360.

O'Malley JP, Ziessman HA,Thrall JH. *Nuclear medicine: the requisites*, 5th ed. Philadelphia, PA: Saunders, 2020:352–353.

26 **Answer A.** A single scintimammography image shows focal uptake in the breast, which is suggestive of a malignancy. In patients with dense breast tissue, this study can be performed to aid in the detection of breast cancer. Generally, 8 to 10 mCi of Tc-99m sestamibi is used. Unfortunately, benign tumors can have increased uptake as well. Detection is not affected by breast density, but sensitivity is decreased for DCIS, cancers <1 cm, and nonpalpable lesions.

Reference: O'Malley JP, Ziessman HA, Thrall JH. *Nuclear medicine: the requisites*, 5th ed. Philadelphia, PA: Saunders, 2020:359.

27 **Answer C.** Immune checkpoint inhibitors are a type of immunotherapy consisting of monoclonal antibodies that block immune checkpoints to augment T–cell-mediated tumor destruction. In current clinical practice, they target cell surface proteins: either programmed cell death protein 1 (PD-1) or cytotoxic T-lymphocyte antigen-4 (CTLA-4) or the PD-1 ligand programmed cell death 1 ligand 1 (PD -L1). CTLA-4 and PD-1 are expressed by T cells. Ipilimumab is a monoclonal antibody that attaches to CTLA-4 and inhibits it. This drug was approved by the FDA in 2011 for melanoma treatment. Nivolumab and pembrolizumab target PD-1, whereas durvalumab targets PD-L1.

References: https://www.cancer.gov/about-cancer/treatment/types/immunotherapy/checkpoint-inhibitors

Wang G, Kurra V, Gainor J, et al. Immune checkpoint inhibitor cancer therapy: spectrum of imaging findings. *RadioGraphics* 2017;37:2132–2144.

28 **Answer A.** Meningiomas are one of the many intracranial tumors that overexpress somatostatin receptors and, as such, are intensely avid on DOTATATE PET imaging. Other intracranial lesions with DOTATATE avidity include pituitary adenoma, carcinoid, hemangioblastoma, medulloblastoma, glioma, and metastasis from neuroendocrine tumors. Primitive neuroectodermal tumors (PNET), glioblastoma, and astrocytoma are primary brain tumors that do not have somatostatin receptors. Due to high levels of expression of the somatostatin receptor subtype 2 in meningiomas and a favorable tumor-to-background ratio, Ga-68 DOTATATE is highly effective in the detection of meningioma. A distinct morphology and location differentiate meningioma from other malignancies. Small meningiomas frequently present with excellent visibility due to their high tracer uptake as well as a typical location adjacent to the meninges (see an example below).

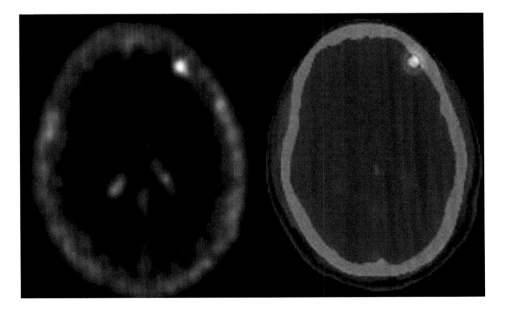

References: Afshar-Oromieh A, et al. Detection of cranial meningiomas: comparison of ^{68}Ga-DOTATOC PET/CT and contrast-enhanced MRI. *Eur J Nucl Med Mol Imaging* 2012;39(9):1409–1415.

Rachinger W, et al. Increased 68Ga-DOTATATE uptake in PET imaging discriminates meningioma and tumor-free tissue. *J Nucl Med* 2015;56(3):347–353.

29 **Answer C.** Axial CT and fused images through the upper mediastinum demonstrate an intensely FDG-avid soft tissue density that conforms to the anterosuperior mediastinal contours and does not exert mass effect on the adjacent structures. Single anterior MIP image demonstrates its characteristic lambda (λ) shape. This appearance is typical for that of thymic hyperplasia. Physiologic uptake of FDG by the thymus is commonly seen in children and young adults. In patients with malignant mediastinal tumors, the thymus may regress during chemotherapy, with possible rebound enlargement after completion of therapy. Metastatic colon cancer, teratoma, and lymphoma do not have the classic appearance of thymic hyperplasia.

References: Ferdinand B, Gupta P, Kramer EL. Spectrum of thymic uptake at 18F-FDG PET. *RadioGraphics* 2004;24(6):1611–1616.

Gawande RS, Khurana A, et al. Differentiation of normal thymus from anterior mediastinal lymphoma and lymphoma recurrence at pediatric PET/CT. *Radiology* 2012;262(2):613–622.

30 **Answer A.** Axial CT, fused, and PET images through the pelvis demonstrate linear areas of moderate to severely increased FDG uptake in the sacrum, medial to sacroiliac joints. This area of abnormal activity corresponds to linear lucencies on the CT scan in keeping with fracture lines that run parallel to the sacroiliac joint with associated surrounding sclerosis (arrows below). The findings are in keeping with abnormal FDG uptake related to inflammatory changes associated with sacral insufficiency fractures. While radiation-induced sarcoma, metastasis, and active Paget disease may have increased F-18 FDG uptake, the appearance is typical for that of sacral insufficiency fracture. Postradiation sarcoma is generally seen after 10 years of radiation therapy. In Paget disease, cortical thickening and coarsened trabecular pattern are seen with expansion of bone on CT.

Sacral insufficiency fractures are commonly seen in elderly female population with osteoporosis without any history of trauma. Other risk factors include pelvic radiation therapy and long-term bisphosphonate use. CT imaging is less sensitive than bone scan and MRI in the diagnosis of sacral insufficiency fractures. A classic Honda sign (uptake in H pattern) on bone scan is diagnostic.

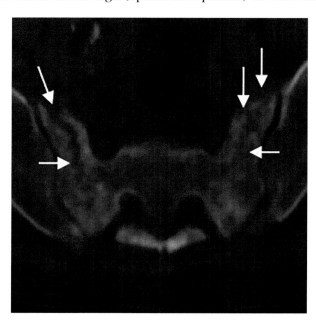

References: Fayad L, Cohade C, Wahl R, et al. Sacral fractures: a potential pitfall of fdg positron emission tomography. *Am J Roentgenol* 2003;181:1239–1243.

Tsuchida T, Kosaka N, Sugimoto K, Itoh H. Sacral insufficiency fracture detected by FDG-PET/CT: report of 2 cases. *Ann Nucl Med* 2006;20(6):445–448.

31 **Answer C.** Axial fused images, CT images, and a single anterior MIP image show an intensely FDG avid mass in the right lung accompanied by intensely FDG avid ipsilateral and contralateral lymph nodes, suspicious for metastatic malignant involvement. No significant FDG uptake is seen in the small right pleural effusion. Also, there is no evidence of focal nodular pleural involvement shown in these pictures. Presence suspicious contralateral lymph node metastasis makes this stage IIIB. Evaluation of lymph node metastasis is an important step in the staging of lung cancer and helps determine whether the patient is offered surgical resection. Presence of metastasis in the contralateral mediastinal or supraclavicular lymph nodes would put the patient in stage IIIB category. Patients with stage IIIB disease are usually treated with a combination of chemotherapy and radiation therapy, with surgery having a little role. As such, identification of metastatic disease in these regions is crucial. F-18 FDG PET/CT is standard in staging investigation of patients with lung carcinoma and is helpful in detection of nodal and unsuspected distant metastases.

Reference: O'Malley JP, Ziessman HA, Thrall JH. *Nuclear medicine: the requisites*, 5th ed. Philadelphia, PA: Saunders, 2020:315–325.

32 **Answer B.** An anterior MIP image demonstrates physiologic distribution of the radiotracer to the pancreas, liver muscle, and the bone marrow. No uptake is seen within the brain, excluding F-18 FDG. This physiologic distribution is seen with F-18 fluciclovine (Axumin®) scan. Fluciclovine is an analog of L-leucine amino acid approved for diagnosis of suspected recurrent prostate cancer based on elevated blood prostate-specific antigen (PSA) levels in patients who have received prior treatment. Normal physiologic amino acid metabolism is responsible for its intense uptake in the pancreas.

Reference: O'Malley JP, Ziessman HA, Thrall JH. *Nuclear medicine: the requisites*, 5th ed. Philadelphia, PA: Saunders, 2020:352–353.

33 **Answer C.** Physiologic distribution in the pancreas, liver, muscles, and bone marrow indicates that this is an F-18 fluciclovine scan. Two foci of intense activity (above that of the bone marrow) are noted in the right hemipelvis. Axial CT, fused PET/CT, and PET images show one of these foci to correspond to a right external iliac/obturator lymph node. In a patient with a history of prostate cancer and a rising PSA level, the findings are most consistent with a recurrent prostate cancer in locoregional lymph nodes. Increased muscular uptake on F-18 FDG scan would be present in patients with exposure to increased endogenous or exogenous insulin or recent exercise. However, lack of physiologic brain uptake excludes F-18 FDG as the radiotracer.

Approximately 20% to 50% of patients with prostate cancer will have biochemical recurrence after initial treatment based on elevated PSA level. The typical sites of nodal recurrence are the pelvic lymph nodes (proximal external iliac, internal iliac and common iliac lymph nodes) and retroperitoneal regions, including para-aortic lymph nodes. For lymph nodes <1 cm in size, the abnormal uptake is defined as that greater than the adjacent blood vessels. For lymph nodes >1 cm in size, the abnormal uptake is defined as that greater than the bone marrow.

References: Gusman M, Aminsharifi JA, Peacock JG, et al. Review of 18F-fluciclovine PET for detection of recurrent prostate cancer. *RadioGraphics*. 2019;39(3):822–841.

Savir-Baruch B, Schuster DM, et al. Fluorine-18-labeled fluciclovine PET/CT in clinical practice: factors affecting the rate of detection of recurrent prostate cancer. *AJR Am J Roentgenol* 2019;213(4):851–858.

12 Physics, Artifacts, NRC, Quality Control, and Safety

QUESTIONS

1   What is the photon energy of the radiopharmaceutical shown below?

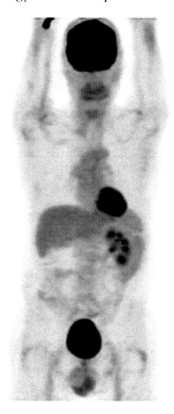

A. 511 keV
B. 1,022 keV
C. 511 MeV
D. 1,022 MeV

2 What collimator was used to acquire these images?

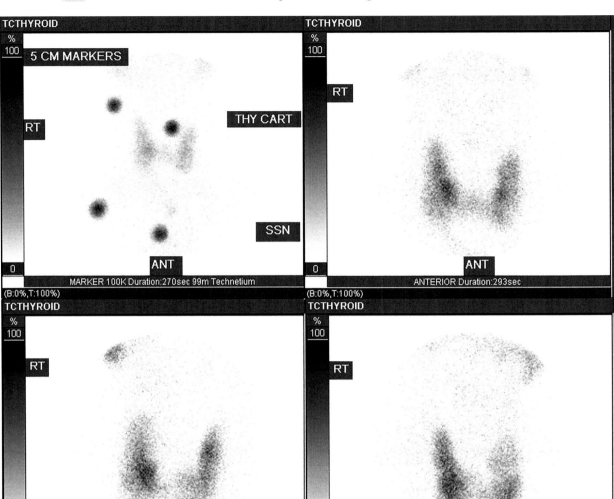

A. Parallel, low energy
B. Parallel, medium energy
C. Parallel, high energy
D. Pinhole

3 A technologist states that there is an unknown radionuclide spilled on the countertop. Which of the following devices could be utilized to identify what radionuclide was spilled?

A. Geiger-Müller counter
B. Ionization survey chamber
C. Dose calibrator
D. Well counter

4 What type of quality control test is being performed on the dose calibrator where a high activity vial of Tc-99m is assayed by the physicist using calibrated lead shields (shown below) to simulate lower levels of radioactivity?

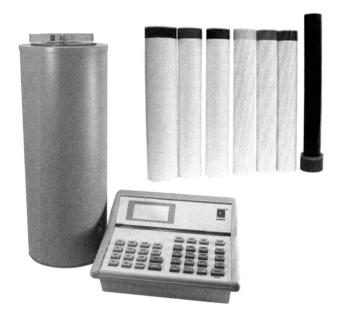

A. Accuracy
B. Constancy
C. Linearity
D. Geometry

5 While performing the morning intrinsic uniformity evaluation, the technologist obtains the following image. What is the most likely etiology?

A. Cracked crystal
B. Damaged collimator
C. Misaligned center of rotation
D. Nonfunctioning photomultiplier tube

6 The following 4- and 24-hour cisternogram images were acquired after intrathecal administration of 500 µCi of In-111 DTPA. Which of the following is the most likely explanation for the degraded image quality at 4 hours compared to that of 24 hours?

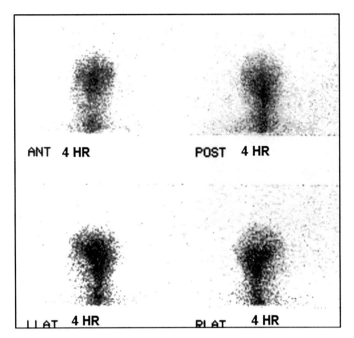

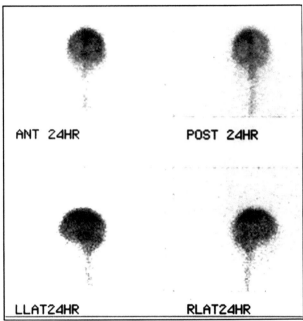

A. Dose infiltration
B. Prior nuclear study
C. Wrong photopeak selected
D. Too little administered activity
E. A patient with In-111 in the adjacent room

7 What is being evaluated on the following quality control image?

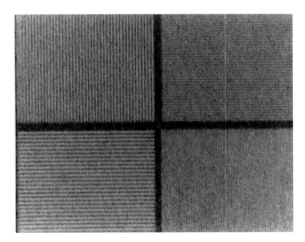

A. Spatial resolution
B. Energy resolution
C. Energy linearity
D. Collimator integrity
E. Uniformity

8 The following anterior images are all from the same gastric emptying study with Tc-99m sulfur colloid. What is the most likely cause of the difference between the top two rows and the bottom two rows of images?

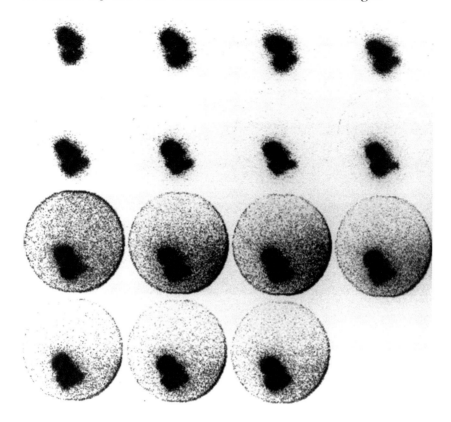

A. Radiotracer decay
B. Dose infiltration
C. Free pertechnetate
D. Nearby radionuclide

9 What is the recommended frequency for acquiring flood uniformity images to assess uniformity on a gamma camera?
A. Daily
B. Weekly
C. Monthly
D. Quarterly
E. Annually

10 What is the maximum allowable molybdenum-99 breakthrough limit in a Mo-99/Tc-99m generator eluate?
A. 0.15 μCi/mCi
B. 1.5 μCi/mCi
C. 0.15 mCi/μCi
D. 1.5 mCi/μCi

11 The following bone scintigraphy was performed to evaluate for osseous metastasis. What is the most likely explanation for the appearance of the images?

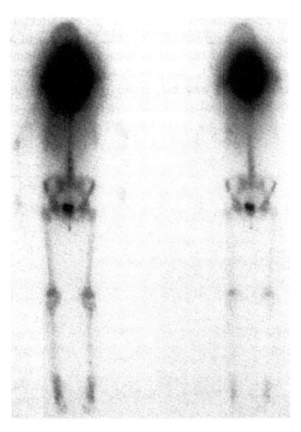

A. Wrong photopeak
B. Thyroiditis
C. Free pertechnetate
D. Prior nuclear study
E. Photomultiplier tube malfunction

12 What is the maximum allowed exposure to other members of the public from a patient who has received an outpatient I-131 therapy?

A. 0.5 mSv
B. 1 mSv
C. 5 mSv
D. 10 mSv
E. 50 mSv

13 What is the annual institutional limit for the amount of radioactive waste (except H-3 and C-14) that can be disposed of in a designated "hot sink"?

A. 1 Ci.
B. 10 Ci.
C. 100 Ci.
D. No limit.
E. One cannot purposefully dispose of radioactive waste down a sink.

14 When reviewing the following CT images from a PET/CT scan of the abdomen, the technologist notices decreased quality of the images when compared to the images from a diagnostic abdominal CT. What is the most likely reason for the decreased image quality?

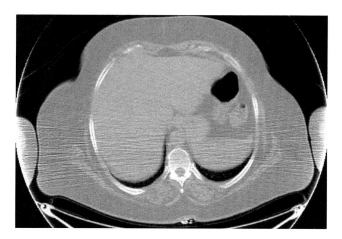

A. Photon starvation
B. Iodinated contrast infiltration
C. FDG dose infiltration
D. Moire interference
E. Dead pixel in the CT detector array

15 After performing a liquid I-131 treatment, a resident physician notices that there is some fluid on the floor. The technologist checks the floor and everyone's shoes and finds that there is contamination of I-131 on both. How long should the contaminated material be stored in isolation prior to further use or disposal?

A. 8 hours
B. 8 days
C. 1 month
D. 80 days
E. 1 year

16 What is the maximum allowable limit of aluminum in an eluate from a molybdenum-99/technetium-99m (Mo-99/Tc-99m) generator in units of μg of aluminum per mL of eluate?

A. <0.1 μg/mL
B. <1 μg/mL
C. <10 μg/mL
D. <100 μg/mL

17 How do radiation regulations of agreement states compare with NRC regulations?

A. They are at least as strict as the NRC regulations.
B. They must be stricter than the NRC regulations.
C. They can be less strict than NRC regulations.
D. They are independent of NRC regulations.

18 What is the maximum allowable dose rate at 1 m from a package with the following placard?

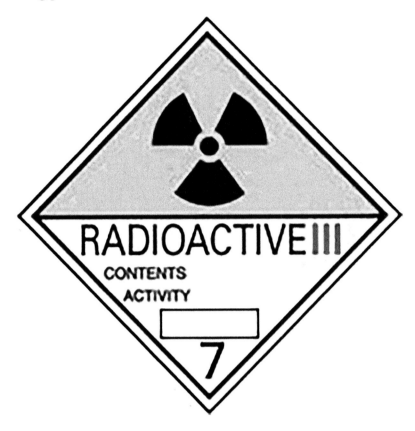

A. 1 mrem/hour
B. 10 mrem/hour
C. 100 mrem/hour
D. 1,000 mrem/hour
E. Indistinguishable from background

19 Why does positron emission tomography (PET) have a higher sensitivity (measured count rate per unit activity) compared to single photon emission computed tomography (SPECT)?

A. Absorptive collimation
B. Electronic collimation
C. Random coincidence
D. Uniformity correction

20 How often should detector uniformity of positron emission tomography (PET) scanners be checked?

A. Daily
B. Weekly
C. Monthly
D. Semiannually
E. Annually

21 What information does the transportation index (TI) on the following placard provide regarding the package containing Mo-99?

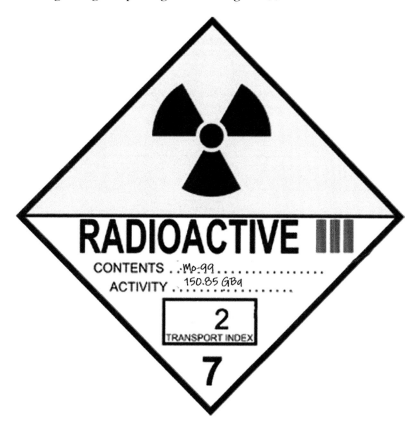

A. Dose rate <2 mrem/hour at package surface.
B. Package contents require 2 weeks to decay to the background.
C. Dose rate <2 mrem/hour at 1 m from the package surface.
D. The driver must remain at least 2 m from the package at all times.

22 What is being checked on the gamma camera when a physicist acquires the full width at half-maximum (FWHM) of Tc-99m, photopeak expressed as a percentage?

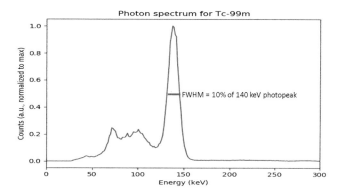

A. Intrinsic uniformity
B. Spatial resolution
C. System sensitivity
D. Energy resolution

23 A postpartum patient undergoes the following examination. If the dose to the nursing infant is to be kept below 1 mSv, how long after the study may the patient resume breast-feeding?

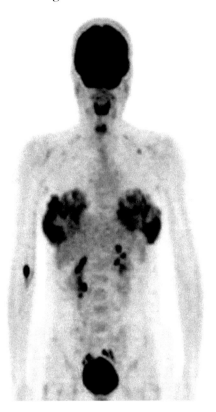

A. No disruption in feeding
B. 4 hours
C. 24 hours
D. Discontinue until next pregnancy

24 What happens when one uses a low-energy collimator to image a medium-energy isotope?

A. Decreased sensitivity
B. Decreased resolution
C. Decreased scatter
D. No difference

25 Mo-99 may be present as a radionuclidic contaminant of Tc-99m. What happens to the relative amount of Mo-99 contamination in a vial of Tc-99m elution or Tc-99m radiopharmaceutical over time?

A. Stays the same with time
B. Decreases with time
C. Increases with time

26 What collimator was most likely used to acquire these Ga-67 gallium citrate images?

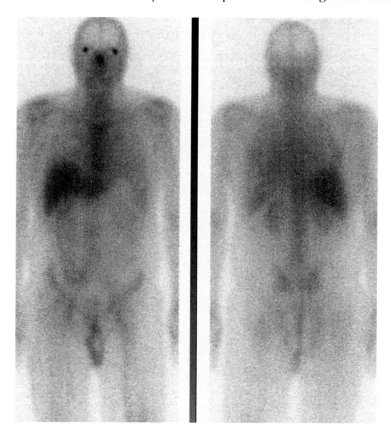

A. Low-energy all-purpose
B. Medium-energy
C. High-energy
D. Diverging
E. Converging

27 A 45-year-old male with a clinical history of a high risk of differentiated thyroid carcinoma underwent radioiodine ablation with 100 mCi of I-131 10 days ago. What collimator was likely used to acquire the posttherapy images shown below?

^{131}I- NaI Thyroid Cancer Posttherapy Scan

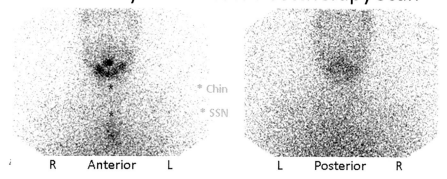

A. Low-energy all-purpose
B. Medium-energy
C. High-energy
D. Pinhole

28 What is the most likely explanation for the differences in the quality of the images shown below?

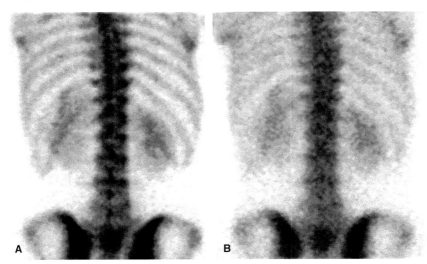

A

B

A. They were acquired with different radiopharmaceuticals.
B. They were acquired at different time points after administration of the radiopharmaceutical.
C. They were acquired at different distances from the collimator.
D. They were acquired with different amounts of the administered radioactivity.

29 A technologist gets called in to do a perfusion scan to evaluate for pulmonary embolism in a patient at night. Instead of making a new Tc-99m MAA, he uses the leftover MAA that was prepared about 12 hours ago. What organ, in addition to the lungs, would be visualized on the images?

A. Brain
B. Heart
C. Liver
D. Thyroid
E. Pancreas

30 Which one of the following issues would result in the cold spots seen at the bottom of the intrinsic uniformity image shown below?

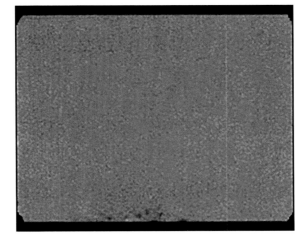

A. Bad photomultiplier tubes
B. Crystal hydration
C. Poor linearity correction
D. Radioactive spill on camera

For Questions 31 through 35, please match the instruments with the appropriate task it is used to perform.

31 The instrument labeled A in the image below is used for which task?

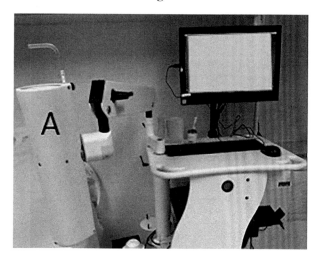

    A. Area survey
    B. Patient release
    C. Radioiodine uptake
    D. Wipe test
    E. Assay of 99mTc-MDP activity

32 The instrument labeled B in the image below is used for which task?

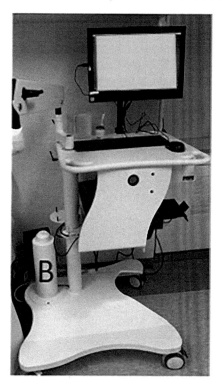

    A. Area survey
    B. Patient release
    C. Radioiodine uptake
    D. Wipe test
    E. Assay of 99mTc-MDP activity

33 For which task is this instrument used?

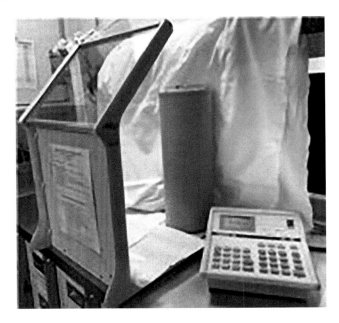

A. Area survey
B. Patient release
C. Radioiodine uptake
D. Wipe test
E. Assay of 99mTc-MDP activity

34 For which task is this instrument used?

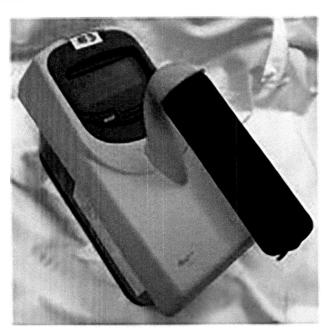

A. Area survey
B. Patient release
C. Radioiodine uptake
D. Wipe test
E. Assay of 99mTc-MDP activity

35 For which task is this instrument used?

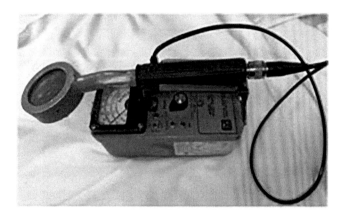

A. Area survey
B. Patient release
C. Radioiodine uptake
D. Wipe test
E. Assay of 99mTc-MDP activity

36 What aspect of tomographic image quality is tested with the SPECT phantom shown in the following image?

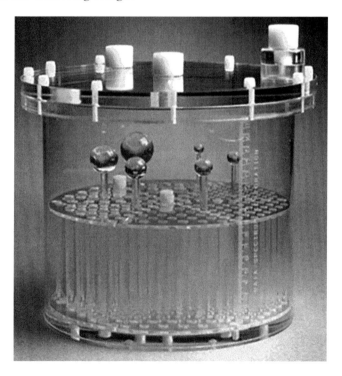

A. Uniformity
B. Spatial resolution
C. Contrast resolution
D. All of the above

37 Match the NRC dose limits in Column A to the corresponding description in Column B.

Column A	Column B
A. 5 mSv	Dose limit to the fetus/embryo over the gestation period for a declared pregnant radiation worker
B. 1 mSv	Annual dose limit for an adult radiation worker
C. 50 mSv	Annual dose limit to lens of the eye for a radiation worker
D. No limit	Dose limit for a patient undergoing a procedure in which ionizing radiation is used
E. 150 mSv	Annual dose limit to the general public and nonradiation workers

38 After I-131 therapy for thyroid cancer, the patient release calculation estimates that the patient's husband (who is the maximally exposed individual [MEI]) will receive an estimated total dose of 2.5 mSv. Which of the following is correct regarding the patient release?

A. The patient cannot be released because the estimated MEI total dose is >1 mSv.

B. The patient can be released because the estimated MEI total dose is <5 mSv.

C. The patient can be released because there is no maximum dose limit if the MEI is an immediate family member.

D. The patient cannot be released until a thyroid bioassay shows no residual I-131 in the patient's thyroid.

39 What is the recommended duration of interruption of breast-feeding after a nuclear medicine study using a Tc-99m imaging agent?

A. No interruption is required.

B. 3 days.

C. 24 hours.

D. Complete cessation for this child.

40 A written directive states: "Patient Andrew Brown to receive 7.4 GBq Lu-177 DOTATATE for the treatment of a somatostatin receptor–positive gastroenteropancreatic neuroendocrine tumor." Which of the following items is also required to be listed on the written directive?

A. The patient's date of birth

B. The patient's pregnancy status

C. The half-life and radioactive emissions of Lu-177

D. The route of administration

41 A written directive is required for which of the following imaging studies?

A. Thyroid cancer posttherapy study using 2 MBq (50 µCi) I-131 sodium iodide

B. Thyroid cancer imaging study using 148 MBq (4 mCi) I-123

C. Prostate cancer imaging study using 222 MBq (6 mCi) In-111 pentetreotide

D. Neuroendocrine cancer imaging study using 259 MBq (7 mCi) Ga-68 DOTATATE

42 What is the most likely reason for the appearance of the posterior bladder on the following CT portion of the SPECT-CT image acquired after the administration of Tc-99m MDP?

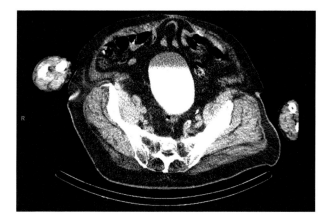

A. Beam-hardening artifact.

B. Secreted Tc-99m MDP into the bladder.

C. The anterior bladder is filled with air, whereas the posterior bladder contains urine.

D. Secreted iodine contrast agent into the bladder.

43 Which of the following best describes the required radiation shielding when converting a SPECT room to a PET/CT room?

A. No shielding is required.

B. Less shielding will be needed.

C. The same amount of shielding will be needed.

D. More shielding will be needed.

44 A medical event occurs at your facility that must be reported to the NRC. When must your facility first notify the NRC that this event has occurred?

A. Within 15 calendar days

B. No later than the next business day

C. Within 15 business days

D. No later than the next calendar day

45 What is being detected to generate the SPECT portion of the following fused SPECT/CT image from a patient who just received Y-90 microsphere therapy?

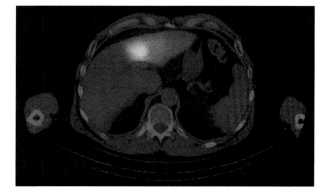

A. Bremsstrahlung x-rays from the CT x-ray tube

B. Bremsstrahlung x-rays from the Y-90 beta radiation

C. 140 keV gamma emissions from decay of Y-90

D. Annihilation photons from Y-90 positrons

46 The written directive for a Y-90 microsphere therapy for hepatocellular carcinoma states that the left liver lobe is to receive 80 Gy (equivalent dose of 80 Sv to the left liver lobe). Due to a technical problem with the delivery system, only half of the prescribed activity was administered, resulting in a left liver lobe dose of 40 Gy (equivalent dose of 40 Sv to left liver lobe). According to NRC regulatory requirements, why must this medical event be reported to the NRC?

A. The delivered dose was less than the planned dose.
B. The undelivered Y-90 activity must be disposed of by the NRC.
C. The therapy delivery system malfunctioned.
D. The delivered and planned doses differed by >20% and by >0.5 Sv.

47 The figure shows the activity Mo-99 and Tc-99m within a Mo-99/Tc-99m generator as a function of time. Assuming the generator was eluted at elapsed time = 0 hours with 100% elution efficiency, at what elapsed time is the activity of Tc-99m highest within the generator?

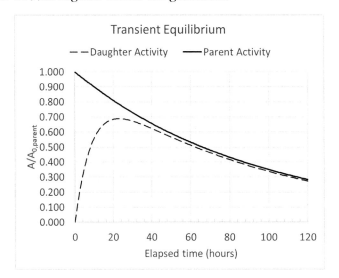

A. 6 hours
B. 13 hours
C. 23 hours
D. 33 hours

48 After a lymphoscintigraphy study using a gamma camera, the patient is transported to the operating room for biopsy of the sentinel lymph node. What radiation detection device is commonly used in the operating room to identify the sentinel lymph node for biopsy?

A. Geiger-Müller counter
B. Handheld gamma probe
C. Thyroid uptake probe
D. Ionization chamber

49 Under NRC regulations, which of the following statements regarding nuclear medicine imaging is true?

A. A written directive must be completed for all imaging studies.
B. An authorized user must administer (e.g., inject) the imaging radiopharmaceutical to the patient.
C. All imaging radiopharmaceuticals must be assayed and labeled prior to administration.
D. A radiolabeling kit can only be used to create an imaging radiopharmaceutical for a single patient.

50 What is the reason for placing limits on the minimum radionuclide purity of an imaging radiopharmaceutical?

A. Excess radionuclide impurities result in severe pharmacologic effects.

B. Excess radionuclide impurities result in significantly different biodistribution.

C. Excess radionuclide impurities result in deterministic effects such as skin erythema at the injection site.

D. Excess radionuclide impurities result in increased patient dose.

51 A dosage of 8 mCi F-18 FDG was actually administered to the patient but was recorded as 10 mCi in error (e.g., because of residual activity left in the syringe). What is the likely effect on SUV measurements in the liver background of an F-18 FDG-PET image secondary to this error?

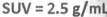

True administered activity = 8 mCi
Administered activity on scanner = 8 mCi
SUV = 2.5 g/mL

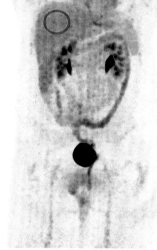

True administered activity = 8 mCi
Administered activity on scanner = 10 mCi
SUV = ??

A

B

A. SUV will be overestimated.

B. SUV will be underestimated.

C. SUV will remain the same.

52 Which gamma camera correction is routinely applied to SPECT studies but is not typically required for planar studies?

A. Extrinsic uniformity correction

B. Spatial linearity correction

C. Center of rotation correction

D. Energy correction

53 The following F-18 FDG-PET images were acquired from the same patient. Which of the following explains the differences between the PET images in A compared to those in B?

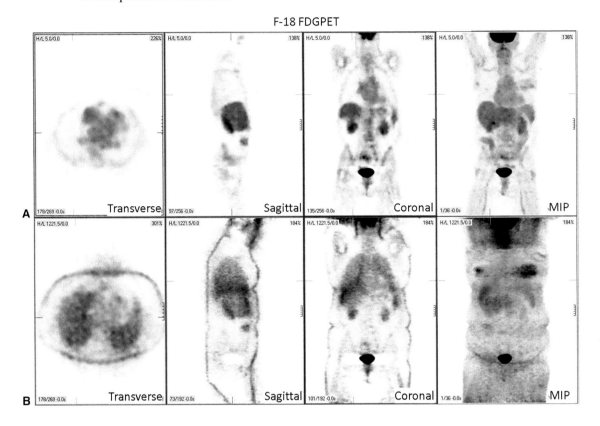

A. Attenuation correction
B. Scatter correction
C. Time-of-flight correction
D. Different radiopharmaceutical

54 When doing SPECT myocardial perfusion imaging (MPI) using a dual-head gamma camera, what detector configuration and rotation arc are typically recommended? Right anterior oblique (RAO), right posterior oblique (RPO), left anterior oblique (LAO), and left posterior oblique (LPO) are relative to the patient's anatomy.

A. 180 degrees "opposing" detector configuration and scan rotation from RAO to LPO
B. 180 degrees "opposing" detector configuration and scan rotation from LAO to RPO
C. 90 degrees "L" detector configuration and scan rotation from RAO to LPO
D. 90 degrees "L" detector configuration and scan rotation from LAO to RPO

55 Images A and B represent transverse slices of the same Tc-99m bicisate (Neurolite ECD) brain perfusion study; however, images A and B were reconstructed with different settings. What reconstruction setting likely caused the change in image quality from image A to image B?

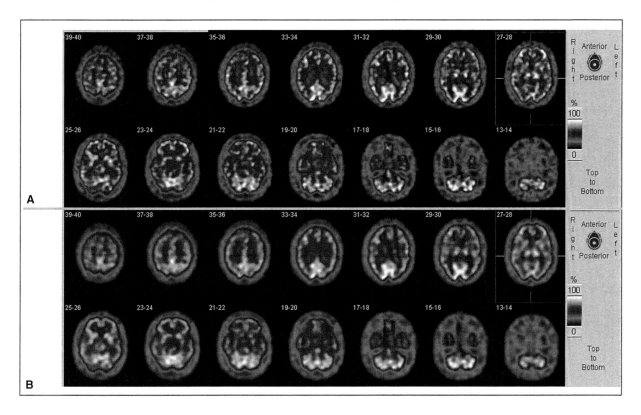

A. Wider smoothing filter used in image B

B. Narrow window width and high window level applied in image B

C. Attenuation correction applied in image B

D. Smaller pixel size used in image B

56 An In-111 OctreoScan SPECT study is usually acquired on a dual-head SPECT scanner with the detectors in 180 degrees opposing configuration and using parallel-hole collimators. Which of the following SPECT protocols is recommended for the best spatial resolution for abdominal imaging tasks?

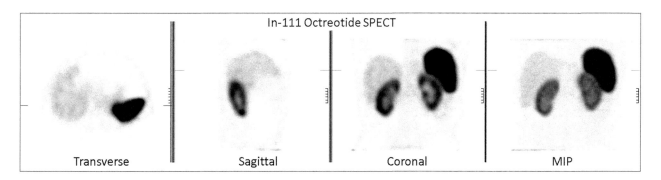

A. Circular orbit (radius of rotation fixed)

B. Noncircular orbit (radius of rotation adapted to body contour)

C. Static images or no orbit (detector does not rotate)

D. Either circular or noncircular orbit (radius of rotation does not matter)

57 What is the most likely cause for the loss of spatial resolution on the Rb-82 RbCl cardiac perfusion images compared to the F-18 FDG metabolism images on this patient who underwent evaluation of myocardial viability with PET/CT?

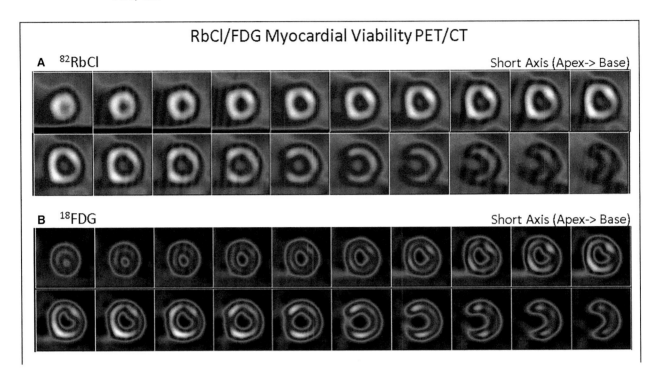

RbCl/FDG Myocardial Viability PET/CT

A ^{82}RbCl   Short Axis (Apex-> Base)

B ^{18}FDG   Short Axis (Apex-> Base)

    A. Lower positron energy of Rb-82
    B. Shorter half-life of Rb-82
    C. Longer positron range of Rb-82
    D. Higher atomic mass of Rb-82

58 F-18 FDG uptake is relatively low in fat. In general, for tumors of similar metabolic activity, the tumor standardized uptake value (SUV) in an overweight patient is _____ the tumor SUV in a thinner patient.

    A. higher than
    B. lower than
    C. equal to
    D. the square root of

59 What is the most likely interpretation for the hot spot on these F-18 FDG-PET/CT images?

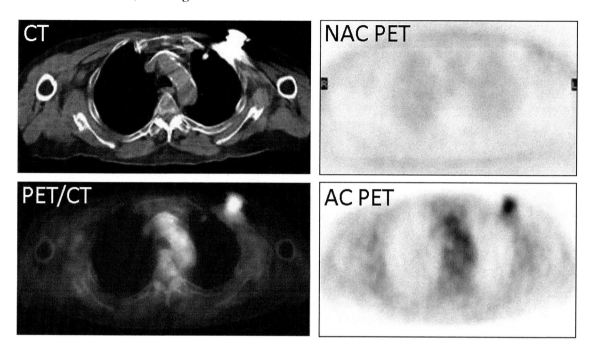

A. Malignant chest wall lesion
B. Artifact resulting from a pacemaker
C. Mispositioned lung lesion due to respiratory motion
D. Inflammation around a surgical scar

60 On the Ga-67 citrate images of the chest/abdomen shown below, what is the most likely cause for the artifact present on the posterior image?

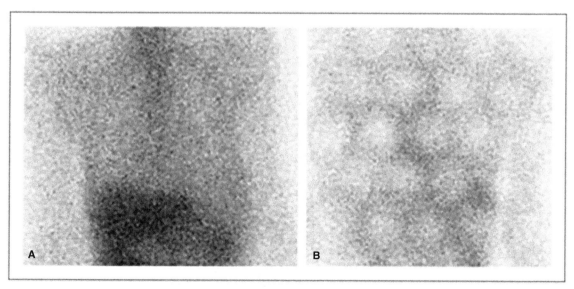

Anterior/Detector 1   Posterior/Detector 2

A. Patient motion
B. Image matrix too coarse
C. Low- rather than medium-energy collimator
D. Bad uniformity correction

61 Why is the hot spot indicated by the arrow localized in the lungs on the attenuation corrected (AC) image but localized in the liver on the non–attenuation corrected (NAC) image?

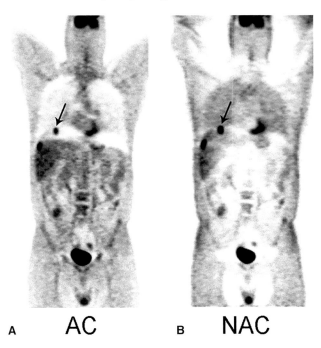

A **AC**   B **NAC**

A. Respiratory motion
B. Contrast media–resulting artifact on the CT AC scan
C. Malfunctioning PET detector block
D. Image matrix shift between AC and NAC images

ANSWERS AND EXPLANATIONS

1 **Answer A.** An anterior maximum intensity projection (MIP) image demonstrates the physiologic distribution of radiopharmaceutical within the gray matter of the brain, lymphoid and glandular tissues of the neck, myocardium, liver, and GI and GU systems. This is an F-18 FDG positron emission tomography (PET) scan. A positron emitted from the F-18 nucleus undergoes annihilation as it interacts with an electron; this annihilation event produces two 511-keV photons, which are detected by a ring of detectors surrounding the patient. Coincidence counting is used to differentiate true events from random events/noise. The diagram below demonstrates a positron annihilation event producing two 511-keV photons.

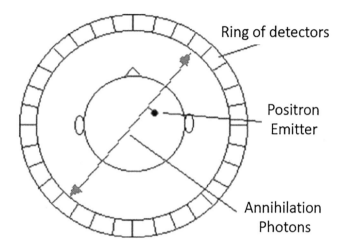

References: Mettler FA, Guiberteau MJ. *Essentials of nuclear medicine imaging*, 7th ed. Philadelphia, PA: Saunders, 2019:38–42.

Saha GB. *Fundamentals of nuclear pharmacy*, 6th ed. New York, NY: Springer, 2010:45. http://users.fmrib.ox.ac.uk/~stuart/thesis/chapter_3/section3_1html

2 **Answer D.** Magnified thyroid images are acquired with a pinhole collimator. Due to their geometry, pinhole collimators can significantly magnify anatomy, so they are used for imaging of small organs such as thyroid and some pediatric examinations (e.g., pediatric hip and pediatric renal imaging using DMSA). A tip that this is a pinhole collimator is the round field of view of the image.

Parallel collimators are used for most examinations and are considered the workhorse of the nuclear medicine department. They do not magnify anatomy. Different parallel hole collimators (low, medium, and high energy) are used depending on the energy of the photons emitted by different radionuclides.

References: Cherry SE, Sorenson JA, Phelps ME. *Physics in nuclear medicine*, 4th ed. Philadelphia, PA: Saunders, 2012:201–204.

Mettler FA, Guiberteau MJ. *Essentials of nuclear medicine imaging*, 7th ed. Philadelphia, PA: Saunders, 2019:23–26.

3 **Answer D.** Well counters are composed of a NaI crystal in the shape of a "well," with the sample placed in the well. This shape enables the well counter to detect very small quantities of radioactivity. However, because of their high detection efficiency and longer dead time, well counters cannot be used with large amounts of radioactivity. Well counter systems typically contain a multichannel analyzer (MCA) to analyze the energy spectrum of photons detected by the well counter. In the case of a spill, a wipe can be used to sample a very small amount of radioactivity. A well counter system can then be used to count the wipe and analyze the energy spectrum to determine the specific radioisotope that was spilled on the countertop.

Geiger-Müller counters are very sensitive handheld instruments that are used to detect small amounts of radioactive contamination. The detector is gas-filled with high voltage applied from the anode to the cathode resulting in a cascade of events from a single gamma ray. They are not energy discriminating (so cannot be used to identify a radioisotope) and have high dead time, which prevents their use in high-radiation areas. Ionization survey chambers are used to measure low or high exposure rates, but they are not as sensitive as a Geiger-Müller counter. They are filled with gas or air and have a relatively low voltage applied from anode to cathode, which means they have shorter dead times and can be used to measure high radiation exposure areas. Dose calibrators are a type of ionization chamber used to assay the amount of activity in vials/syringes from a known radiopharmaceutical. Ion survey chambers and dose calibrators are not energy discriminating, so they cannot be used to identify a specific radioisotope.

Reference: Mettler FA, Guiberteau MJ. *Essentials of nuclear medicine imaging*, 7th ed. Philadelphia, PA: Saunders, 2019:19–23, 522–523.

4 **Answer C.** The physicist is checking the linearity of the dose calibrator. Linearity (see diagram below) is the ability of the dose calibrator to accurately measure radioactivity at all clinically applicable levels (lowest to highest). This can be evaluated by one of the two following methods: (1) Assay a high-activity vial of Tc-99m multiple times over a time period sufficient for the radioactivity to decay from the highest quantity of radioactivity administered to a patient to below 30 µCi or (2) assay a high-activity vial of Tc-99m using calibrated lead shields to simulate lower levels of radioactivity that would have occurred with radioactive decay. Linearity is checked at installation and then quarterly. The lead shield method should only be used after the linearity has been evaluated using the decay method.

The response of a dose calibrator is dependent on the position, size, shape, and material of the source container as well as the volume of the source because of geometric efficiency. Geometric efficiency is the fraction of emitted radioactivity that is incident on the detection portion of the counter. The quality assurance test that assesses the effect due to the volume and location of the source in the dose calibrator is called the geometry test. In this case, the same amount of radioactivity is measured in different volumes to test whether or not there is a change in the response of the dose calibrator. This test is performed at installation, after a repair, after recalibration, or upon moving the instrument.

Accuracy refers to the ability of the dose calibrator to accurately assay samples at all clinically relevant radionuclide energies (low, medium, and high). Typically, two energies are checked (e.g., 662 keV with Cs-137 and 122 keV with Co-57). Accuracy is checked at installation and then annually.

Constancy measures the instrument's precision of the dose calibrator and is intended to show the reproducibility of measurements. A long-lived source such as Cs-137 is measured daily, and the measurements should be within ±5%. Constancy is tested at installation and daily.

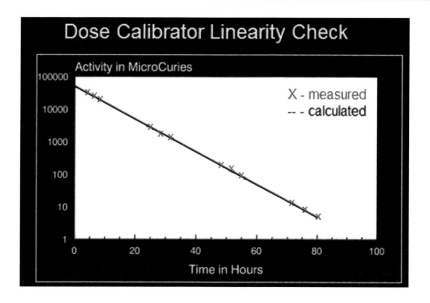

References: Carey JE, et al. *AAPM Report 181: the selection, use, calibration, and quality assurance of radionuclide calibrators used in nuclear medicine.* 2012. https://www.aapm.org/pubs/reports/detail.asp?docid=137

O'Malley JP, Ziessman HA, Thrall JH. *Nuclear medicine: the requisites,* 5th ed. Philadelphia, PA: Saunders, 2020:61.

Zanzonico P. Routine quality control of clinical nuclear medicine instrumentation: a brief review. *J Nucl Med* 2008;49(7):1114–1131.

5 **Answer D.** The image demonstrates a circular-shaped defect on the flood uniformity image, which is classic for a nonfunctioning photomultiplier tube. Intrinsic uniformity is evaluated without the collimator on the camera head, so this artifact cannot be due to a damaged collimator. In addition, damage to a collimator is very unlikely to have a round shape and often has a more linear shape (see image below). A cracked crystal (image below) also would not be round in shape but would be in the shape of a crack. Center of rotation (COR) errors are seen on reconstructed SPECT images and not on planar images. With small COR errors, a point source appears blurred, and with large COR errors, point source would appear as a doughnut on the reconstructed SPECT images (image below).

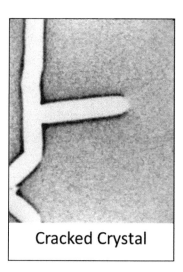

Cracked Crystal

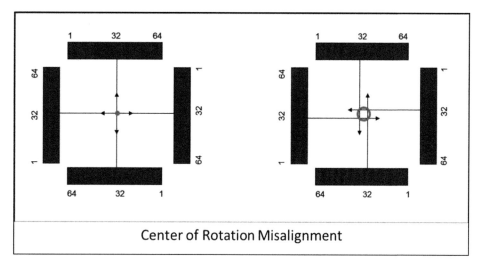

Center of Rotation Misalignment

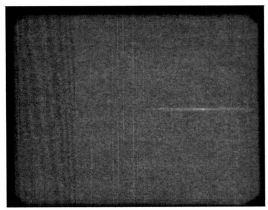

Extrinsic flood uniformity image of camera head with damaged collimator. Note linear appearance of damage to collimator

Reference: Mettler FA, Guiberteau MJ. *Essentials of nuclear medicine imaging*, 7th ed. Philadelphia, PA: Saunders, 2019:47–51.

6 **Answer C.** Significantly poor image quality is present with poor count statistics on the 4-hour images. The 24-hour images demonstrate better quality and better count statistics. The findings are consistent with the use of a photopeak other than that of In-111 on the 4-hour scan. The correct photopeak was selected on the subsequent 24-hour scan. Acquisition at a wrong photopeak could result in degraded contrast and detail resolution depending on the window selected and peak energy of the radiopharmaceutical. For example, higher energy In-111 photons (photopeaks at 172 and 245 keV) lose energy upon scattering in the patient. These lower energy scattered photons will be detected in the incorrectly selected lower energy window, such as 140 keV (Tc-99m). This increased scatter detection would result in degraded image quality.

While too little administered activity (e.g., due to dose infiltration) would result in higher noise due to poor count statistics, the statistical noise would be similar on 24-hour images and would not explain better images at the 24-hour time point. Having a patient scanned in an adjacent room with a high-energy radiopharmaceutical such as F-18 FDG can cause image degradation; however, this would not occur with In-111 since the medium-energy collimator used for this In-111 DTPA examination would reject most photons from a patient with In-111 in an adjacent room. There is no evidence of a prior nuclear study as there is no evidence of altered biodistribution.

Reference: Habibian M, et al. *Nuclear medicine imaging: a teaching file*, 2nd ed. Philadelphia, PA: Lippincott Williams & Wilkins, 2009:516–521.

7 **Answer A.** Bar phantoms are used to evaluate spatial resolution and spatial linearity on a weekly basis. The bars in each quadrant are different widths and separated by linear gaps of size equal to the bars. The ability of the system to clearly resolve the bars is representative of the spatial resolution of the system. Spatial linearity is assessed by determining if the linear bars appear straight or wavy. The resolution pattern in each quadrant of the camera can be checked by using a combination of rotating and flipping of the phantom.

The energy resolution is evaluated by measuring the width (full width at half-maximum) of a photopeak (often 140 keV photopeak of Tc-99m) expressed as a percentage of the photopeak energy. Energy linearity is measured by testing multiple radionuclide photopeaks being within ±5% of true value. Collimator integrity is tested by acquiring a high-count flood uniformity image and looking for defects. Uniformity is checked by acquiring images of a source that uniformly irradiates the entire detector face, not a bar phantom.

References: Halama JR, et al. *AAPM TG 177: acceptance testing and annual physics survey recommendations for gamma camera, SPECT, and SPECT/CT systems.* 2019. https://www. aapm.org/pubs/reports/detail.asp?docid=184

Mettler FA, Guiberteau MJ. *Essentials of nuclear medicine imaging*, 7th ed. Philadelphia, PA: Saunders, 2019:47–51.

8 **Answer D.** The bottom two rows of images demonstrate a significant increase in the background activity. This is due to scattering from high-energy photons from a nearby radioactive source. In this case, a patient who had an earlier PET scan (511 keV photons) walked into the adjacent room. These high-energy photons significantly penetrate the collimator and the shielding of the camera head, resulting in increased background counts.

The half-life of Tc-99m is 6 hours; there is not enough decay over the course of the examination to cause degradation in the images. Also, the counts that are acquired are corrected to adjust for decay to ensure that gastric emptying percentages are accurate. In addition, radiotracer decay would not cause an increase in the background activity. Gastric emptying studies are performed using an oral meal; therefore, it is not possible for the dose to infiltrate. Free pertechnetate would demonstrate uptake in the stomach and thyroid and would not be expected to contribute to background activity, nor would the amount of background activity be expected to change.

Reference: Habibian M, et al. *Nuclear medicine imaging: a teaching file*, 2nd ed. Philadelphia, PA: Lippincott Williams & Wilkins, 2009:516–521.

9 **Answer A.** Flood uniformity images should be obtained daily to evaluate the intrinsic function of the camera and, if the flood is extrinsic, the integrity of the collimator. If extrinsic floods are not acquired daily, then the collimator should be visually inspected each day. All cameras have some degree of field inhomogeneity, which can usually be corrected by acquiring a high count uniformity correction image. The use of a camera with an inhomogeneous field could result in misinterpretation of scan findings.

References: Halama JR, et al. *AAPM TG 177: acceptance testing and annual physics survey recommendations for gamma camera, SPECT, and SPECT/CT systems.* 2019. https://www. aapm.org/pubs/reports/detail.asp?docid=184

Mettler FA, Guiberteau MJ. *Essentials of nuclear medicine imaging*, 7th ed. Philadelphia, PA: Saunders, 2019:47–51.

10 **Answer A.** The maximum allowable limit of molybdenum-99 (Mo-99) breakthrough is 0.15 µCi Mo-99 per mCi of Tc-99m (0.15 Bq of Mo-99 per kBq of Tc-99m) at the time of radiopharmaceutical administration. Mo-99 in the Tc-99m eluate is an example of radionuclide impurity. Excess Mo-99 leads to an unnecessary increase in patient radiation dose. Over time, the amount of Mo-99 breakthrough increases in a sample due to its longer half-life (66 hours for Mo-99 compared to 6 hours for Tc-99m). Quality control testing for the Mo-99 breakthrough is performed by placing the eluate in a 6-mm-thick lead container (inside a dose calibrator), which stops all 140-keV photons from Tc-99m while the 740- and 780-keV photons from Mo-99 are able to penetrate the lead container allowing the dose calibrator to assay only the activity of the Mo-99 contaminant.

References: Mettler FA, Guiberteau MJ. *Essentials of nuclear medicine imaging*, 7th ed. Philadelphia, PA: Saunders, 2019:14–15.

Saha GB. *Fundamentals of nuclear pharmacy*, 6th ed. New York, NY: Springer, 2010:77.

11 **Answer D.** The study demonstrates intense uptake ballooning out from the neck region because the patient recently underwent an I-131 radioiodine therapy. Compton scatter from the I-131 photons (and to a lesser extent photons that penetrate the septa of the low-energy collimator) in the thyroid are detected in the 140 keV Tc-99m energy window used during the bone scintigraphy examination. This created the appearance of intense uptake emanating from the neck region. When a scan has an abnormal biodistribution, one should consider the possibility of the presence of interfering medications or the patient having had a recent nuclear medicine study.

The degree of uptake is too intense for free Tc-99m pertechnetate. Also, lack of physiologic uptake in the stomach goes against free Tc-99mm pertechnetate as the cause. Bone scintigraphy agents do not localize in the thyroid gland and, as such, would not image thyroiditis. Selection of the wrong photopeak would result in reduced contrast of bone and soft tissue and poor resolution but would not cause the intense uptake seen in the neck. Since the radiopharmaceuticals are administered by peripheral intravenous access, infiltrations in the neck would be atypical. A malfunctioned photomultiplier tube would cause a linear cold defect on whole-body images or a round cold spot in static images, not a large hot artifact.

Reference: Habibian M, et al. *Nuclear medicine imaging: a teaching file*, 2nd ed. Philadelphia, PA: Lippincott Williams & Wilkins, 2009:516–521.

12 **Answer C.** According to current regulations, NRC 10 CFR 35.75, a patient may be released from the medical facility if the authorized user physician determines that the effective dose equivalent to the maximally exposed individual (often a family member or caregiver) will not exceed 5 mSv (0.5 rem) from a single radioisotope treatment. The NRC maintains that its current release criteria are based on sound radiation protection principles and are sufficient to protect public health and safety. These release criteria result in reduced health care costs and allow patients to be in the comfort of their homes.

References: NRC.gov. 10CFR§35.75. Release of individuals containing unsealed byproduct material or implants containing byproduct material. https://www.nrc.gov/reading-rm/doc-collections/cfr/part035/part035-0075.html

NRC Regulatory guide 8.39. Release of patients administered radioactive materials. https://www.nrc.gov/reading-rm/doc-collections/reg-guides/occupational-health/rg/division-8/division-8-2.html

NUREG 1556, Vol. 9, Rev. 3. Appendix U: Release of patients or human research subjects administered radioactive materials. https://www.nrc.gov/reading-rm/doc-collections/nuregs/staff/sr1556/v9/

13 **Answer A.** Per NRC regulation, the annual institutional limit for the summed amount of radioactivity from all isotopes (except H-3 and C-14) that can be disposed of in a designated sink, toilet, or other release point is 1 Ci (37 GBq). In addition to the 1 Ci of radioactivity mentioned above, an additional 5 Ci (185 GBq) of H-3 and 1 Ci (37 GBq) of C-14 can be disposed of in a designated sink, toilet, or other release points on an annual basis. This type of waste disposal is referred to as "Disposal of Liquids into Sanitary Sewage." One sink in each laboratory may be designated as a "hot sink." This is the only permissible location for disposing of radioactive liquid waste in the department. A logbook should be set up so that each liquid waste disposal is documented by the radioisotope, amount, date, and the initials of the people involved. One or more toilets may be designated "hot toilets" for use by individuals undergoing medical diagnosis or therapy with radioactive material. Note that excreta from individuals undergoing medical diagnosis or therapy with radioactive material are not subject to these limitations on total disposed activity.

References: Mettler FA, Guiberteau MJ. *Essentials of nuclear medicine imaging*, 7th ed. Philadelphia, PA: Saunders, 2019:398.

NRC.gov. 10CFR§20.2003. Disposal by release into sanitary sewerage. http://www.nrc.gov/reading-rm/doc-collections/cfr/part020/part020-2003.html

NUREG 1556, Vol. 11, Rev. 1. Appendix O: Model waste management procedures. https://www.nrc.gov/reading-rm/doc-collections/nuregs/staff/sr1556/v11/

14 **Answer A.** A single axial CT image demonstrates a significant streak artifact due to photon starvation from imaging with the patient's arms down. Photon starvation occurs when an insufficient number of photons reach the detector. This occurs most often when the photon beam travels through high-attenuating portions of the patient, such as the upper abdomen with arms held down at their sides. An insufficient number of photons being detected results in noisy projection data, and CT reconstruction enhances noise, so streaks appear in the image. In this case, the thickest portion of the patient is in the lateral direction, and so the streaks are horizontal. This artifact can be exacerbated in CT imaging used with PET imaging for attenuation correction because the tube current (mAs) is lower compared to the diagnostic CT. This image also displays a truncation (out-of-field) artifact at the edges of the field of view in the patient's arms. This artifact presents as bright pixels that appear to have much higher HU values (more attenuating) than you would expect in soft tissue. This effect occurs because the HU values for each voxel of soft tissue located outside the field of view is added to the voxels in the arm located just inside the field of view.

Contrast infiltration would result in high-HU regions in the CT image at locations in the body where iodinated contrast leaves the intravascular compartment and enters the surrounding soft tissue (this is often seen at the injection site where extravasation occurs). FDG contrast infiltration would change the appearance of the PET images but would not be visible on the CT image. A dead pixel in the CT detector array would result in a ring artifact. Moire interference is represented by the wavy appearance of the images. An example of Moire interference for a bar-phantom image is shown below.

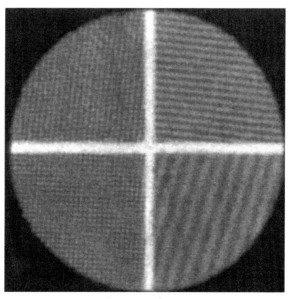

Moire Interference

References: Barrett JF, Keat N. Artifacts in CT: recognition and avoidance. *Radiographics* 2017;24(6):1679–1691.

Bushberg JT, et al. *The essential physics of medical imaging*, 2nd ed. Philadelphia, PA: LWW, 2002:369–371. http://www.displaymate.com/moire.html

Hsieh J. *Computed tomography: principles, design, artifacts, and recent advances*, 2nd ed. Hoboken, NJ: Wiley Interscience; SPIE Press, 2012. Chapter 7.

15 **Answer D.** Medical waste contaminated with radioactive isotopes with a physical half-life of <120 days can be kept on site using the "decay in storage" method of radioactive waste disposal. The radioactive waste can be disposed of as nonradioactive waste or returned to use when the radioactive material has decayed to undetectable levels. A general rule of thumb is that the radioactive waste must be stored for at least 10 half-lives; after 10 half-lives, the radioactive materials on contaminated waste will typically have decayed to undetectable levels. Since the half-life of iodine is 8 days, this would require the contaminated material to be kept in storage for 80 days. In general, nuclear waste is separated according to the half-life of the radiopharmaceutical and stored in a shielded area. The image below shows "decay in storage," with multiple sharps containers that are separated by half-lives and surrounded by lead bricks.

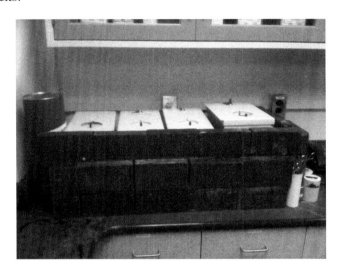

References: Mettler FA, Guiberteau MJ. *Essentials of nuclear medicine imaging*, 7th ed. Philadelphia, PA: Saunders, 2019:398.

NRC.gov. 10CFR§35.92. Decay-in-storage. https://www.nrc.gov/reading-rm/doc-collections/cfr/part035/part035-0092.html

NUREG 1556, Vol. 11, Rev. 1. Appendix O: Model waste management procedures. https://www.nrc.gov/reading-rm/doc-collections/nuregs/staff/sr1556/v11/

16 **Answer C.** The maximum amount of aluminum allowed in an eluate is 10 μg of aluminum per mL of Tc-99m eluate. Mo-99/Tc-99m generators contain an elution column made of alumina (Al_2O_3). Aluminum that becomes detached from the column and infiltrates the Tc-99m eluate is known as an aluminum breakthrough. This affects the chemical purity of the radiopharmaceutical and can affect biodistribution and image quality (e.g., excess aluminum in the standard Tc-99m MDP kit results in the formation of Tc-Al colloidal particles, which can be visualized as hepatic uptake). The amount of aluminum in the eluate can be measured using paper colorimetric test strips during radiopharmaceutical quality control tests for chemical purity.

References: Mettler FA, Guiberteau MJ. *Essentials of nuclear medicine imaging*, 7th ed. Philadelphia, PA: Saunders, 2019:14–15.

Saha G. *Fundamentals of nuclear pharmacy*, 7th ed. New York, NY: Springer, 2017:87.

17 **Answer A.** Many states have an agreement with the NRC to accept the responsibility for regulating by-product, source, and special nuclear materials within their jurisdiction. These are known as agreement states, and their radiation regulations are required to be at least as strict as the NRC regulations. It is possible for agreement states to have stricter regulations than the NRC, but it is not required. The NRC provides assistance to states expressing interest in establishing programs to assume NRC regulatory authority under the Atomic Energy Act of 1954, as amended. For specific information regarding radioactive material license and use in the state in which you practice, please consult the following references.

References: Mettler FA, Guiberteau MJ. *Essentials of nuclear medicine imaging*, 7th ed. Philadelphia, PA: Saunders, 2019:384–384.

NRC.gov. Agreement State Program websites. https://www.nrc.gov/about-nrc/state-tribal/agreement-states.html; https://scp.nrc.gov/rulemaking.html

18 **Answer B.** This is a yellow III label with a maximum allowable transport index (TI) of 10 mrem/hour at 1 m. Labels rely principally on symbols to indicate the type of hazard and the level of hazard contained in a package. The label required on the package is based on the radiation hazard OUTSIDE the package; however, the type of package required for transporting radioactive material is based on the activity INSIDE the package.

Radioactive materials have three possible labels depending on the relative radiation levels external to the package. The label must include the transport index (TI), which is the highest radiation level at 1 m from the surface of the package. In addition to the TI, the label must include the contents (radionuclides) and the activity of contents. The three labels are commonly called White I, Yellow II, and Yellow III, referring to the color of the label and the Roman numeral prominently displayed. A specific label is required if the surface radiation limit and the limit at 1 m satisfy the following requirements:

Label	Surface Radiation Level		Radiation Level at 1 m
White I	<0.5 mrem/h		Not applicable
Yellow II	<50 mrem/h	AND	<1 mrem/h
Yellow III	>50 mrem/h but <200 mrem/h	OR	>1 mrem/h but <10 mrem/h

Since the TI is the radiation level at 1 m, it is clear that a White I label has no TI. A Yellow II must have a TI < 1, and a Yellow III may have a TI between 1 and 10. If the TI is above 10, the package must be transported in a closed exclusive-use vehicle.

References: eCFR.gov. 49CFR§172.403. Class 7 (radioactive) material. https://www.ecfr.gov/cgi-bin/text-idx?SID=a0d4cdcb60217fc322b2816f9ebf9548&mc=true&node=se49.2.172_1403&rgn=div8

Mettler FA, Guiberteau MJ. *Essentials of nuclear medicine imaging*, 7th ed. Philadelphia, PA: Saunders, 2019:390–391.

19 **Answer B.** PET uses electronic collimation, where an energy window and a coincidence timing window are used to limit the counting of photons that are not true primary events (e.g., scattered coincident photons, random coincidences from single events), which may arrive at the detector at lower energy or at a later time than true primary coincident photons. Electronic collimation allows more emitted primary photons to reach the detector for PET imaging compared to SPECT, which uses absorptive collimations with many lead or tungsten septa placed perpendicularly over the detectors to stop the scattered photons. There is no absorptive collimation in most PET imaging or a few annular-shaped septa are used between detector rings to further reduce scatter in "2D mode" PET imaging. As such, the sensitivity (count rate detected per unit activity) of PET is many times higher in 3D mode without septa compared to 2D mode, and sensitivity of PET imaging is several orders of magnitude higher than that for SPECT.

Absorptive collimation reduces the detection of events that are not traveling parallel to the direction of the septa. The lead septa of the collimator block oblique primary and scattered photons from reaching the detector. Absorptive collimation reduces scatter but also attenuates some of the primary (unscattered) photons from reaching the detector surface, which leads to decreased detection of the counts and decreases the sensitivity. Random coincidence events detected by PET systems degrade the image quality in PET. Random coincidence events do not occur for SPECT. Uniformity corrections improve the image quality in both PET and SPECT by correcting for relative differences in count performance and detector response across the field of view of the detector.

References: Cherry SR, Sorenson JA, Phelps ME. *Physics in nuclear medicine*, 4th ed. Philadelphia, PA: Saunders, 2012:322.

Mettler FA, Guiberteau MJ. *Essentials of nuclear medicine imaging*, 7th ed. Philadelphia, PA: Saunders, 2019:38–47.

20 **Answer A.** Both gamma cameras and positron emission tomography (PET) scanners should have their detector uniformity checked daily. The detectors are irradiated with a uniform radiation field (i.e., flood source). The images are then evaluated quantitatively and qualitatively to detect nonuniformities in the images that could develop due to expected causes like drifts in the relative response between regions of the detector over time or due to unexpected causes like incorrect calibrations, component failure, or software errors.

Weekly and monthly quality control (QC) of PET scanners typically are determined by the manufacturer and may include calibrations such as gain adjustments of the PET detector and detector normalization calibration. Semiannual QC is also typically determined by the manufacturer and includes preventative maintenance repairs by the manufacturer's field service engineers, and emission correction factor calibrations may be recommended either semiannually or annually. Physics testing of PET is typically performed annually. Audits of the QC program and PET image quality QC testing (e.g., ACR phantom testing) are typically checked quarterly for PET scanners. Licensing agencies and accrediting organizations may impact the frequency of these tests.

References: Bushberg JT, et al. *The essential physics of medical imaging*, 3rd ed. Philadelphia, PA: Lippincott Williams & Wilkins, 2012:735.

Mettler FA, Guiberteau MJ. *Essentials of nuclear medicine imaging*, 7th ed. Philadelphia, PA: Saunders, 2019:47–49.

Saha GB. *Basics of PET imaging: physics, chemistry and regulations*, New York, NY: Springer, 2004:101.

21 **Answer C.** The transportation index (TI) indicates the maximum radiation level in mrem/hour at a distance of 1 m from the external surface of a package or container. In this example, the TI of 2 indicates that at 1 m from the package, the radiation intensity that is measured should be <2 mrem/hour, which is equivalent to 0.02 mSv/hour. If the radiation exposure of a received package at 1 m is greater than what is listed on the placard, one should consider if the shielding was damaged, if the wrong radiopharmaceutical was shipped, or if the label is wrong. If the measured TI is greater than the indicated TI, the radiation safety officer and/or committee at your institution should be notified to assess the situation and should follow up with the courier/sender.

The TI does not provide any information on how long it will take for the package contents to decay to the background or on the distance the driver should maintain between himself or herself and the package.

References: eCFR.gov. 49CFR§ 72.403. Class 7 (radioactive) material. https://www.ecfr.gov/cgi-bin/text-idx?SID=a0d4cdcb60217fc322b2816f9ebf9548&mc=true&node=se49.2.172_1403&rgn=div8

Mettler FA, Guiberteau MJ. *Essentials of nuclear medicine imaging*, 7th ed. Philadelphia, PA: Saunders, 2019:390–392.

NRC.gov. 10CFR§71.4. Definitions. https://www.nrc.gov/reading-rm/doc-collections/cfr/part071/full-text.html

NRC.gov. https://www.nrc.gov/reading-rm/basic-ref/students/for-educators/labeling.html

22 **Answer D.** The radionuclide photopeak is qualitatively evaluated for energy shifts and energy offsets daily by checking the energy spectrum. Annually, the photopeak is quantitatively evaluated by measuring the energy resolution. The energy resolution is measured as the full width at half-maximum (FWHM) of the photopeak in the energy spectrum and is expressed as a percentage of the photopeak energy. For example, the measured FWHM is typically 14 keV for the 140 photopeak of Tc-99m. This results in an energy resolution of 10% at FHWM.

The intrinsic uniformity test evaluates differences in detector response across the field of view (FOV) by calculating the relative differences in the number of counts recorded at each image pixel when a flood source irradiates the detector with the collimators removed. Uniformity is expressed as the differential uniformity difference in small groups of adjacent pixels and the integral uniformity difference across all pixels in the entire detector (UFOV) or the center 50% of the detector (CFOV). Spatial resolution is checked using a bar phantom and is typically done weekly. Some camera manufacturers do not require this test to be done during routine weekly QC; spatial resolution is also evaluated annually during physics testing. Sensitivity is a measurement of the camera's ability to detect activity and convert it into a signal and is expressed as the count rate per unit of radioactivity. This test is typically done annually.

References: Cherry SR, Sorenson JA, Phelps ME. *Physics in nuclear medicine*, 4th ed. Philadelphia, PA: Saunders, 2012:148–150.

Mettler FA, Guiberteau MJ. *Essentials of nuclear medicine imaging*, 7th ed. Philadelphia, PA: Saunders, 2019:47–51.

23 **Answer B.** The anterior F-18 FDG-PET image demonstrates physiologic activity in the brain, salivary and lymphoid tissues of the neck, vocal cords, liver, and GI and GU systems. Intense uptake is noted in the breasts, which is from physiologic glandular uptake in this postpartum patient. However, F-18 FDG is not excreted into breast milk. As such, the main source of potential radiation hazard to a breast-feeding infant is from close proximity to the breast (external) rather than the ingestion of milk (internal). As a result, the Advisory Committee on Medical Uses of Isotopes (ACMUI) advises the patient to suspend breast-feeding for 4 hours after the injection in order to reduce the dose to the nursing infant to below 1 mSv.

If the radiopharmaceutical is not excreted, the duration of breast-feeding suspension or cessation primarily depends on the half-life of the radiopharmaceutical, type of emission (e.g., gamma, alpha, or beta), the energy of radioactive emission, and the administered activity. The duration of breast-feeding suspension or cessation depends heavily on the residence time in the infant tissues if the radiopharmaceutical is excreted in breast milk. Four hours of interruption of breast-feeding is recommended for F-18 FDG at diagnostic activities (2 to 20 mCi) because the half-life of F-18 FDG is relatively short (F-18 physical half-life 110 minutes). Tc-99m has lower energy gamma emissions, but the longer half-life results in a longer recommended interruption of 24 hours. A 3-day interruption is recommended after administration of the short-lived I-123 NaI radiopharmaceutical because NaI is expressed in breast milk. Discontinuation of breast-feeding until the next pregnancy is recommended after administration of radiopharmaceuticals labeled with long-lived isotopes and isotopes that emit high-energy photons or beta particles, such as I-131, I-124, and Lu-177, or labeled with an alpha emitter, such as Ra-223.

Isotope(s)	Duration of Interruption of Breast-Feeding
I-124 NaI, I-131 NaI, Lu-177 OCTREOTATE, and Ra-223 (and all other alpha emitters)	Complete cessation of breast-feeding for the current child (can resume breast-feeding for future children)
I-123 NaI	3 d
Tc-99m radiopharmaceuticals	24 h
F-18 radiopharmaceuticals	4 h
O-15 and Rb-82 radiopharmaceuticals	No discontinuation

References: ACMUI Subcommittee on "Nursing Mother Guidelines for the Medical Administration of Radioactive Materials." June 2018. https://www.nrc.gov/docs/ML1817/ML18177A451.pdf

NRC Regulatory guide 8.39 (Draft guide DG-8057). July 2019. https://www.nrc.gov/docs/ML1910/ML19108A463.pdf

24 **Answer B.** Gamma cameras localize the source of activity by using collimators. Collimators prevent photons traveling in the wrong direction from reaching the detector (e.g., oblique primary photons and scattered photons). Medium- and high-energy collimators have thicker and longer septa, while lower-energy collimators have thinner septa and smaller holes. If a low-energy collimator is used to image a higher energy radioisotope, there will be increased septal penetration with the resultant decrease in spatial resolution.

For a given medium-energy isotope, the measured sensitivity, or counts per unit activity, of the gamma camera increases due to the septal penetration when low-energy collimators are used, compared to when medium-energy collimators are used. Fewer of the medium-energy photons are stopped by the thinner septa of the low-energy collimator, so more photons are detected for medium-energy isotopes compared to low-energy isotopes due to increased scatter. Therefore, the relative scatter with a low-energy collimator will increase with medium-energy isotopes compared to low-energy isotopes. Energy resolution in typical scintillation gamma cameras depends on the Poisson statistical fluctuation in the amount of scintillation light produced when photons are detected. This statistical fluctuation becomes relatively smaller when more scintillation light is produced, and more scintillation light is produced when the photopeak energy of the isotope increases. Therefore, the energy resolution of the photopeak typically improves for medium-energy isotopes compared to low-energy isotopes.

References: Mettler FA, Guiberteau MJ. *Essentials of nuclear medicine imaging*, 7th ed. Philadelphia, PA: Saunders, 2019:23–26.

O'Malley JP, Ziessman HA, Thrall JH. *Nuclear medicine: the requisites*, 5th ed. Philadelphia, PA: Saunders, 2020:21–23.

25 **Answer C.** The half-life of Mo-99 is 66 hours, which is more than 10 times longer than that of Tc-99m, which has a half-life of 6 hours. The amount of Mo-99m will decrease at a much slower rate than the amount of Tc-99m. As a result, the relative amount of Mo-99 contamination increases with time. For example, a sample containing 0.001% Mo-99 contamination at the time of elution will contain 0.012% Mo-99 contamination 24 hours later. The NRC regulatory limit for Mo-99 contamination or "Mo-99 breakthrough" is 0.015% or 0.15 μCi Mo-99 per 1 mCi Tc-99m at the time of administration. This is why Tc-99m radiopharmaceutical doses should be prepared and administered within 24 hours of the time that the Tc-99m was eluted from the generator.

References: Mettler FA, Guiberteau MJ. *Essentials of nuclear medicine imaging*, 7th ed. Philadelphia, PA: Elsevier, 2019:1–19.

Saha GB. *Fundamentals of nuclear pharmacy*, 6th ed. New York, NY: Springer, 2010:128.

26 **Answer B.** The anterior and posterior images demonstrate the physiologic distribution of the radiopharmaceutical to the lacrimal glands, nasal mucosa, liver, kidneys, bowel, and bone marrow. This is a Ga-67 scan. The Ga-67 is imaged with a medium-energy collimator with a 20% window over 93, 185 and 300 keV photopeaks. Medium-energy collimators have a maximum suggested energy of about 300 keV.

Low-energy collimators are generally used to image energy up to 150 keV, such as Tc-99m-labeled agents (photopeak 140 keV). Using a low-energy collimator to image Ga-67 would result in loss of spatial resolution and loss of contrast in the images. This is because of the septal penetration by scatter and primary photons at oblique angles (i.e., not parallel to the collimator septa). The small lacrimal glands would likely not be resolved as well because of the loss of spatial resolution, and subtle contrast difference between soft tissue and skeletal uptake would not be visible because of increased background counts in the images. High-energy collimators are used to image isotopes with gamma energies in excess of 300 keV, such as I-131 (photopeak 365 keV). High-energy collimators have thicker septa and larger holes than do medium-energy collimators, so spatial resolution would be degraded for a Ga-67 examination.

Converging collimators are used to produce magnified images of small objects in the body (e.g., heart or brain). These collimators have converging holes that are all aimed at a focal spot in front of the detector face and produce a magnified image of a single region of the body. Converging collimators are rarely used today for clinical imaging and have been replaced with multifocal collimators for cardiac imaging tasks. Fan beam collimators are a special type of converging collimators that have holes that converge only in the x-axis. They are used for brain tomography. Converging collimators have a limited field of view (FOV) and were never used for whole-body imaging, where the camera is scanned in a cranial–caudal or caudal–cranial direction along the length of the patient. Diverging collimators have holes that are all aimed at a focal spot behind the detector face and produce minified images or large objects. Divergent collimators were once used for imaging when the dimensions of the gamma camera detectors were much smaller than the diameter of the patient's body. Diverging collimators are never used today for clinical imaging on modern gamma cameras.

References: Bushberg JT, et al. *The essential physics of medical imaging*, 3rd ed. Philadelphia, PA: Lippincott Williams & Wilkins, 2012:677–681.

Mettler FA, Guiberteau MJ. *Essentials of nuclear medicine imaging*, 7th ed. Philadelphia, PA: Saunders, 2019:23–26.

O'Malley JP, Ziessman HA, Thrall JH. *Nuclear medicine: the requisites*, 5th ed. Philadelphia, PA: Saunders, 2020:21–23.

27 Answer C. High-energy collimator is used to image I-131 because I-131 emits a high energy gamma of 365 keV (83% of decays), and 637-and 722-keV gammas are also emitted (7% and 2% of decays). High-energy collimators are used to image isotopes with gamma energies in excess of 300 keV.

Low-energy all-purpose collimators are used to image isotopes with gamma and x-ray energies <150 keV, such as Tc-99m (140 keV). Medium-energy collimators are used to image isotopes of gamma energies >150 keV and up to 300 keV, such as In-111 (171 keV, 245 keV). Posttherapy imaging of differentiated thyroid cancer includes scans of the thyroid bed and nodes for evidence of residual disease and/or metastases, which is not feasible with a pinhole collimator. A pinhole collimator is used to magnify very small objects such as the thyroid but have a very limited field of view and would typically only be able to show the thyroid organ and a small region of the neck.

References: Mettler FA, Guiberteau MJ. *Essentials of nuclear medicine imaging*, 7th ed. Philadelphia, PA: Saunders, 2019:23–26.

O'Malley JP, Ziessman HA, Thrall JH. *Nuclear medicine: the requisites*, 5th ed. Philadelphia, PA: Saunders, 2020:21–23.

28 Answer C. The posterior planar image on the right is much blurrier than the image on the left; it is because the camera (detector/collimator) was further away from the patient during the acquisition of image B compared to image A. The spatial resolution of the gamma camera degrades as the target gets further away from the detector/collimator. It is crucial to acquire images with the detectors as close to the patient as possible and target organ(s) in the center of the field of view.

The use of different radiopharmaceuticals would have resulted in a different physiologic distribution. Acquisition at different time points would result in images with varying numbers of counts in soft tissue compared to the bone, which is not the case here. While lower administered activity would result in a noisier image, it would not affect its resolution.

References: Chandra R. *Nuclear medicine physics: the basics*, 8th ed. Philadelphia, PA: Lippincott, Williams & Williams, 2012:149–150.

Cherry SE, Sorenson JA, Phelps ME. *Physics in nuclear medicine*, 4th ed. Philadelphia, PA: Saunders, 2012:222–228.

Naddaf SY, Collier BD, Elgazzar AH, et al. Technical errors in planar bone scanning. *J Nucl Med Technol* 2004;32(3):148–153.

29 Answer D. The thyroid would be visualized because of free pertechnetate in the Tc-99m MAA. Tc-99m MAA is unstable, and the probability of free Tc-99m pertechnetate and MAA agglomeration increases with time. As such, it is preferable to use Tc-99m MAA soon after its preparation and no later than 6 hours postpreparation. Free Tc-99m pertechnetate localizes to the thyroid and stomach.

Brain, liver, heart, and pancreatic uptake are unusual in Tc99m-MAA studies unless there is a physiologic abnormality, such as cardiac or pulmonary shunting resulting in brain, kidneys, and liver uptake.

Reference: Parker JA, Coleman RE, et al. SNM practice guideline for lung scintigraphy 4.0. *J Nucl Med Technol* 2012;40(1):57–65.

30 Answer B. Crystal hydration typically appears as cold spots or "measling" near the edge of the field of view on a uniformity image. Artifact related to hydration is usually present in the periphery as it usually begins at/near the outer edge of the camera NaI crystal. Hydration results in reduced light output, so the spots are cold/dark. A hydrated crystal should be replaced as soon as possible.

A bad photomultiplier tube would usually appear as a large, cold/dark circle on the image (see question 5). Without a linearity correction, the image would appear very nonuniform, with all of the PMTs visible. A radioactive spill would likely result in splotchy hot/bright spots in the region of the field of view where the spill had occurred, not as cold spots.

Reference: *IAEA Quality Control Atlas for Scintillation Camera Systems*. Vienna, Austria: IAEA, 2003.

For Questions 31 through 35, please match the instruments with the appropriate task it is used to perform.

31 **Answer C.** Radioiodine (I-131 or I-123) uptake is best accomplished with an organ uptake probe. Uptake probes are used almost exclusively for measuring thyroid uptake, so they are commonly referred to as thyroid uptake probes. An uptake probe consists of a wide-aperture collimator, scintillation crystal, photomultiplier tube, multichannel analyzer, and gantry/stand. The open end of the probe (collimator) is placed over/near the thyroid, and counts are acquired for a fixed amount of time. These are compared to that of a standard capsule and background over the patient's thigh to determine the radioiodine uptake by the thyroid gland.

References: Mettler FA, Guiberteau MJ. *Essentials of nuclear medicine imaging*, 7th ed. Philadelphia, PA: Saunders, 2019:19–23.

Zanzonico P. Routine quality control of clinical nuclear medicine instrumentation: a brief review. *J Nucl Med* 2008;49(7):1114–1131.

32 **Answer D.** Wipe test is best accomplished with a well counter. The well counters are composed of a NaI crystal in the shape of a "well," with the sample placed in the well. This shape provides a geometric efficiency of nearly 100%, enabling the well counter to detect minimal quantities of radioactivity. They operate best when counting activities <37 kBq (1 µCi). Greater activities will result in increased dead time and significant count losses. To prevent count losses, even at low activities, well counters should be operated using live time, which increases the counting time by the amount of dead time encountered during the sample counting. The well counters are often used in conjunction with a multichannel analyzer (MCA) to analyze the energy spectrum of photons detected by the well counter. A wipe can be used to sample a minute amount of radioactivity from a surface. A well counter + MCA can then be used to count the wipe and analyze the energy spectrum to determine the specific radioisotope and amount of radioactivity that was wiped off of (i.e., removed from) that surface.

References: Mettler FA, Guiberteau MJ. *Essentials of nuclear medicine imaging*, 7th ed. Philadelphia, PA: Saunders, 2019:19–23.

Zanzonico P. Routine quality control of clinical nuclear medicine instrumentation: a brief review. *J Nucl Med* 2008;49(7):1114–1131.

33 **Answer E.** Assay of 99mTc-MDP activity for a bone scan is best accomplished with a dose calibrator. A dose calibrator is a cylindrical ionization chamber (usually filled with pressurized, inert argon) with a central well that can measure activities in the microcurie, millicurie, and even curie ranges. Vials or syringes containing activity from known radiopharmaceuticals are placed in the well of the dose calibrator and assayed before patient administration.

References: Mettler FA, Guiberteau MJ. *Essentials of nuclear medicine imaging*, 7th ed. Philadelphia, PA: Saunders, 2019:19–23.

Zanzonico P. Routine quality control of clinical nuclear medicine instrumentation: a brief review. *J Nucl Med* 2008;49(7):1114–1131.

34 Answer B. The patient release is best accomplished with an ion chamber survey meter. Ionization survey chambers measure high or low exposure rates, although they are not as sensitive as GM meters. Ion chamber survey meters are filled with gas or air and have a relatively low voltage applied from anode to cathode. This prevents the cascade events seen with GM, resulting in shorter dead times. As such, they are used to measure high radiation exposure areas. Importantly, ion chamber survey meters have a signal that is directly related to the exposure rate for all radionuclides, which is NOT the case for GM meters. This is why ion chamber survey meters should be used to measure the exposure rate at 1 meter from the patient in order to determine whether or not the patient can be released from the hospital.

References: Mettler FA, Guiberteau MJ. *Essentials of nuclear medicine imaging*, 7th ed. Philadelphia, PA: Saunders, 2019:19–23.

Zanzonico P. Routine quality control of clinical nuclear medicine instrumentation: a brief review. *J Nucl Med* 2008;49(7):1114–1131.

35 Answer A. Area survey is best accomplished with a Geiger-Müller (GM) meter. A GM meter is a very sensitive handheld instrument used to detect small amounts of radioactive contamination, making it a useful device for an area survey. The detector is gas-filled with a high voltage applied from the anode to the cathode resulting in a cascade of events from a single gamma ray hitting the detector. They are not energy discriminating (cannot be used to identify a radioisotope) and have high dead time (preventing their use in high-radiation areas).

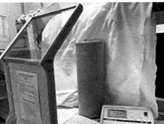
Dose calibrator

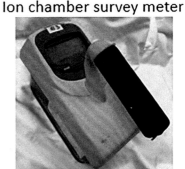
Ion chamber survey meter

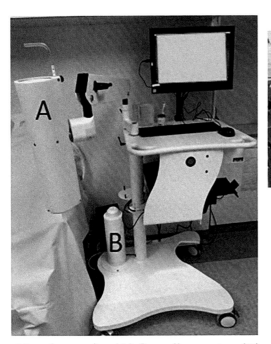
Uptake probe (A) & well counter (B)

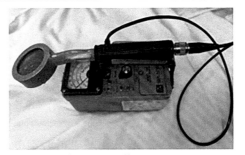
Geiger-Muller meter

References: Mettler FA, Guiberteau MJ. *Essentials of nuclear medicine imaging*, 7th ed. Philadelphia, PA: Saunders, 2019:19–23.

Zanzonico P. Routine quality control of clinical nuclear medicine instrumentation: a brief review. *J Nucl Med* 2008;49(7):1114–1131.

36 Answer D. This is a picture of the Jaszczak or ACR SPECT phantom. This phantom is used to assess the overall performance of a SPECT system, which should be tested quarterly. This cylindrical, acrylic phantom is filled with Tc-99m. It contains different sections and inserts consisting of cold/nonradioactive acrylic spheres and rods surrounded by an aqueous solution of radioactivity. The various sections of the phantom are designed to assess the tomographic uniformity, contrast, and resolution (see images below) as well as the attenuation correction accuracy of a SPECT imaging system.

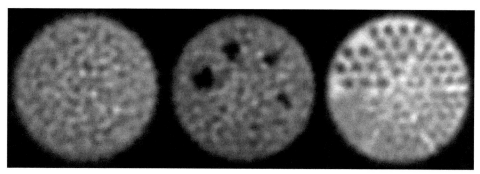

Images of the ACR phantom used to assess tomographic uniformity (*left*), contrast (*middle*), and resolution (*right*).

References: Halama JR, et al. *AAPM TG 177: acceptance testing and annual physics survey recommendations for gamma camera, SPECT, and SPECT/CT systems.* 2019. https://www.aapm.org/pubs/reports/detail.asp?docid=184

Mettler FA, Guiberteau MJ. *Essentials of nuclear medicine imaging,* 7th ed. Philadelphia, PA: Saunders, 2019:19–59.

Zanzonico P. Routine quality control of clinical nuclear medicine instrumentation: a brief review. *J Nucl Med* 2008;49(7):1114–1131.

37 Answer:

A. 5 mSv	Dose limit to the fetus/embryo over the gestation period for a declared pregnant radiation worker
C. 50 mSv	Annual dose limit for an adult radiation worker
E. 150 mSv	Annual dose limit to lens of the eye for a radiation worker
D. No limit	Dose limit for a patient undergoing a procedure in which ionizing radiation is used
B. 1 mSv	Annual dose limit to the general public and nonradiation workers

The annual occupational dose limit for the general public and nonradiation workers is 1 mSv (0.01 rem).

The dose to the embryo/fetus during the entire pregnancy from the occupational exposure of a declared pregnant radiation worker should not exceed 5 mSv (0.5 rem), which is 10% of the adult limit. This only applies to a radiation worker who has declared her pregnancy; there is no fetal dose limit if the pregnancy is not declared to the employer. Efforts should be made to avoid substantial variation above a uniform monthly exposure rate in a declared pregnancy (e.g., avoid exposure >0.5 mSv/month).

The annual occupational dose limit for a whole-body dose for an adult radiation worker is 50 mSv (5 rem).

The annual occupational dose limit for the lens of the eye for an adult radiation worker is 150 mSv (15 rem).

There is no limit on the amount of dose received by a patient as prescribed by a physician during a procedure in which ionizing radiation is used for medical diagnosis or therapy.

While not listed in the chart above, the NRC dose limits also include the following: the annual occupational dose limits for minors are 10% the adult limits; the annual occupational dose limit for an adult radiation worker to any individual organ or tissue other than the lens of the eye is 500 mSv (50 rem); the annual occupational dose limit for an adult radiation worker to the skin of the whole body or to the skin of any extremity is 500 mSv (50 rem).

References: Mettler FA, Guiberteau MJ. *Essentials of nuclear medicine imaging*, 7th ed. Philadelphia, PA: Saunders, 2019:385.

NRC.gov. 10CFR§20.1201. Scope. https://www.nrc.gov/reading-rm/doc-collections/cfr/part020/part020-1002.html

NRC.gov. 10CFR§20.1201. Occupational dose limits for adults. https://www.nrc.gov/reading-rm/doc-collections/cfr/part020/part020-1201.html

NRC.gov. 10CFR§20.1207. Occupational dose limits for minors. https://www.nrc.gov/reading-rm/doc-collections/cfr/part020/part020-1207.html

NRC.gov. 10CFR§20.1208. Dose equivalent to an embryo/fetus. https://www.nrc.gov/reading-rm/doc-collections/cfr/part020/part020-1208.html

38 **Answer B.** The patient can be released because the estimated total dose to the maximally exposed individual (MEI) is <5 mSv. Per federal regulation, patients who have been administered unsealed radioactive material (such as I-131 for thyroid cancer treatment) can be released if a physician determines that the total radiation dose from the patient to any other individual is not likely to exceed 5 mSv. Because the estimated dose to the MEI is >1 mSv, the released individual must be provided with instructions, including written instructions, on actions recommended to reduce exposure to other individuals as low as is reasonably achievable. The NRC maintains that its current release criteria are based on sound radiation protection principles and are sufficient to protect public health and safety. These release criteria result in reduced health care costs and allow patients to be in the comfort of their homes.

The dose limit for the general public and nonradiation workers is 1 mSv; however, in the case of MEI, it is increased to 5 mSv. The patient release is determined on a case-by-case basis by the physician, and release depends only on the calculated dose to individuals near the patient. There is no constant time or activity limit in the thyroid that requires a patient to stay at the hospital. In many instances, radionuclide therapies are outpatient procedures with no hospital stay.

References: Mettler FA, Guiberteau MJ. *Essentials of nuclear medicine imaging*, 7th ed. Philadelphia, PA: Saunders, 2019:394–396.

NRC.gov. https://www.nrc.gov/reading-rm/doc-collections/cfr/part035/part035-0075.html

NRC.gov. 10CFR§35.75. Release of individuals containing unsealed byproduct material or implants containing byproduct material. https://www.nrc.gov/reading-rm/doc-collections/cfr/part035/part035-0075.html

NRC Regulatory guide 8.39. Release of patients administered radioactive materials. https://www.nrc.gov/reading-rm/doc-collections/reg-guides/occupational-health/rg/division-8/division-8-2.html

NUREG 1556, Vol. 9, Rev. 3. Appendix U: Release of patients or human research subjects administered radioactive materials. https://www.nrc.gov/reading-rm/doc-collections/nuregs/staff/sr1556/v9/

39 **Answer C.** For a patient who is nursing, interruption of breast-feeding for 24 hours is recommended after administration of a Tc-99m labeled radionuclide. The table with guidance for the duration of interruption of breast-feeding is provided in answer 23. Per NRC and ACMUI guidance, the duration of the interruption of breast-feeding is chosen to reduce the dose to the breast-feeding infant to <1 mSv. Note that the NRC and ACMUI recommend but do not require the 1-mSv dose limit for infants and children; the official NRC regulatory release criteria of 5 mSv to the maximally exposed individual (MEI) still applies even if the MEI is an infant or child. Per NRC regulation, if the dose to a breast-feeding child is likely to exceed 1 mSv with no interruption of breast-feeding, (1) written guidance must be provided on the interruption/cessation of breast-feeding and (2) information must be provided on the consequences of failure to follow this guidance.

References: Advisory Committee on Medical Uses of Isotopes (ACMUI) Sub-Committee on nursing mother guidelines for the medical administration of radioactive materials. https://www.nrc.gov/reading-rm/doc-collections/acmui/reports/#2018

NRC Draft regulatory guide 8.39. Release of patients administered radioactive materials. pp. 11–13. https://www.nrc.gov/reading-rm/doc-collections/reg-guides/occupational-health/draft-index.html

NRC.gov. 10CFR§35.75. Release of individuals containing unsealed byproduct material or implants containing byproduct material. https://www.nrc.gov/reading-rm/doc-collections/cfr/part035/part035-0075.html

40 **Answer D.** The route of administration also needs to be included in the written directive. Per NRC regulation, the written directive must contain the following four items for the administration of an unsealed radionuclide therapy:

1. Patient or human research subject name
2. The radioactive drug
3. The dosage (this is the activity to be administered)
4. The route of administration

The written directive must also be signed and dated by an authorized user. Note: For radioiodine (I-131 NaI), the route of administration is assumed to be oral and not required.

The patient's date of birth and pregnancy status are important considerations that may contraindicate radionuclide therapy but are not required to be on a written directive per the NRC. Therapeutic procedures are not typically performed on pregnant women. The half-life and radioactive emissions of the radionuclide used for therapy are known from listing of the radioactive drug.

References: NRC.gov. 10CFR§35.40. Written directives. https://www.nrc.gov/reading-rm/doc-collections/cfr/part035/part035-0040.htm

Saha G. *Fundamentals of nuclear pharmacy*, 7th ed. New York, NY: Springer, 2017:244.

41 **Answer A.** Of the answer options provided, only I-131 sodium iodide meets the criteria to require a written directive. I-131 sodium iodide is the only imaging agent that requires a written directive, and the written directive is only required when the administered activity of I-131 sodium iodide is >1.11 MBq (30 μCi). Per NRC federal regulation, a written directive is required for the administration of

- I-131 sodium iodide with activity >1.11 MBq (30 μCi) OR
- Any therapeutic dosage of unsealed by-product material OR
- Any therapeutic dose of radiation from by-product material

References: NRC.gov. 10CFR§35.40. Written directives. https://www.nrc.gov/reading-rm/doc-collections/cfr/part035/part035-0040.htm

Saha G. *Fundamentals of nuclear pharmacy*, 7th ed. New York, NY: Springer, 2017:244.

42 **Answer D.** Sometimes, the patients undergo imaging procedures with iodinated contrast before undergoing nuclear medicine imaging. The kidneys excrete the iodinated contrast agents into the bladder. Consequently, urine containing iodinated contrast will appear hyperattenuating on the CT images.

Because urine containing iodinated contrast was excreted during the time the patient is lying supine and is denser than normal urine, it settled in the posterior region of the bladder.

Even though Tc-99m MDP is cleared by the kidneys, trace amounts are administered, and the concentration of Tc-99m MDP in urine will not affect its appearance on the CT scan. A large air bubble within the bladder would have a similar appearance to the air outside the body (black on CT image). The normal urine would have a similar density as water and not appear hyperattenuating. Beam-hardening artifacts occur due to the preferential attenuation of low-energy photons in the polychromatic x-ray beam and generally present as dark bands between two highly attenuating structures or as streaking from high-density structures. Injected contrast media can cause beam-hardening artifacts, but beam-hardening artifacts do not appear in the posterior bladder.

Reference: Bushberg JT. *The essential physics of medical imaging*. Philadelphia, PA: Wolters Kluwer Health/Lippincott Williams & Wilkins, 2012. Chapter 10.

43 Answer D. PET scanners detect 511 keV annihilation photons while SPECT scanners mostly detect 140-keV photons (from Tc-99m based radiopharmaceuticals). The higher energy photons used in PET require substantially more shielding than do those used in SPECT. The PET/CT system also has a CT scan, which generates x-rays; the room shielding must provide sufficient protection from both the PET annihilation photons and from scatter and leakage radiation during CT scanning. For PET/CT systems that use CT primarily for attenuation scans, the amount of shielding required for the PET studies will also be sufficient for CT imaging. This is because (1) attenuation correction scans are low workload (low output of radiation), and (2) the average energy of CT scatter and leakage radiation is much less than that of the 511-keV annihilation photons. If the system was upgraded from SPECT to SPECT/CT, it is likely that more room shielding would be required as well.

References: Cherry SR, et al. *Physics in nuclear medicine*, 4th ed. Philadelphia, PA: Elsevier/Saunders, 2012:434–437.

Madsen MT, et al. AAPM TG 108: PET and PET/CT shielding requirements. *Med Phys* 2006;33:4–15.

44 Answer D. If a medical event is discovered, the NRC must be notified no later than the next calendar day by telephone. A written report must be provided to the NRC within 15 calendar days. If the licensee is an agreement state, the initial notification and the written report is made to the appropriate regulatory office in that state.

References: Mettler FA, Guiberteau MJ. *Essentials of nuclear medicine imaging*, 7th ed. Philadelphia, PA: Saunders, 2019:389–390.

NRC.gov. 10CFR§35.3045. Report and notification of a medical event. https://www.nrc.gov/reading-rm/doc-collections/cfr/part035/part035-3045.htm

45 Answer B. Y-90 is a high-energy beta emitter (2.28 MeV). These high-energy beta particles interact with matter in the patient's body and produce bremsstrahlung ("braking radiation") x-rays. With an appropriate energy window (e.g., 65 keV ± 100%), the bremsstrahlung x-rays can be detected during SPECT imaging in order to verify the activity distribution of Y-90 microspheres posttherapy.

The Bremsstrahlung x-rays from the CT x-ray tube are used to create projection images for the creation of the CT data set images. The CT x-ray tube cannot be used to generate SPECT images. Y-90 is a beta emitter and does not emit 140 keV gamma emission photons during decay. A small fraction of Y-90 decay results in the emission of positrons (~32 positrons emitted per 106 Y-90 decays). However, imaging of the Y-90 annihilation photons requires the use of a PET scanner.

Reference: Mettler FA, Guiberteau MJ. *Essentials of nuclear medicine imaging*, 7th ed. Philadelphia, PA: Saunders, 2019:325–326.

46 **Answer D.** The delivered and planned doses differed by >20% and by >0.5 Sv, meeting the criteria of a medical event that must be reported to the NRC as defined in 10CFR§35.3045. Per NRC regulation relevant to any therapy, including Y-90 therapy, a licensee must report medical events to the NRC if any of the following four criteria are met:

1. Dose differs from prescribed dose by >50 mSv (5 rem) whole body or >500 mSv (50 rem) to an organ, tissue or skin AND the total dose or activity delivered from the dose differs from the prescribed dose or activity by >20% or falls outside of the prescribed dose range, OR
2. Dose exceeds the prescribed dose by >50 mSv whole body or >500 mSv to an organ, tissue, or skin due to administration of the wrong radioactive drug; through the wrong route; to the wrong individual; or using the wrong mode of treatment, OR
3. Dose to any organ, tissue, or skin other than the treatment site that exceeds the prescribed or calculated dose by >500 mSv (50 rem) AND is >50% of the dose expected to that site defined in the written directive, OR
4. Any event resulting from an intervention in an individual in which the administration of radioactive material or radiation from radioactive material results (or will result in) unintended permanent functional damage to an organ or a physiologic system, as determined by a physician.

The NRC does not need to be notified when the delivered dose is greater than (or less than) the planned dose if the dose difference does not meet the criteria of 10CFR§35.3045. There is no requirement that the NRC must dispose of undelivered Y-90 microsphere therapy doses; Y-90 has a half-life of 64 hours and can be safely disposed of on-site using the decay in storage method. The NRC does not need to be notified of malfunctioning therapy delivery systems unless they result in a medical event that meets the criteria of 10CFR§35.3045.

References: Mettler FA, Guiberteau MJ. *Essentials of nuclear medicine imaging*, 7th ed. Philadelphia, PA: Saunders, 2019:389–390.

NRC.gov. 10CFR§35.3045 Report. and notification of a medical event. https://www.nrc.gov/reading-rm/doc-collections/cfr/part035/part035-3045.html

47 **Answer C.** Tc-99m is produced via the decay of Mo-99. If a generator at time t = 0 hours contains only Mo-99, the maximum activity of Tc-99m within the generator will occur at t = 23 hours. This is approximately four half-lives of Tc-99m and explains why generators are eluted daily at approximately the same time.

The generator can be eluted at any time other than 23 hours; however, this will just result in a yield of Tc-99m that is less than the yield obtained at 23 hours.

Note from the graph that after the maximum activity of Tc-99m is reached, the two isotopes are in transient equilibrium. Also, note that the activity of Tc-99m within the generator will always be less than the activity of Mo-99 because the yield of Tc-99m from Mo-99 is 0.876; 87.6% of Mo-99m decays to Tc-99m, and the remainder decays to Tc-99. Tc-99m produced in the generator is constantly decaying to Tc-99, which is a carrier, and so the generator elution is not carrier free. Generators that have not been eluted for several days have a significant buildup of this carrier, Tc-99, which can compete with Tc-99m and adversely affect the radiopharmaceutical labeling efficiency. As such, it is best practice to elute a generator daily, including the weekends, even if the dose will not be used.

References: Cherry SR, et al. *Physics in nuclear medicine*, 4th ed. Philadelphia, PA: Elsevier/Saunders, 2012:50–53.

Mettler FA, Guiberteau MJ. *Essentials of nuclear medicine imaging*, 7th ed. Philadelphia, PA: Saunders, 2019:5–6.

Saha G. *Fundamentals of nuclear pharmacy*, 7th ed. New York, NY: Springer, 2017:77–92.

48 **Answer B.** After injection of filtered Tc-99m sulfur colloid or Lymphoseek, gamma camera imaging may be used to identify the sentinel lymph node (lymph node to receive drainage from tumor site). The patient is then transported to the operating room, and the sentinel lymph node is confirmed for excision using a handheld gamma probe. These probes have a narrow field of view (about 3 to 15 mm) that is ideal for the precise localization of radioactive lymph nodes. The design of the gamma probe depends on the gamma-ray energy of the radionuclide. In cases with predictable lymphatic drainage, such as axilla in breast cancer or groin in lower extremity melanoma, imaging using a gamma camera may not be required.

Geiger-Müller counters, thyroid uptake probes, and ionization chambers are all heavily utilized radiation detectors used in the nuclear medicine department. However, they are not used intraoperatively to help localize the sentinel lymph node.

References: Cherry SR, Sorenson JA, Phelps ME. *Physics in nuclear medicine*, 4th ed. Philadelphia, PA: Saunders, 2012:192–194.

Mettler FA, Guiberteau MJ. *Essentials of nuclear medicine imaging*, 7th ed. Philadelphia, PA: Saunders, 2019:322–324.

49 **Answer C.** All radioactive drugs must be assayed and labeled prior to patient administration. Per NRC regulation, each syringe and vial that contains unsealed by-product material for patient use must be assayed and then labeled to identify the radioactive drug. Each syringe shield and vial shield must also be labeled unless the label on the syringe or vial is visible when shielded.

Written directives are only required for the administration of >1.11 MBq (30 µCi) of I-131 for imaging or therapy, any therapeutic dosage of unsealed by-product material, or any therapeutic dose from by-product material. Imaging-only studies, except I-131 with activity >30 µCi, do not require a written directive.

There is no federal regulation that requires an authorized user to administer a radioactive drug for imaging or therapy. Properly trained nuclear medicine technologists generally perform administrations under the supervision of an authorized user. The level of supervision (e.g., direct or remote) is specified in the license. Depending on an institution's license and policy and local and state regulation, an authorized user may be required to perform the administration (e.g., a given hospital may have a policy in place that requires an authorized user to administer the dose for Y-90 microsphere or Ra-223 dichloride therapy).

Many kits (e.g., sestamibi) are made into multiuse vials with high activities of the radionuclide. Then, rather than making and performing quality control on a new kit for each patient, the dosage to be administered can be withdrawn from a single kit for many patients. Note that under new USP 825 standards, very specific conditions must be met by the radiopharmacy for the preparation and use of multiuse vials.

References: NRC.gov. 10CFR§35.69. Labeling of vials and syringes. https://www.nrc.gov/reading-rm/doc-collections/cfr/part035/part035-0069.html

NRC.gov. 10CFR§35.27. Supervision. https://www.nrc.gov/reading-rm/doc-collections/cfr/part035/part035-0027.html

Saha G. *Fundamentals of nuclear pharmacy*, 7th ed. New York, NY: Springer, 2017:246.

USP General Chapter <825>. Radiopharmaceuticals—preparation, compounding, dispensing, and repackaging. https://www.usp.org/chemical-medicines/general-chapter-82

50 **Answer D.** Radionuclide impurities will result in increased patient dose. Radionuclide impurities are radionuclides other than the imaging radionuclide that are contained within the radiopharmaceutical. An example of this is Mo-99 in a Tc-99m labeled radiopharmaceutical. Unwanted radionuclides in the radiopharmaceutical cause increased radiation dose to the patient with either no gain or degradation of image quality.

The concentration of radionuclide impurities will be very low compared to the desired radionuclide, which is already injected in trace amounts that are below the concentration thresholds to cause pharmacologic or deterministic effects. As such, the risk for a pharmacologic effect from a radionuclide impurity is essentially nonexistent since the risk of pharmacologic effects from the imaging radionuclide is essentially nonexistent. It is possible for some impurities (e.g., the chemical impurity of alumina breakthrough) to affect the biodistribution of the radiopharmaceutical through the formation of colloids, reduction of labeling efficiency, or decomposition of the radiopharmaceutical. However, the expected alteration of biodistribution for radionuclide impurities is low due to the trace concentrations. Any radiation effects from increased dose from radionuclide impurities will be stochastic in nature.

Reference: Saha G. *Fundamentals of nuclear pharmacy*, 7th ed. New York, NY: Springer, 2017:164–176.

51 **Answer B.** The SUV in each image pixel is calculated using the equation:

$$\text{SUV} = (\text{Image pixel value}/\text{Administered activity}) \times (\text{Patient weight})$$

From the above SUV equation, we see that if the "Administered activity" is overestimated by 25% in error, the SUV in all image pixels will decrease by 25%, and SUV measurements in the liver will likewise be underestimated by 25%. SUV values can be affected by errors in recording the administered activity (e.g., errors during dose assay, neglecting to measure and subtract residual activity in the syringe, or mistyping of the administered dose) or dose extravasation. Errors in SUV measurements are inversely proportional to the errors in recording the "Administered activity." Likewise, errors in the recording of the patient weight directly affect the calculated SUV. Additionally, errors in the camera activity calibration factors that convert image pixel values from counts to MBq/mL can also lead to errors in the SUV measurements in images.

References: Bailey DL, Townsend DW, Valk PE, et al. *Positron emission tomography: basic sciences*. London: Springer, 2005:288.

Mettler FA, Guiberteau MJ. *Essentials of nuclear medicine imaging*, 7th ed. Philadelphia, PA: Saunders, 2019:341–342.

52 **Answer C.** Center of rotation correction is applied to SPECT studies to correct for small deviations between the mechanical center of rotation of the detectors and the center of the reconstructed image caused by sagging or wobbling of the detectors as they rotate around the patient. Center of rotation correction is not applied to planar imaging studies because the detectors do not rotate during the data acquisition.

Extrinsic uniformity correction, spatial linearity correction, and energy correction are applied to all imaging data acquired on gamma cameras, which includes both SPECT and planar images. Extrinsic uniformity correction is done to correct for regional variations in the detector response across the detector face. Spatial linearity corrections and energy corrections are also applied to all imaging data acquired on gamma cameras. Spatial linearity correction is applied to correct for nonlinear detection efficiency at different spatial locations on the detector. Energy correction adjusts for the difference in energy recorded for events that occur between the photomultiplier tubes versus the energy recorded for events directly under the photomultiplier tube.

References: Cherry SR, Sorenson JA, Phelps ME. *Physics in nuclear medicine*, 4th ed. Philadelphia, PA: Saunders, 2012:228–229, 302–304.

Samei E, et al. *Hendee's physics of medical imaging*. Hoboken, NJ: John Wiley & Sons, Inc., 2019:285–286.

SNMMI procedure standard for myocardial perfusion imaging 3.3. http://s3.amazonaws.com/rdcms-snmmi/files/production/public/docs/Parathyroid_Scintigraphy_V4_0_FINAL.pdf

SNMMI procedure standard for gated equilibrium radionuclide ventriculography 3.0. http://s3.amazonaws.com/rdcms-snmmi/files/production/public/docs/Gated%20Equilibrium%20Radionuclide%20Ventriculography%203.0.pdf

53 **Answer A.** These are F-18 FDG PET images of the same patient. The top, image A, is the attenuation corrected image (AC) and the bottom, image B, is the non–attenuation corrected image (NAC). In order to reach the ring of PET detectors, annihilation photons must travel through different amounts and types of tissue depending on where the annihilation occurred in the body. This results in different amounts of photons reaching the detectors due to attenuation, depending on the location of the annihilation and characteristics of overlying tissues. For example, more photons from the surface and from areas with no significant attenuating tissues such as lungs would reach the detectors, making them look more intense than more centrally located structures surrounded by dense organs. Attenuation correction corrects for these differences. Most modern scanners utilize CT based attenuation correction algorithms for the correction. Note the increased skin activity, hot lungs, nonuniform liver uptake, and reduced activity in the central portion of the body on NAC images, which are all corrected on the AC image. Skin lesions, including malignancy such as melanoma, are better seen on NAC data because of the generalized "subtraction" of counts from the surface related to the absence of attenuation there compared to deeper structures. Also, in the presence of prosthesis, reviewing NAC data is crucial to avoid attenuation correction artifacts.

Scatter correction could improve image contrast, but the effect of scattering is not associated with the "hot" lung artifact seen on the images. Time of flight (TOF) correction could improve image contrast because knowing the relative time difference between arrivals of each photon of the coincident pair within the timing window allows annihilation events to be localized within a smaller region of the line of response between the coincident PET detectors. However, TOF correction is not associated with the "hot lung" artifacts seen in the coronal images. Different radiopharmaceuticals would result in different physiologic distributions, which is not the case for these two images.

References: Cherry SR, Sorenson JA, Phelps ME. *Physics in nuclear medicine*, 4th ed. Philadelphia, PA: Saunders, 2012:309, 310, 335–340, 356–360.

Mettler FA, Guiberteau MJ. *Essentials of nuclear medicine imaging*, 7th ed. Philadelphia, PA: Saunders, 2019:44–45.

Surti S. Update on time-of-flight PET imaging. *J Nucl Med* 2015;56(1):98–104.

54 **Answer C.** The SPECT protocols with 90 degrees "L" detector configuration and scan rotation from a right anterior oblique (RAO) to a left posterior oblique (LPO) are recommended for acquiring myocardial perfusion imaging (MPI) SPECT and SPECT/CT studies. The heart is typically located in the anterior left hemithorax, so scan rotation from the RAO to the LPO is recommended during SPECT, as the detectors will be as close as possible to the organ and result in the best spatial resolution. This scan rotation also adequately samples all the projection angles needed for accurate tomographic reconstruction of the left hemithorax thorax and heart. It should be noted that with the dual detectors in the 90 degrees or "L" configuration, the leading detector will sample the projections from the LAO to the LPO positions, and the trailing detector will sample the projections from the RAO view to the LAO from the start to the end of the data acquisition.

A scanner protocol with a 180-degree "opposing" detector configuration will take twice as long to sample all the projection angles needed for accurate tomographic reconstruction. When the detectors are in the "opposing" configuration, the gantry must complete a half rotation for either detector to see all angles between RAO to LPO, but in the L configuration of the detectors, the gantry only needs a one-fourth rotation for either detector to see all angles between RAO to LPO. The faster L configuration image acquisition protocol is recommended for SPECT MPI examinations to reduce patient motion. A rotation arc from the left anterior oblique (LAO) to the right posterior oblique (RPO) is not recommended during SPECT of the heart because of the loss of spatial resolution that results from the increased distance of the detectors from the heart.

References: Dorbala S, et al. SNMMI/ASNC/SCCT guideline for cardiac SPECT/CT and PET/CT 1.0. *J Nucl Med* 2013;54(8):1485–1507.

Dorbala S, et al. Single photon emission computed tomography (SPECT) myocardial perfusion imaging guidelines: instrumentation, acquisition, processing, and interpretation. *J Nucl Cardiol* 2018;25:1784–1846.

55 **Answer A.** Image B appears less noisy but blurrier than image A. Increasing the FWHM of the gaussian filter causes the smoother image appearance seen in image B. The gaussian reconstruction filter reduces image noise or variations between neighboring image pixels. Increasing the full width at half maximum (FWHM) setting of the filter from 3 mm FWHM in image A to 7 mm FWHM in image B causes increased smoothing between pixels and a less noisy appearance of the image B.

The window width and window level display settings are the same between images A and B, as can be seen in the similar appearance between high- and low-contrast regions on the images. The color bars on the left also show that the window widths and window levels are similar. Attenuation correction was applied during the reconstruction of image A and image B. Attenuation depends on the distance the gamma ray travels through tissue before reaching the detector; therefore, the center of objects would appear to have fewer counts than the periphery. Both images A and B appear to have similar count density in the perfused structures at the center compared to the count density at the periphery of the brain. Smaller pixel size would typically increase the apparent noise in the image; however, image B appears less noisy than does image A. Smaller pixel size is usually achieved by using an image matrix with more pixels per slice. Images with smaller pixel sizes and more pixels would appear noisier and have higher statistical variation between pixels because each pixel contains fewer counts when the same fixed total number of counts is distributed among many more pixels. A similar consequence of increased noise occurs for image volumes reconstructed with thinner slices.

References: Cherry SE, Sorenson JA, Phelps ME. *Physics in nuclear medicine*, 4th ed. Philadelphia, PA: Saunders, 2012:270–273, 293–299, 373.

Hutton BF, et al. Review and current status of SPECT scatter correction. *Phys Med Biol* 2011;56:R85–R112.

Ishii K, et al. Impact of CT attenuation correction by SPECT/CT in brain perfusion images. *Ann Nucl Med* 2012;26:241–247.

56 **Answer B.** A noncircular or "body-contour" orbit is recommended for SPECT image acquisition of the abdomen to achieve the best spatial resolution. For gamma cameras with parallel-hole collimators, the system spatial resolution degrades with increasing distance between the detector and the patient. Therefore, a noncircular orbit is recommended to bring the detectors as close as possible to the patient at all angles of rotation during any SPECT imaging of the abdomen.

A circular orbit will result in degraded spatial resolution as the distance between the detector and the patient will be too large for all angles except the lateral views. SPECT images cannot be reconstructed from static imaging where the detectors do not rotate. In tomographic imaging, data must be acquired for ≥180 degrees around the patient to adequately sample the projections for accurate tomographic image reconstruction. However, in most body SPECT studies, the detectors are arranged in the opposing configuration and acquire data for 360 degrees (180 degrees for each detector) around the patient. This simultaneous acquisition of opposing views (conjugate counting) improves the image quality of SPECT reconstruction by reducing variations in attenuation and resolution that occur because tissue and organs are at different depths in the body and depth relative to the detector changes across the projection angles.

References: Balon HR, et al. The SNM practice guideline for somatostatin receptor scintigraphy 2.0. *J Nucl Med Technol* 2011;39(4):317–324.

Hutton B. Angular sampling necessary for clinical SPECT. *J Nucl Med* 1996;37(11):1915–1916.

57 **Answer C.** The loss of spatial resolution on Rb-82 image is the result of higher positron energy of Rb-82 resulting in the longer positron range or distance before it undergoes an annihilation event to create the PET coincident photons. The spatial spreading out of the annihilation events, relative to the location of the radiotracer uptake and positron emission, depends on the energy of that emitted positron. The effect of positron range on spatial resolution is negligible for the lower energy positron emissions of F-18, which has an average positron energy of 0.2 MeV and a short average positron range of 0.4 mm, which is an order of magnitude smaller than the FWHM spatial resolution of the PET scanner. By comparison, the average positron energy of Rb-82 is 1.5 MeV, and the average positron range is 4 mm, which is on the same order of magnitude as the spatial resolution of the PET scanner. As such, the spatial resolution of PET images acquired using Rb-82 RbCl are degraded compared to the sharp appearance of the F-18 FDG images of the myocardium.

The shorter 1.3-minute half-life of Rb-82 compared to the 110-minute half-life of F-18 does not affect the spatial resolution of RbCl/FDG myocardial images. Statistical noise in images can affect spatial resolution, especially in low count studies; however, the Rb-82 and the F-18 myocardial images shown above have similar count densities in the images and similar levels of noise. The Rb-82 RbCl perfusion image is acquired 1 to 2 minutes after intravenous administration of approximately 40 mCi Rb-82 RbCl. This is then followed by intravenous administration of approximately 8 mCi F-18 FDG, and the F-18 FDG metabolism images are acquired 1 hour later using similar PET/CT image acquisition and processing scanner parameters. The higher atomic mass of Rb-82 has no direct effect on positron energy or positron range and so does not affect spatial resolution in the images.

References: Dilsizian V, et al. ASNC imaging guidelines/SNMMI procedure standard for positron emission tomography (PET) nuclear cardiology procedures. *J Nucl Cardiol* 2016;23:1187–1226.

Dorbala S, et al. SNMMI/ASNC/SCCT guideline for cardiac SPECT/CT and PET/CT 1.0. *J Nucl Med* 2013;54(8):1485–1507.

Moses SS. Fundamental limits of spatial resolution in PET. *Nucl Instrum Methods Phys Res A* 2011;648(Suppl 1):S236–S240.

58 **Answer A.** The standardized uptake value (SUV) is the tissue radioactivity concentration in each pixel measured by a PET scanner divided by the administered radioactivity multiplied by the patient body weight, as shown in the equation below. Body composition and habitus can have significant effects on SUV because SUV normalizes by body mass. Generally, fat has a much lower uptake of F-18 FDG than do other tissues. An overweight patient has more fat and higher body mass than does a thin, lower weight patient. Consequently, SUV values tend to be elevated in overweight patients. Although less common, SUV can be normalized by lean body mass (SUVLBM) or body surface area (SUVBSA), and these SUV metrics are less dependent on body habitus. Accordingly, it is recommended to use SUVLBM to gauge tumor response with PET imaging with the so-called PERCIST criteria. The SUV in each image pixel is calculated using the equation:

$$SUV = (\text{Image pixel value/Administered activity}) \times (\text{Patient weight})$$

References: Keyes JW. SUV: standardized uptake or silly useless value? *J Nucl Med* 1995;36:1836–1839.

Mettler FA, Guiberteau MJ. *Essentials of nuclear medicine imaging*, 7th ed. Philadelphia, PA: Saunders, 2019:341–342.

Wahl RL, Jacene H, Kasamon Y, et al. From RECIST to PERCIST: evolving considerations for PET response criteria in solid tumors. *J Nucl Med* 2009;50(Suppl 1):122S–150S.

59 **Answer B.** The hot spot is an attenuation correction artifact resulting from a metallic pacemaker. The metal in the pacemaker results in very high CT Hounsfield numbers (compared to normal tissue) and streaking artifacts on the associated CT scan that is used for attenuation correction of the PET data. These high CT Hounsfield numbers and CT artifacts cause the attenuation correction algorithm to overcorrect the PET data resulting in artificially high FDG uptake in the location of the metal pacemaker. Note that this artifact is NOT present on the non–attenuation correction (NAC) images. High-density materials such as metal and barium in the colon can cause errors/artifacts on the attenuation corrected images, so both the AC and NAC images should be examined when reading the PET/CT examination.

Normal uptake in that region on the NAC images rules out a malignant chest wall lesion, a mispositioned lung lesion, and inflammation around a surgical scar.

Reference: Yao LL, Gay SB, Vu QDM, et al. *PET/CT basics*. University of Virginia Health Sciences Center, Department of Radiology. https://www.med-ed.virginia.edu/courses/rad/PETCT/Metal.html

60 **Answer D.** On the posterior image, there are circular areas of photopenia corresponding to the outlines of the photomultiplier tubes (PMTs). This is due to the corruption of the uniformity correction for detector 2. The uniformity correction for detector 1 is fine, so there is no artifact on the anterior image. A missing or corrupted uniformity correction often causes circular outlines of the PMTs.

A motion could result in the mislocation of certain anatomical features or increase blur in the image, but the motion would not cause circular photopenic areas. An image matrix that is too coarse (e.g., 64×64 rather than 128×128) would degrade spatial resolution but would not cause circular photopenic areas. For Ga-67, the use of a low-energy (rather than medium-energy) collimator would likely result in an image with increased scatter and overall degraded image quality, but it would not cause circular photopenic areas.

Reference: Glaser JE, Song N, Jaini S, et al. Photomultiplier tube artifacts on Ga-67 citrate imaging caused by loss of correction floods due to an off-peak status of one head of a dual-head γ-camera. *J Nucl Med Technol* 2012;40(4):278–280.

61 **Answer A.** Respiratory motion during scanning is a common source of attenuation correction artifacts on the PET/CT imaging. Artifacts stem from the discrepancy between the chest position on the CT image and that on the PET image. The CT scan is acquired quickly during a specific phase of the breathing cycle, while the PET scan involves a long acquisition time over many respiratory cycles. The difference in respiratory motion between the PET and CT scans causes breathing-related artifacts on PET/CT images. In this example, the CT scan was acquired at full inspiration with downward displacement of the diaphragm and liver. At full inspiration, the regions that normally contain the diaphragm and superior liver (higher attenuation) now contain lung tissue (low attenuation). Consequently, the attenuation correction of the PET data is underestimated in this region, which produces a curvilinear cold area at the lung/diaphragm/liver interface. The AC image suffers from this artifact, and the hot lesion is incorrectly localized in the lungs. However, this artifact is not present on the NAC image (since there is no attenuation correction) where the lesion is correctly localized in the superior liver. Due to the possibility of artifacts, both the AC and NAC images should be examined when reading a PET study.

Contrast media present in the CT scan used for attenuation correction could result in overestimation of activity in the AC image (which is not the case in these images), but it is unlikely to cause mislocalization of an anatomical feature in the AC image. In addition, contrast media is rarely used during the low-dose attenuation correction CT.

PET scanners have many detector blocks, and a single malfunctioning detector block would result in little, if any, degradation of image quality. Furthermore, a malfunctioning detector block would not result in different locations of anatomical features in AC versus NAC images.

PET data is reconstructed onto an image matrix to create an NAC image. Both the NAC and AC images are reconstructed onto the same matrix, so the matrix cannot shift between the two images. However, due to motion, the anatomy may shift between the collection of the PET and CT data (used for attenuation correction), which would result in artifacts in the AC image.

Reference: Sureshbabu W, Mawlawi O. PET/CT Imaging Artifacts. *J Nucl Med Technol* 2005;33(3):156–161.